D0971274

THE OKINAWA DIET PLAN

BY THE SAME AUTHORS

The Okinawa Program:
How the World's Longest-Lived People
Achieve Everlasting Health—and How You Can Too

THE OKINAWA DIET PLAN

Get Leaner, Live Longer, and Never Feel Hungry

Bradley J. Willcox, M.D.

D. Craig Willcox, Ph.D.

Makoto Suzuki, M.D.

WITH LEAH FELDON

CONTRIBUTIONS BY HIDEMI TODORIKI, PH.D.
RECIPES BY SAYAKA MITSUHASHI

Clarkson Potter/Publishers
New York

Copyright © 2004 by Bradley J. Willcox and D. Craig Willcox

All rights reserved. No part of this book may be reproduced
or transmitted in any form or by any means, electronic or
mechanical, including photocopying, recording, or by any
information storage and retrieval system, without permission
in writing from the publisher.

Published by Clarkson Potter/Publishers, New York, New York.
Member of the Crown Publishing Group,
a division of Random House, Inc.
www.crownpublishing.com

CLARKSON N. POTTER is a trademark and POTTER and
colophon are registered trademarks of Random House, Inc.

Printed in the United States of America

Design by Caitlin Daniels Israel

Library of Congress Cataloging-in-Publication Data
Willcox, Bradley J.
    The Okinawa diet plan : get leaner, live longer, and never feel
hungry / Bradley J. Willcox, D. Craig Willcox.
    1. Longevity.   2. Aging—Prevention.   3. Longevity—
Nutritional aspects.   4. Diet.   I. Willcox, D. Craig.   II. Title.
RA776.5.W493   2004
613.2'5—dc22   2003023285

ISBN 1-4000-4953-9

10   9   8   7   6   5   4   3   2   1

FIRST EDITION

Acknowledgments

We are indebted to many more people than we could possibly mention in a few short words for helping us to bring you a new and exciting approach to the science of healthy weight and healthy aging.

Stedman Mays of Clausen, Mays and Tahan Literary Agency was key in motivating us from beginning to end. His steady guidance and that of Mary Tahan helped make this book a reality. Leah Feldon was very helpful in making the science literate, understandable, and engaging. Our editors, Annetta Hanna and Pam Krauss, devoted their time and considerable skills throughout the editorial process, as did the whole team at Clarkson Potter. We thank them for their commitment to academic excellence and truth. We also thank our research assistant and nutritional anthropologist, Sayaka Mitsuhashi, who created and analyzed most of the recipes in conjunction with many of the great Okinawan chefs of the world. Sayaka continues to improve our nutritional database and invent wonderful new ways to enjoy healthy and delicious blends of Eastern and Western cuisine for many restaurants, books, and magazines. We also appreciate the beautiful illustrations of Miki Kato-Starr, visiting lecturer at Macalester College, St. Paul, Minnesota.

Many researchers contributed essential information to this project and helped build the Okinawa Centenarian Study database, only a small number of whom we were able to include in this book. These researchers form a key part of the Okinawa collaborative network on successful aging, and we are greatly indebted to their stellar work. In particular we would like to thank Dr. Hidemi Todoriki, Dr. Seizo Sakihara, Dr. Hiroko Sho, Dr. Masafumi Akisaka, Dr. Ikuya Ashitomi, Dr. Kazuhiko Taira, and Professor Liu Asato of the University of the Ryukyus, Faculty of Medicine and School of Health Sciences. Our collaborators from the Tokyo Centenarian Study in particular deserve our thanks, including Dr. Nobuyose Hirose. New collaborations, such as those with Dr. Leonard Poon, director of the Georgia Centenarian Study and the father of U.S. centenarian studies, Dr. Peter

Martin, director of the Iowa Centenarian Study and the International Centenarian Study Consortium, continue to enrich our work.

The Pacific Health Research Institute (PHRI) and the University of Hawaii have been instrumental in providing a home, full of the spirit of aloha, for the U.S. base of our research. First and foremost, we thank Dr. David Curb, former associate director of the National Institute on Aging (Epidemiology, Biometry, and Demography) and current CEO and medical director of Pacific Health Research Institute and chief of Clinical Epidemiology and Geriatrics Research at the University of Hawaii, for his superb mentorship and support. Others who have been very helpful and to whom we owe much gratitude include research assistant Brandi Tanaka, Dr. Katsuhiko Yano, Vicki Shambaugh, Dr. Beatriz Rodriguez, Dr. Rob Abbott, Dr. John Grove, Dr. Tim Donlon, Dr. Qimei He, Dr. Kamal Masaki, Dr. Lon White, Dr. Helen Petrovich, Dr. Web Ross, Dr. Chien-Wen Tseng, Randi Chen and our other talented programmers, our IT department, Proposal Prep department, and all the other talented team members who make PHRI the leading independent, non-profit medical research institute in Hawaii.

We are indebted to our dieticians both in Okinawa and abroad, in particular to Mayo Clinic dietician Kristine Kuhnert for her careful review of the recipes. We also appreciate the valuable assistance of Drs. Hisashi Tauchi and Yuichiro Gotoh and members of the Tokyo Metropolitan Institute of Gerontology for their help over the years. We thank Dr. Satoshi Sasaki of the Japan National Nutrition Institute for his helpful comments.

Several experts read the manuscript at various stages and contributed valuable suggestions. Expert epidemiologist Dr. KatsuhikoYano, who has been an inspiration to us for years, provided many helpful comments, as did integrative medicine expert Dr. Andrew Weil and epidemiologist Dr. Yoshihide Kinjo. We also thank Professors Eitetsu Yamaguchi, Takashi Tsuha, and Seishin Akamine for their remarkable insight and helpful advice regarding Okinawan history and culture. Dr. Hiroko Sho's work in nutrition, aging, and culture has been a source of inspiration for us from the beginning of our nutritional studies in Okinawa, and we thank her for her continuing efforts in promoting the health of all citizens of Okinawa.

Many researchers and academics from the University of Toronto, the alma mater of both Bradley and Craig Willcox, deserve our gratitude and thanks. These include Dr. David Jenkins and Dr. Thomas Wolever of the Department of Nutritional Sciences, Faculty of Medicine. Their discovery of the Glycemic Index led to much of the current thinking about dietary links among high glycemic index carbohydrates, insulin, and chronic disease. Dr. Jenkins's mentorship and his support for our first research trip to Okinawa in the early 1990s was instrumental in our forming collaborative links that exist to this day. We are grateful to Professor Richard Lee of the Department of Anthropology for laying the groundwork for the field of nutritional anthropology. His work has spawned a generation of work in studies of the health and nutritional status of hunter-gatherer societies. We also thank Okinawa International University, Pacific Health Research Institute, the University of Hawaii, Kuakini Medical Center, Okinawa Prefectural University–College of Nursing, the Mayo Clinic, Harvard Medical School, Beth Israel Deaconess Medical Center, and the Hebrew Rehabilitation Center for Aged for helping support our research.

Our colleagues at Harvard University and Harvard Medical School deserve our gratitude and praise for their help. Dr. Walter Willet of the Harvard School of Public Health has been very supportive over the years and continues to be a powerful force for nutritional change, particularly in the field of nutritional epidemiology. Dr. Edward Giovannucci and Dr. Eric Rimm continue to be a source of inspiration and many helpful discussions. Our colleagues in the Harvard Division on Aging represent the cutting edge of research in gerontology and geriatric medicine. We are indebted to Dr. Thomas Perls and Dr. Margery Silver for their help in establishing an international collaboration between Boston University's New England Centenarian Study and the Okinawa Centenarian Study. We thank Dr. Lewis Lipsitz, Head of the Division on Aging at Harvard Medical School in particular for his continued support.

Various foundations and organizations have supported our research, to which we are very grateful. These include Japan Ministry of Health, Labour and Welfare, Japan Ministry of Education, Culture, Sports, Science and Technology, Japan Foundation for Aging and Health, Japan Foundation, Tokyo Metropolitan Institute of Gerontology, University of Toronto, Mayo Clinic, Harvard University, Hebrew Rehabilitation Center for Aged, Medical Research Council of Canada, Natural Sciences and Engineering Research Council of Canada, Pacific Health Research Institute, National Institutes of Health (NIH), and National Institute on Aging (NIA). Winnie Rossi, our program administrator at the NIA, has been a wonderful source of support and encouragement, as has Dr. Evan Hadley, director of the Clinical Gerontology and Geriatrics Division at the NIA.

In particular, we thank the centenarians, other elders, and their family members and local government and village officials who have participated in our study for so many years, as well as the many members of our research team in the Department of Community Medicine at Ryukyus University Hospital and the Okinawa Longevity Science Research Center. Without their assistance there would be no Okinawa Centenarian Study.

Most of all, we express our gratitude and dedicate this book to our parents, spouses, and other family members for their understanding, patience, support, and helpful advice throughout the writing of this book: They made it all possible.

Contents

THE OKINAWA DIET PLAN

Chapter 1

OKINAWA: LEAN PEOPLE, LONG, HEALTHY LIVES

N'kashin tchu nu kutuba ya, amari fusuko neran.
The wisdom of the ancients is still true and applicable.

Far off in the East China Sea, between the main islands of Japan and Taiwan, is an archipelago of 161 beautiful, lush green islands known as Okinawa. The beaches are a dazzling powdery white; the waters are crystal turquoise, and the pristine subtropical rain forests house a huge variety of exotic flora and fauna. But while Okinawa has all the makings of a tropical paradise, it is in fact something even more special—Okinawa is more like a "real-life Shangri-la."[1] Why?

Because the islands are home to the longest-lived population in the world.[2] It's a place where the aging process seems to have slowed and age-related diseases common in the West are kept to a minimum (see figure 1.1). Great-grandfathers practice martial arts. Energetic great-grandmothers garden and perform traditional dance. And some centenarians of both sexes even run businesses and lead socially fulfilling and wonderfully independent lives. You can see them daily as you stroll the streets. Here, a lean, wiry woman who appears to be sixty walks with a container of freshly made Okinawan tofu perched on her head—she's ninety-nine years old. There, a slender, tanned "seventy-something" woman sells traditional bright red, yellow, and blue Okinawan kimonos in the thriving marketplace—she's actually 101. And there, a spry woman pushing an over-loaded wheelbarrow collects bottles for her recycling company—she's 102 years old. And over there, a fit-looking, older man with a floppy straw hat threshes sugarcane. He is 103 years old. This is life as usual in Okinawa.

> I hope to live to 120 . . . To tell the truth, I really only feel like eighty.
> *Ushi Okushima, 100 years old*

Okinawa, in fact, has the highest concentration of centenarians worldwide, some of them 110 years old and older, including the world's oldest living citizen, Kamato Hongo, still going at age 116.[3] These so-called supercentenarians now account for more than 15 percent of the world's documented living super-centenarians—despite Okinawa's paltry 0.0002 percent contribution to the world's population.[4] When you consider that the United States counts only about 10 centenarians per 100,000 people, while Okinawa has 40 per 100,000, you begin to see the significance of these numbers.[5]

My brother and I first began investigating this amazing phenomenon a decade ago when we joined Dr. Makoto Suzuki as part of the research team for the landmark Okinawa Centenarian Study, which had been established in 1976 to uncover the secrets of the elders' successful aging. But we had been fascinated by reports of unusually hale and hearty Okinawan elders all through our university days. It was in 1994, in fact, upon meeting one of these elders, Mr. Toku Oyakawa, while doing a research project as medical and graduate students at the University of Toronto that we initially felt compelled to go to Okinawa.

We had been studying the impact of body fat on hormone-associated cancers, and because the Japanese had among the lowest risks of breast, prostate, and colon cancers in the world, we had wanted to include as many Japanese (and Japanese-Canadians) in our study as possible.[6] Mr. Oyakawa, who had been raised in Okinawa and had immigrated to Canada more than half a century earlier, graciously agreed to an interview. At the time, he was 105 years old and likely the oldest man in Canada.

When we arrived at his home in the Ontario countryside, Mr. Oyakawa was just coming back from fishing—one of his regular favorite pastimes. As he walked over to greet us, fresh catch in hand, we were flabbergasted. This 105-year-old man was lean and vital. He had twinkly eyes and tan, supple skin, and he moved with a grace and ease that any seventy-year-old would envy. After talking with him for only a few minutes, it was obvious that his mind was as youthful as his body.

As Mr. Oyakawa recounted stories of his unusually long life and told us about Okinawa, we were more fascinated than ever. One fact that especially caught our attention was that Mr. Oyakawa and his ninety-two-year-old wife (who was also in incredible shape) had maintained a near-traditional Okinawan

Figure 1.1

AGE-ADJUSTED DEATH RATES IN THE U.S. AND OKINAWA

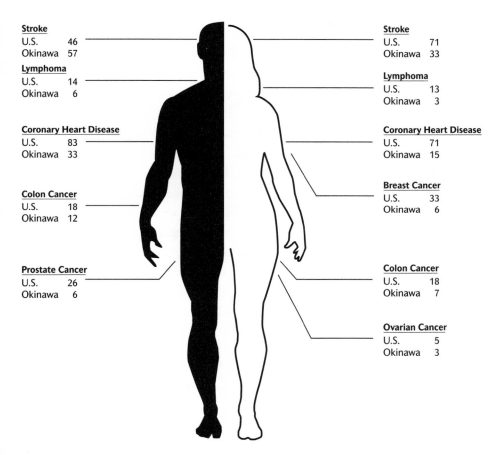

Stroke
U.S.   46
Okinawa 57

Lymphoma
U.S.   14
Okinawa   6

Coronary Heart Disease
U.S.   83
Okinawa   33

Colon Cancer
U.S.   18
Okinawa   12

Prostate Cancer
U.S.   26
Okinawa   6

Stroke
U.S.   71
Okinawa   33

Lymphoma
U.S.   13
Okinawa   3

Coronary Heart Disease
U.S.   71
Okinawa   15

Breast Cancer
U.S.   33
Okinawa   6

Colon Cancer
U.S.   18
Okinawa   7

Ovarian Cancer
U.S.   5
Okinawa   3

Note: All of these diseases have been linked to dietary habits, especially calorie intake. Data from Okinawa Prefectural Government, Department of Health and Welfare; Japan Ministry of Health, Labour and Welfare, 1996 (Statistics and Information Division for year 1995); World Health Statistics Annual for 1995 (publication year 1996, WHO, Geneva). Age-standardized to world standard population. Numbers are deaths per hundred thousand persons per year.

diet during all their years in Canada. Dietary habits were an important part of our study, and if indeed there was an entire population of people who had the same eating patterns as Mr. Oyakawa and were as fit, slim, and healthy as he was, we absolutely needed to find out more. With the help of a research grant from the Medical Research Council of Canada, we were soon on our way to the East China Sea.

Okinawa has been a big part of our lives ever since—and it's even more magical for us now than it was in the beginning. Amid the physical beauty of the islands, we've discovered a rich, wondrous culture with fascinating shamanistic traditions and inspiring holistic beliefs. It's a land where good health is viewed as a natural right, women play the dominant role in religion, the elderly are honored and revered, and ancient healing herbs and tonics are smoothly integrated with Western medicines. And the people are truly exceptional.

The men and women we've met, interviewed, and befriended over the years—many of whom we introduced to you in our last book, *The Okinawa Program*—are remarkable individuals in their eighties, nineties, and beyond, who in many ways are much like Mr. Oyakawa. Their minds are lucid, their bodies are slim, their movements are fluid, and their zest for life is infectious. And, of course, their health is superb for their years. Not only do these long-lived people have among the lowest rates of the West's leading killers—cancer, heart disease, and stroke—but they also have the world's longest *disability-free life expectancy.*[7] While Americans have about seven years of disability at the end of their lives, Okinawans have only 2.6 years of disability—*even though they live longer than Americans.* This means that Okinawans are not just living longer but living longer *in good health*—and that's really the secret to successful aging. I think we'd all agree that longevity tends to lose its appeal if it means years of infirmity and dependency.

Other Shangri-la Contenders

Of course, we've heard stories of such Shangri-la populations before. Long-lived people supposedly lived in abundance in Pakistan's Hunza Valley, in the mountainous village of Vilcabamba in Ecuador, and in the Caucasus region of the former Soviet Union, where yogurt was supposed to be the magic elixir. (The TV commercial featuring an ancient Soviet Georgian crone sweetly coaxing her octogenarian son to eat his yogurt is a classic.) Unfortunately, none of those longevity claims held up to scientific scrutiny.[8] On close examination, it turned out that age exaggeration was rampant and that birth certificates—the sine qua non of credibility in studies of long-lived people—were few and far between.

Okinawa, however, is a different story. Every town, city, and village has an official family register system *(koseki)* that has been recording all births, marriages, and deaths since 1879. Pertinent data, including birth certificates, are highly reliable. There's no doubt that Okinawan centenarians have beaten the odds to ascend the peak of the world's longevity scale. The question is, How did they do it.

The Okinawa Centenarian Study

That question continues to be addressed and answered by the Okinawa Centenarian Study. The study, now entering its twenty-eighth year, is the world's longest-running population-based study of centenarians and has spawned more than two hundred scientific papers.[9] Over the years, we've interviewed and examined more than seven hundred Okinawan centenarians and hundreds of "youngsters" in their seventies, eighties, and nineties, looking for any and all commonalities in their diets, exercise habits, genetics, psychospiritual practices, and social structures that could possibly explain their long-term vitality and exceptionally healthy longevity. And we've found many of them.

We shared a good number of these discoveries with you in *The Okinawa Program* as we explored the elders' life-affirming worldviews, supportive social structures, and inspiring psychospiritual practices, examined their restorative eating and exercise habits, and developed a holistic health program geared toward healthy longevity.[10] Now we have more to share with you. Since the highly successful publication of that book, our ongoing study has continued to reveal even more secrets of the Okinawans' healthy lifestyle. Our latest findings are not only among the most outstanding—they could make a huge difference in your life.

DISCOVERY: OKINAWAN ELDERS ARE LEAN FOR LIFE

We've always been impressed by how slim and fit the Okinawan elders are, but recently we discovered something even more impressive. The Okinawans are not just lean; they are *lean for life.* Okinawan elders constitute one of the only known adequately nourished large-scale populations that *have not gained significant weight with age.*[11,12] While most of us struggle daily to keep off the pounds, the Okinawan elders have done it naturally all their lives, without dieting and without giving it a second thought. In fact, many of the healthy, slim centenarians we've interviewed over the years are not even familiar with the concept of dieting.

This was a startling discovery as well as a watershed in gerontology research. To get accurate data on a population's long-term weight gain and eating habits, researchers have to carefully follow a group of people over a long period and check them at regular intervals. That's why these kinds of studies are expensive and rarely undertaken. But the ancestors must have been smiling on us with the Okinawans. Like the fortunate existence of birth certificates that verified their ages, we found records that gave us impressive data on the Okinawans' health and dietary statistics over the years.

Our search first took us back to early Japanese government dietary surveys, which we meticulously studied and compared with the dietary surveys of elder Okinawans we ourselves had compiled over twenty-eight years in our Okinawa Centenarian Study. Then we flew to Washington, D.C., and pored over thousands of documents from the National Archives for health and nutrition data on the Okinawans. (Because Okinawa was an American territory from 1945 to 1972, the National Archives are a storehouse of useful historical data.) All our weeks in the paper trenches paid off. We discovered stacks of records listing the actual kinds of foods Okinawans ate, its caloric content, and the heights and weights of the people surveyed.

Figure 1.2

WEIGHT GAIN WITH AGE IN AMERICANS AND OKINAWANS ON DIFFERENT DIETS

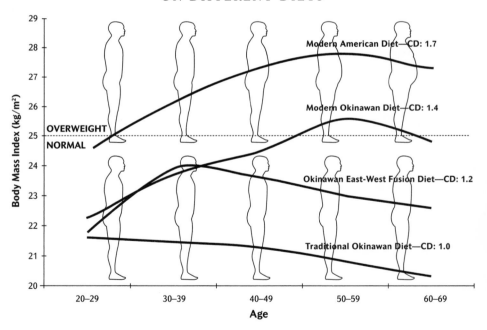

Note: Body Mass Index (BMI) is a measure of your weight (body mass) adjusted for your height and is a rough measure of overweight and obesity. You can determine your BMI with this equation:

$$BMI = \left\{ \frac{\text{Weight (lbs.)}}{\text{Height (in.)}^2} \right\} \times 703$$

BMI of 18.5 is considered a healthy weight, 25 to 30 is considered overweight, above 30 is considered obese. Health risks rise with increasing BMI, particularly as BMI exceeds 25 and substantially as BMI exceeds 27. As you can see, the more the traditional Okinawan diet becomes like the Western (American) diet, the higher the caloric density (CD) becomes and the more Okinawans tend to gain weight as they age. On both the Okinawan traditional (1950s) and East-West fusion diets (1960s), body weight peaks in young adulthood and declines with age thereafter.[12]

This was an awesome find. Joining this treasure trove with other data we had collected from old anthropological records and the modern data we've been collecting since the 1970s, we were able to piece together fascinating statistics that all led to the same conclusion: Unlike the rest of us, Okinawans who followed their traditional diet simply did not gain weight as they aged.[11,12] No matter how we ran the numbers, that conclusion was inescapable. While the Harvard Alumni Study,[13] one of the best ongoing, long-term exercise- and weight-related gerontology studies, revealed that American men gain an average of twenty-two pounds between the ages of twenty and sixty and the Cooper Clinic studies showed that American women average a twelve-pound gain,[13] our statistics showed that Okinawans actually *lost* about five pounds during those years, consistent with the fact that older people require fewer calories as they age (see figure 1.2).

This discovery promises enormous potential benefits for all of us fighting the battle of the bulge. Once we establish exactly *how* Okinawan elders stay lean all their lives, we can do it too—and greatly reduce our risk for weight- and age-related diseases such as coronary heart disease, stroke, diabetes, and cancer. We'll have a potential solution to America's epidemic obesity problem, and we'll be able to get off the psychologically debilitating dieting treadmill that has us running from one trendy weight-loss plan to another, only to end up right back where we started—or even heavier. Eating the Okinawa way could be the answer to our prayers.

EATING THE OKINAWA WAY

So how exactly do the Okinawans manage to keep off the pounds and stay so healthy for so long? Well, as we analyzed and reanalyzed our nutrition data, we found that the elders shared an important dietary factor—one that gerontologists have been studying for decades, and the only one shown to consistently increase life span in multiple species: caloric restriction.[14] Every piece of data we came across lent further support to the conclusion that Okinawan elders are a naturally calorically restricted population, particularly when we plotted their weight gain over time. In other words, they consume fewer calories over the span of their lifetime than other populations. This was an intriguing finding because we knew the Okinawans weren't malnourished, starving, or hungry. On the contrary, food and cooking have a tremendously important place in their cultural tradition, and traditional Okinawan cuisine is often touted as one of the last undiscovered gourmet pleasures.

Fewer Calories Slows Aging

Scientifically speaking, the fact that these extraordinarily long-lived people consume fewer calories made perfect sense. Although we're only now beginning to appreciate how important calorie intake is to human health and longevity, we've known about the benefits of caloric restriction in animals for quite some time. Dr. Clive McCay's studies at Cornell University in the 1930s demonstrated that rats fed 30 percent fewer calories than they would normally eat given free access to food aged more slowly, looked younger, and lived 30 percent longer than the control rats in the studies.[15] Depending on how strict the diet is, calorie restriction can increase maximum animal lifespan by up to 50 percent. That would be the equivalent to humans living 150 to 160 years!

Since those first studies, experiments have been carried out on dozens of species and they repeatedly show that calorie-restricted (CR) animals live longer. Even simple CR rotifers (aquatic organisms) live longer—all through dietary manipulation. The bonus is that CR animals are *functionally* younger as well. The fur of elderly CR animals retains its sheen; the age-related loss of calcium from their bones is slowed; and CR mice can run mazes at a clip equal to others half their age.

Now nonhuman primates—primarily rhesus monkeys—kept on CR diets are showing similar results.[16] Ongoing studies at four institutions, including the National Institute on Aging (NIA), are showing the same early adaptations in the primates on low-cal diets that have been seen in other species. The monkeys already show remarkable changes that point to lower risk for chronic age-related diseases. They have slower age-related declines in blood DHEA levels (DHEA is a hormone from adrenal glands that steadily declines as we age), lower blood sugar levels, lower insulin levels, and reduced risk for diabetes. As you'll see in the upcoming chapters, lower blood sugar and insulin levels are important factors in healthy weight control as well as for lower disease risk and slower aging.

If the usual rules of biology and physiology hold across species—and in this case they almost certainly do—the primates on the CR diet will outlive their well-fed counterparts, and do so in far better health. Indeed, the NIA now houses the longest-lived rhesus monkey ever known.[17] C-58 (an unfortunate name, we know), an erstwhile alpha male who's had his calories carefully allotted all his life, is thirty-nine years old—the equivalent of 114 in human years. While his beard is graying and he's somewhat less rambunctious than he was in his younger days (passersby no longer have to worry about getting grabbed), he's still quite energetic, and—other than a touch of arthritis and a cataract—is in excellent health.

Biological Versus Chronological Age

Not surprisingly, the human population whose calorie allocation is most like that of these healthy CR primates is the Okinawans.[12] We've found that their low-cal diet is not only key to their lifelong leanness but also an important element of their successful aging. It's a good part of how they have managed to slow the aging process and why so many of them *look* half their age and are able to function like younger people. It's helped keep their faces less wrinkled, their skin less saggy, their eyes brighter, and their bodies more mobile and healthy. While of course they age chronologically like the rest of us, the Okinawa diet has helped keep them physiologically and biologically many years younger than their actual ages.[18]

As you'll see when we introduce you to biomarkers of longevity in the next chapter, we now have ways to measure how quickly we're aging. By measuring the stiffness of our arteries, blood pressure levels, cholesterol levels, hormonal levels, and several other functions, we can gauge our biological age, a much better indicator of where we stand in the aging process than our calendar age.[19] The elder Okinawans' young biomarkers continue to astound us. They are extraordinarily young relative to their actual age in almost every area measured.

THE SCIENCE

The science behind caloric restriction and its ability to help keep the body slim, healthy, and youthful is fascinating. The most plausible theoretical mechanism is a reduction in the production of cell-damaging free radicals, which are generated primarily by metabolizing food for energy—if you eat less food, you generate fewer free radicals. Lower free radical production in turn minimizes potential damage to cellular machinery, such as DNA and mitochondria (cell power generators), which ultimately results in slower aging at the cellular level. In essence, reducing calories increases the body's metabolic efficiency. It allows your body to process its fuel (blood sugar) more efficiently as it generates energy, which results in lower blood sugar levels and less damage to cells and tissues from a process called *glycation*. (When glycation occurs, sugar sticks to cells and their components, sort of like an old sticky piece of candy in your pocket would, literally gumming up the works.) When you consume a large quantity of calories, you are, in effect, turning up your thermostat and creating more friction as your body generates energy. Your whole system runs hotter and is likelier to burn out before its time.

From the standpoint of evolutionary theory, it's been proposed that limiting calories kicks into play an "adaptive response," the same kind animals use when faced by episodic periods of food shortage in the wild. They simply shift their allocation of energy from growth and reproduction to maintenance and repair and thus survive the period of deprivation, becoming even stronger in the process.[19] It's an intriguing mechanism and, judging by the Okinawan longevity phenomenon, it seems to work as well in humans. This should send a loud wake-up call to Americans, because while the long-lived Okinawans have naturally limited their calories and thrived, Americans' approach to food is the polar opposite.

OVERFED AMERICANS

Americans consume way too many calories. According to data from the U.S. Department of Agriculture and the National Center for Health Statistics from the mid-1990s, we eat about 2,500 calories per day compared to the Okinawans' 1,800 calories, and this surplus of calories has turned the United States into a fat nation.[20,26] According to a recent U.S. Surgeon General's report, more than 61 percent of American adults are overweight, and 27 percent of us—*50 million people*—are obese.[21]

Our children are in serious trouble too. The percentage of overweight six- to eleven-year-olds has nearly doubled in two decades, and it has tripled for adolescents. In the next decade, weight-related illnesses threaten to overwhelm the health-care system. New evidence from the Framingham Heart Study shows that obesity *doubles* the risk of heart failure and *triples* the risk of breast cancer in women.[22] A man with twenty-two extra pounds—the average weight gain during middle age—has a 75 percent greater chance of having a heart attack than he would at a healthy weight. Gaining just fifteen pounds doubles the risk of developing Type II diabetes, an illness that has increased by nearly 50 percent in the past decade.

These kinds of statistics point out how crucial healthy weight maintenance is to our overall health and well-being. By staying fit and lean, we greatly reduce our risk of life-threatening diseases; our bodies operate more efficiently; we feel lighter and more energetic; and we may add ten or more *disability-free* years to our lives, and possibly much more than that, as we will show you later on.[23] Simply put, we have a considerably better quality of life. The good news is that we now better understand the mechanism behind lifelong weight maintenance. We know what it takes to lead a happier, healthier life. The Okinawans have shown us the way. Now all we have to do is follow them.

Calorie Restriction Without the Restriction

While the benefits of calorie restriction are undeniable, the concept itself may not sound especially appealing. The very word *restriction* tends to send a collective shiver up our back and conjure up visions of rabbit food, constant hunger, and deprivation. But trust us, we are in no way suggesting you nibble on nothing but romaine the rest of your life. When the calorie restriction principle is applied properly—done the Okinawa way—it's anything but deprivation. It's not even a diet. You could think of eating the Okinawa way as *unrestricted calorie restriction*. You can eat wonderfully tasty food—and a lot of it—and still reduce your calorie intake. That's what the Okinawan elders do. They enjoy fabulous food and rarely gain a pound. Weight is never a concern.

When you try the recipes in the book, you'll see that Okinawan fusion cooking, often referred to as "Japanese food with salsa," is a delicious blend of East and West—the best of both worlds. It's a variation of the kind of Asian fusion cuisine that's rapidly gaining in popularity across the United States and is already a media-touted phenomenon in California, Hawaii, Seattle, New York, and other areas with significant Asian populations. In fact, two Asian fusion culinary superstars, both rated among the best chefs in the world, have Okinawa connections. Chef Nobu Matsuhisa, who cooks for the stars at Nobu in New York and Matsuhisa in Los Angeles (among his other restaurants), was greatly influenced by Okinawan cooking when he spent the early part of his career in Peru, which has one of the largest Okinawan immigrant populations worldwide. Chef Roy Yamaguchi, who now owns a string of Roy's restaurants around the world, learned to cook from his Okinawan mother. Okinawan specialties are among his signature dishes at Roy's in Hawaii, and within months after it opened, Mimi Sheraton chose it as one of *Conde Nast Traveler*'s top fifty American restaurants. To see Chef Roy in action, watch him on *Hawaii Cooks*, his hit PBS series—where he's been known to rave about his mother's wonderful Okinawan cooking. Okinawans are so adept at creating wonderful meals that they once owned over 80 percent of Honolulu's restaurants and are still a culinary force in Hawaii.

Need we say more? You can see we're not exaggerating when we talk about how delicious Asian fusion and Okinawan fusion cooking is. Now imagine being able to enjoy this kind of wonderful food without gaining weight—that's *eating the Okinawa way.* The principles behind Okinawan low-cal cooking can also be used effectively to create wonderful westernized dishes, as you'll see in chapters 7 and 8. So even if you're not ready to take the culinary leap across the Pacific, you can still eat well and reap the health benefits of the Okinawa diet.

Eat More, Weigh Less

Here's the topper: Not only is the food terrific but also you can eat a good deal of it and still keep your figure. One of the most startling findings of our latest research is that while Okinawan elders have consumed fewer calories through-out their lives than Americans, they have actually eaten more food—that is, the food on their plates actually weighed more than that on the plates of typical Americans. From data provided by the landmark Seven Countries Study, we were able to calculate the content of a traditional American diet in the 1960s, which we then computed and compared to Okinawans' traditional diet during

Figure 1.3

HOW TO EAT MORE, FEEL FULLER, AND WEIGH LESS
EATING THE OKINAWA WAY

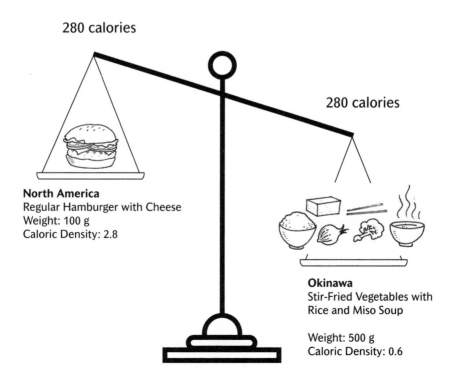

280 calories

280 calories

North America
Regular Hamburger with Cheese
Weight: 100 g
Caloric Density: 2.8

Okinawa
Stir-Fried Vegetables with
Rice and Miso Soup

Weight: 500 g
Caloric Density: 0.6

the same period. It turned out that Americans were eating about 2,100 calories per day, which amounted to about two pounds of food. The Okinawans, on the other hand, were eating only about 1,600 calories per day—that's 500 calories less—but their food weighed about 2.5 pounds—a half pound more. In other words, it wasn't *how much* the Okinawans ate that resulted in their lifelong lean-ness but rather the *kinds* of foods they ate. The Okinawans were, in fact, eating more food but consuming fewer calories.

To figure out how they were able to do that, we analyzed the amount of car-bohydrates, fat, and protein they consumed and computed the balance of these nutrients, factoring in the differences in exercise habits between the young and the old. After we crunched and recrunched the numbers, we found that it was not the amount of carbs, fat, protein, or some complicated balance of these fac-tors. The Okinawan elders were not hitting some magical calorie-burning zone. What they were doing was intuitively making the right food choices based on years of healthy habit. The foods they were choosing were nutrient-rich, but the amount of calories per gram of food was very low. By eating foods low in *caloric density*—remember those magic words—the Okinawans could eat until they were satisfied and not gain weight. This was the key we had been searching for —and a big part of what we now call eating the Okinawa way.

Caloric Density—The Key to Eating the Okinawa Way

Caloric density (CD) is closely associated with the calorie restriction principle that works so efficiently in foraging animals when they shift their energy alloca-tion from growth to maintenance and repair during times of food shortage. It's also the subject of a great deal of ongoing scientific research, including our own. It's become such a hot topic, in fact, that the *Wall Street Journal* recently reported it as a cover story,[17] and the National Institute on Aging has invested heavily in studies geared to learning more about the mechanisms involved.[24] Most of these studies are reaching the same conclusion we have: Limiting calorie intake is the healthiest approach to eating.

Technically, *caloric density* refers to the number of calories in a specific amount of any given food—it's usually based on a 1-gram unit. The fewer calo-ries in 1 gram of food, the more of that food you can eat and still maintain your weight. The more calories in 1 gram of a specific food, the less of it you can eat without gaining weight. In our program, we call low–caloric density foods *lightweights*—those are the foods you can eat with impunity—and we call high–caloric density foods *heavyweights*—those you have to considerably moderate or eliminate. There's a caloric density scale as well as a caloric density food pyramid in chapter 3 that makes it ultra-easy to tell one from the other. We'll talk about how to use the scale, specific foods, and delicious lightweight recipes in the following chapters. Suffice it to say here that the caloric density principle allows you to thoroughly enjoy your food and eat a satisfying amount of it without gaining weight. It also allows you to lose weight efficiently, without hunger or feelings of deprivation, should that be your goal.

Interestingly, we're programmed to eat about the same amount of food regardless of how many calories it contains. Studies done by experts in Great Britain, the Netherlands, and the United States have all come to the same conclusion. People eat about two to three pounds of food daily. A recent study by Dr. Barbara Rolls, a nutrition and obesity expert at Pennsylvania State University, showed that women, when served pasta with vegetables in low–, medium–, or high–caloric density meals, ate the same weight of food no matter whether it was a CD lightweight or heavyweight meal.[25] Lightweight meals (more vegetables and less pasta) resulted in a 30 percent lower caloric intake but no reported difference in fullness or satisfaction. Obviously, depending on your food choices and their caloric density, this could result in a vastly different caloric intake—and a different size waistline. Again, comparing the traditional Okinawan diet to the average American diet illustrates the point.

The American Versus the Okinawan Diet

The traditional Okinawan diet, which we'll discuss at length in the following chapters, contains a good percentage of caloric lightweights—mostly plant-based foods and low-glycemic-index carbohydrates. These are foods that contain more water, such as soups and stews, and more fiber, such as vegetables. Most foods are peppered with the delicious calorie-free spices of the Orient.

Standard American fare, on the other hand, contains seriously high-caloric heavyweights: burgers, fries, soft drinks, white bread, sugar-laden cookies, doughnuts, candy, fatty sauces, salad dressings—and the list goes on. If you eat a "satisfying" amount of that kind of food, kiss your waistline good-bye, not to mention your health and perhaps decades of your life. That's exactly what typical Americans are doing.

Even as we obsess about controlling our weight, we're eating more calories per bite than our ancestors, *and* the foods are increasingly laden with refined sugar and fat. The USDA's dietary intake surveys show a 236-calorie-per-person increase in our daily calorie consumption between 1987 and 1995—that theoretically adds an average of twenty-four pounds to our waistlines every year![26] Our only saving grace is that as we pack on the pounds, our body's thermostat—called its *basal metabolic rate* (BMR)—runs hotter and actually burns more calories, so most of us can still fit in a single airplane seat.[26,27] But the extra damage our bodies accrue from running the furnace so hot takes its toll on our health. More about that in the next chapter.

Not surprisingly, 39 percent of the extra calories we consume, and the weight gain they produce, comes from refined grains (such as white bread, white rice, low-fat but sugar-laden cookies, and crackers); 32 percent from added fats such as cooking oils, salad oils, and French-fried potatoes; and 24 percent simply from more sugar.[20] It may seem incredible, but Americans actually eat an average of 27 teaspoons of sugar per person per day. About a third comes from soft drinks, but sugar is also found in a huge number of foods. Even foods like lunch meat, sausages, microwave pizza, many breads, soup, crackers, spaghetti sauce, canned fruit and vegetables, fruit drinks, yogurt, catsup, and mayonnaise have more than their fair share.

To make matters even worse, at the same time the nutritional value of our food has gone downhill, the portion size of snacks and meals has soared upward.[28] McDonald's original burger, fries, and 12-ounce Coke provided a hefty 590 calories but now a supersize Extra Value Meal, which includes a quarter-pounder with cheese, supersize fries, and drink, packs an incredible 1,550 calories! In the 1950s movie theater popcorn averaged three cups, but a *medium*-size popcorn today is sixteen cups in the same theater—an extra 700 calories. 7-Eleven's 64-ounce Double Gulp soda weighs in at almost *ten* times the calories as the original 6.5-ounce bottle of Coca-Cola! You can see the problem.

Marketing Versus Common Sense

Studies by the Center for Science in the Public Interest indicate that fast-food outfits often entice customers with supersize items by pushing "value."[29] The pitch: A lot more food for just a little more money equals "good value for your dollar." And hey, who can resist a good deal? Cinnabon, a pastry chain, sells their 3-ounce Minibon for about $2.00, but for another half dollar you can gorge on an 8-ouncer. While great for your wallet, it more than doubles the calories. Value marketing also results in "bargain meals." For example, at McDonald's a quarter-pounder with cheese, medium fries, and soft drink costs an average of $5.03. The exact same items packed into an Extra Value Meal cost only $3.74. Wendy's plays the same game where a Classic Double Cheese Old-Fashioned Combo Meal costs $4.89 and weighs in at 1,360 calories but for only 39 cents more, you can eat a walloping 1,540 calories in a "biggie" meal. The scary thing is that when these supersize, biggie, "value" portions are in front of us, our instincts tell us to eat it.

This was clearly demonstrated by a study done at Pennsylvania State University.[30] The subjects were lean young men already shown to exhibit good calorie control. They were given different-size portions of macaroni and cheese for lunch on different days. When presented with 16 ounces on their plates, they ate 10 ounces. But here's the scoop—when presented with a 25-ounce "jumbo lunch," they packed away 15 ounces. That's 50 percent more food than they had felt was satisfactory the last go-round. Sound familiar?

But we're not just dealing with clever marketing, we're also struggling against biology. Throughout most of human history, food was scarce, and it required a great deal of physical energy to acquire it. Those who ate the most calories staved off famine and had the energy to reproduce. Those who ate fewer calories perished. As a result, we humans are hard-wired to prefer calorie-rich diets high in fat and sugar. The problem, of course, is that today there's a complete mismatch between biology and the environment. Our physiology tells us to eat food whenever it's available. But food is *always* available. Food is so plentiful in the United States that an average of 3,800 calories per person per day is available.[26] Yet most of us need less than half that amount to thrive.

Strangely, people seem to have disconnected the relationship between food availability, eating behavior, and their rapidly growing waistlines. Americans seem to operate with little awareness about how much they're actually eating. An American Institute of Cancer Research study in the year 2000 revealed that 62 percent of participants felt that restaurant portions are the same size or smaller than they were a decade ago.[31] Only a few routinely measured food portions, and most could not correctly estimate serving sizes. Most admitted to being overweight. In a similar Harvard study, most participants were overweight, but 78 percent did not see this as a health problem.[32] Cancer and heart disease were viewed as important health problems but obesity was not—yet obesity increases the risk for both heart disease and cancer *and* cuts an average seven years off a life. In fact, being obese is equivalent to being a lifelong smoker—and having both health problems cuts an average fourteen years off your life.[33]

All these misconceptions are really not that surprising. Nutrition advice has been all over the map—low fat versus the "right fat"; low protein versus high protein; low carbohydrate versus high carbohydrate. People are more confused than ever, and that makes them vulnerable to any slickly marketed diet plan that comes down the pike, whether they're ketogenic low-carbohydrate diets like the Atkins and Protein Power diets or mythical Zone diets like Barry Sears's. Plus, various medical organizations offer different, sometimes divergent dietary advice. You've got the American Heart Association focusing on dietary fat and cholesterol; the American Diabetes Association concentrating on carbohydrates and blood sugar; and the National Cancer Institute recommending those five-a-day fruit/veggie diets for cancer prevention, just to name a few.[34]

Unified Dietary Guidelines

Thankfully, the recent creation of the Unified Dietary Guidelines should help clarify and simplify dietary advice and put matters into perspective.[35] The guidelines, a joint effort of the National Cancer Institute, American Heart Association, American Dietetic Association, and the National Institutes of Health, suggest six simple rules for healthy eating. The rules emphasize a varied, plant-based diet, high in complex carbohydrates (more than 55 percent of total calories), low in fat (less than 30 percent of total calories, with an emphasis on mono/poly/sat fat, in that order), five to six servings a day each of grains and vegetables/fruits, and no more than 6 grams of salt per day. As you'll see when you read chapter 4, these guidelines are remarkably similar to the diet traditional Okinawans have been following their entire lives. It seems that the elders have been right all along.

The bottom line is that excess calories not only contribute to age-associated maladies but also have a huge impact on the aging process itself.[14] Consuming too many calories makes you look older and actually age faster. The only credible way to slow the aging process is to cut the excess calories, and our twenty-eight years of research shows that the easiest, most enjoyable, and healthiest way to do that is by eating the Okinawa way.

Naturally, other factors contribute to optimum health and successful aging. There's no longer any question that our lifestyle and attitudes have a considerable bearing on health and longevity—for the Okinawans and ourselves. We need to keep our activity level up and our stress level down, and we'll address these factors later in the book. We strongly believe that achieving good health and longevity is a holistic endeavor—and we will honor that approach, as we did in *The Okinawa Program*. But in this book we want to concentrate on diet because it's an area where so many of us go wrong so often. We want to help you lose the weight you want to lose in the healthiest way possible and keep it off all through your life without dieting—just like the Okinawan elders.

Chapter 2

NEW FINDINGS FOR
HEALTHY WEIGHT

To lengthen thy life, lessen thy meals.
—Cicero (Roman orator, 103–43 B.C.)

For many years, excess weight was considered relatively unimportant in terms of health. It was viewed mainly as a red flag: If someone was overweight, his or her doctor would check for high cholesterol and other factors that might increase the risk for heart disease. Because our study was focused primarily on healthy aging, we concentrated on how weight affected age-related diseases that influenced longevity.[1] But as science has progressed and we've become more sophisticated in our research techniques, it's become clear that weight gain and longevity are flip sides of the same coin—extreme excess weight simply negates longevity. Simply put, overweight people don't live as long as slim people. Overweight (and obesity) is not just a warning sign but rather a complex multifactorial disease in and of itself as well as a precursor to other life-threatening diseases such as diabetes, heart disease, stroke, many cancers, and even aging itself. In fact, the Rand Institute equated being obese with aging prematurely by twenty years![2]

Why does excess weight present such a risk? The reason, incredible as it may sound, is that fat is actually now considered by leading scientists to be an endocrine organ.[3] As you probably know, the endocrine system consists of a number of organs, including the thyroid, pituitary gland, pancreas, and sex glands, that secrete hormones that act as messengers and tell other organs or systems what to do. Well, fat appears to be the latest addition to the endocrine club. It sends messages just like the other members. Fat doesn't just hang around your waist like a spare tire; it actually produces many messenger hormones. For example, fat cells secrete hormones such as leptin, which helps regulate appetite and helps tell your body how much energy to burn. Fat cells respond to hormones such as insulin that tell them to store fat. They also send signals to genes that control uncoupling proteins, which tell mitochondria (the cell's energy furnaces) how much of your calorie intake should be burned off as heat, how much should be stored as fat, or how much to use ASAP. Fat cells even produce estrogen. In fact, after menopause, body fat becomes the major source of a woman's estrogen. That's why estrogen-dependent cancers, such as endometrial cancer and breast cancer, are more common in obese women—more fat means more estrogen production.[4]

The common links between body fat and longevity, particularly in regard to the hormones involved in both processes, have renewed interest among gerontologists to search for biomarkers, or physiological signs of aging[5]—and we've found some fascinating ones, including a great many that are weight-related.[6] Some of the healthy biomarkers we've found in the lean, long-lived Okinawan elders are directly related to their low–caloric density diet, which we'll be talking about in depth in the next chapter as we show you how to incorporate the principles of caloric density in your everyday life.

But first we'd like to share some of our other key discoveries with you: biomarkers and other findings that leave no doubt that health, longevity, and weight are closely linked and even share some of the same biological factors—both genetic and lifestyle-related.

KEY FINDING #1
Lifestyle Trumps Genes

One of the things we're frequently asked about the Okinawans' extraordinary longevity and lifelong leanness is, "How do you know it's not genetic?" Well, to a small degree it *is* genetic.[7] The more we learn about genes, the more we understand their importance. There's no longer any doubt that genes play a part in successful aging, body weight, and overall health. In fact, landmark discoveries in the past decade have connected more than 250 genes or genetic markers to obesity, including the OB gene (Obesity Gene), a defect associated with increased body fat in certain people; insulin, leptin, and grehlin, hormones that help control appetite and metabolism; and neuropeptides such as Neuropeptide Y, a hormone found in both the gut and the brain that influences appetite and obesity.[8] Scientists can now even genetically engineer a mouse to be obese by giving it two copies of a superfat OB gene.[9]

But mice aside, the real question is how relevant genes are in terms of the average person's weight. How do genes affect you? The truth is, only marginally —if you follow a healthy lifestyle. During the years between 1991 and 1998, there was a 50 percent rise in obesity in the United States.[10] Genes? Certainly human genes hadn't changed dramatically—if, indeed, at all—during those eight years. In fact, for most of human history, obesity was a non-issue. It occurred only among royalty—which, not coincidentally, was the only group that could afford our modern obesity-prone lifestyles.

The fact is that for the most part, genes involved in weight gain don't directly cause corpulence but rather increase susceptibility to it in those who possess the genes when they are exposed to modern obesity-friendly environments—which is most of the time.[11] Any environment that features an overabundance of high–caloric density food and discourages regular hearty physical activity is considered to be obesity-friendly. Sound familiar? It should, as most of you reading this are living in modern fast-food nations. The bottom line: If we all lived a healthy lifestyle, the percentage of us who would *not* be able to maintain a healthy weight would be in the single digits. Which naturally brings us to the Okinawans.

GOOD GENES HELP, BUT LIFESTYLE COUNTS MORE

While genetic research on body weight, obesity, and aging is still in its infancy, the bulk of our evidence shows that the very old Okinawans have *some* genetic protection that helps them stay lean and healthy and live longer. But lifestyle factors—what they eat, what they do, and what they think—have considerably greater significance.[7]

First the genes: By current estimates, we have about 30,000 genes in our bodies, spread out across the forty-six chromosomes (twenty-three pairs) found in the nucleus of most of our cells. Our genes tell our cells when to make copies of themselves and what kinds of proteins and other substances to manufacture to keep the body running smoothly. Genes even tell a cell when to self-destruct (if it's injured or malfunctioning, for instance) and instruct our body how to respond to stresses like receiving inadequate amounts of food—or getting too much of it.

One example of genes that can help or hurt your battle with body fat and affect you in many other areas are the HLA genes. HLA (human leukocyte antigen) genes constitute a group of about 150 genes located on chromosome number 6 (which contains genes that control your body's response to insulin and affect your body fat level, among other functions)—and they are very important to our overall health.[12] Some of the genes in this group are linked to diseases of the immune system, such as diabetes, and to chronic inflammatory diseases like rheumatoid arthritis and SLE (lupus). New studies also suggest that HLA genes may be linked to obesity, coronary heart disease, and aging itself.[12] We've found that Okinawan centenarians are more likely to have low-risk HLA gene profiles (or "elite" genes)—which means, in effect, that they have a better than average chance of avoiding problems in these areas.[7]

But another interesting finding emerged from our genetic studies—and this is the one you want to pay close attention to. We found that *some centenarians did not possess the low-risk genes.* In fact, some even had high-risk genes. This means some Okinawans remained slim, healthy, and robust for a full century *despite* "bad genes" or the absence of good ones.

This remarkable finding strongly suggests that genes, environment (including lifestyle), and, to a degree, chance interact to determine your health status. If you have an average set of genes (as most of us do), it's your lifestyle that becomes the most important determinant in your ability to stay lean, healthy, and live to a ripe old age (see table below). Needless to say, having both good genes and a healthy lifestyle would be the most desirable, but genes are the luck of the draw and beyond our control (for the time being, anyway.) Lifestyle, on the other hand, is entirely within our control. Make good choices, and you've got a better than average shot at staying lean for all your long, healthy life—just like the Okinawans.

Do You Need Elite Genes to Be Lean, Long-Lived, and Healthy?

Gene Quality	Good[1]	Average[2]	Poor[3]	Total
% Centenarians	6.1	85.4	8.5	100
% Total Population	0.0	69.2	30.8	100

DR1: protective gene; DRw9: deleterious gene.
[1]DR1 (+), DRw9 (−)
[2]DR1 (−), DRw9 (−)
[3]DR1 (−), DRw9 (+)

Note: In this example of important HLA genes, only 6.1 percent of centenarians had elite (good) genes, most had average genes, and 8.5 percent even had high-risk (poor) genes yet still lived to one hundred. This finding is consistent with other genetic studies that suggest that it is not just how well designed your body is but how you treat it that determines your weight and health. Adapted from the Okinawa Centenarian Study *Genetics of Longevity Database* (see note 7 for more information).

OKINAWANS IN BRAZIL: PARADISE LOST?

Our study is not the only one to demonstrate that lifestyle is a far more important contributor to the Okinawan elders' lifelong leanness and healthy longevity. Migration studies by our colleague Dr. Yukio Yamori from the World Health

Organization–Collaborating Center for Research on the Primary Prevention of Cardiovascular Disease at Kyoto University in Japan show that Okinawans who grow up in Brazil and abandon traditional Okinawan lifestyle patterns get significantly fatter, suffer higher death rates from all causes, and have a much shorter lifespan than those who grow up in Okinawa.[13]

The differences between traditional Okinawans and Brazilian Okinawans are truly impressive. Almost every cause of death, especially heart disease and cancer of the colon, breast, and prostate, goes up dramatically when Okinawans leave their protective Shangri-la for Brazil.[13] Perhaps even more alarming is that they lose seventeen years of life expectancy. While this may pale in comparison to the fate of the lithe beauty in James Hilton's book *Lost Horizon,* who instantaneously ages a hundred years and turns to dust when she leaves her Shangri-la, it does tell us something loud and clear: Genes aren't the answer. The Okinawans in Brazil, with their elevated chronic disease rates and shorter life expectancy, have the same genes as the robust, long-lived, slim Okinawan elders. All the study subjects were first-, second-, or third-generation Okinawan Brazilians, and three generations are but a blink in evolutionary history. Their genes hadn't changed—their lifestyles had. This pretty much blows a hole in the it's-all-in-their-genes theory.

The most likely explanation for the health discrepancy is diet. When Okinawans grow up in Brazil they tend not to eat the Okinawa way but rather adopt the Brazilian way, which is all too close to the American way. They consume eighteen times more meat, including double the processed meats like Spam, triple the sugar and milk, a third fewer vegetables and less fish.[13] As if this was not enough, they sprinkle 20 percent more salt on their plates. This dietary pattern (more fat and simple sugars) significantly increases the number of calories in their diet, even when they eat the same *amount* of food as their Okinawa-based brethren, and puts them at higher risk for obesity, diabetes, heart disease, and cancer—all diseases linked by higher insulin levels and largely determined by high calorie intake and inadequate physical activity. Okinawans, alas, have much less likelihood of reaching a ripe old age in Brazil (see figure 2.1).

OKINAWA'S NEXT GENERATION

There is one more case in point we want to make regarding genetics, although we've touched on it briefly before, and that's the young Okinawans. They add considerable weight—literally—to the lifestyle-over-genes debate. While

Okinawans were once the leanest Japanese, the current generation is now the heaviest.[14] The stereotypic image of the lean Okinawan, the norm until only a few decades ago, is fast disappearing from the Japanese collective consciousness. Again, this obviously has nothing to do with genes and everything to do with lifestyle. We humans have been evolving a very long time, making it highly unlikely that a three-decade progression from lean to fat is some sort of spontaneous, maladaptive evolutionary leap. If anything, it may be a case of success breeding complacency; the healthy example of the Okinawan elders seems to have been lost on the young.

Again, diet is most certainly the major culprit in the turnaround. The transition occurred in parallel with many changes in the traditional Okinawan diet. Around 1960, it was noticed that young Okinawans were eating about 40 percent fewer calories than their Japanese counterparts.[15] The government deemed them underweight and instituted a new school lunch program that was much higher in fat and refined carbs to solve the perceived problem. Full-fat milk and refined white bread replaced a low-calorie plant-based diet centered on vegetables, unprocessed grains, soy foods, fish, and occasional lean pork. At the time, the new diet seemed a luxury—but predictably, once the traditional way of eating was superseded, the eating habits of the once slim Okinawan children tilted too much toward the Western model, and they gained weight accordingly,

Figure 2.1

BMI AND CENTENARIAN PREVALENCE IN OKINAWANS IN OKINAWA VS. BRAZIL

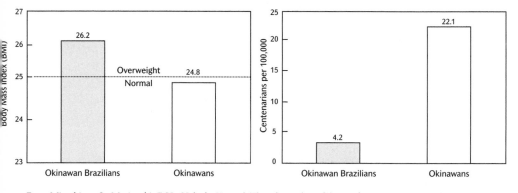

From Mizushima, S., Moriguchi, E.H., Hakada, Y., et al. The relationship of dietary factors to cardiovascular diseases among Japanese in Okinawa and Japanese immigrants, originally from Okinawa, in Brazil. *Hypertension Res* 1992: 15:45–55.

soon surpassing the rest of the Japanese (see figure 2.2). Their weight gain was exacerbated as adults. Now all Okinawans up until about age seventy have a higher body mass index (BMI) than other Japanese.[16] To be fair, we should mention that some of the other changes initiated after World War II were quite beneficial—near eradication of infectious diseases, much lower infant mortality rates, and, for a while, anyway, a more balanced diet with a wider variety of foods. But that was then, this is now.

Today, the dietary patterns of the general Okinawan population (excluding the elders) have shifted significantly from the traditional diet of vegetables, fruit, soybeans, whole grains, fish, and limited amounts of lean meats to one much heavier in meat, processed grains (e.g. white rice), and fast food.[17] The shift has markedly increased the caloric density of the diet and led to higher consumption of calories. At the same time, daily physical activity has diminished. This deadly combination is an all-too-familiar story. The same scenario has been cast with native Hawaiians, Pima Indians, and many other traditional peoples whose diets and lifestyles were rapidly westernized. Those cultures suffer epidemics of obesity, diabetes, heart disease, and associated complications—just like in the rest of America.[18]

Figure 2.2

BODY WEIGHT TRENDS IN TWELVE-YEAR-OLD FEMALES IN OKINAWA AND JAPAN IN THE PAST FIFTY YEARS

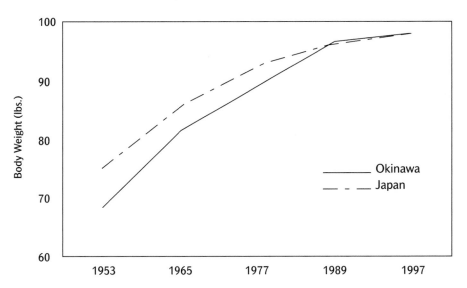

Adapted from Todoriki, H., Willcox, D.C., and Kinjo, Y., et al., 2002.[16]

KEY FINDING #2
Energy Balance Is Crucial for Healthy Weight Control

It may be hard to imagine, but most adults eat close to a ton of food a year. Yes, a ton! Yet our average weight fluctuation during the year averages only a few pounds. The reason all that food doesn't settle in and turn us into truck-size monsters is energy balance. *Energy balance is the equilibrium that's reached when your calorie intake equals the number of calories you expend in energy.* When you maintain an energy balance or energy homeostasis your body weight remains stable, your body's furnace runs efficiently, you're healthier and leaner, and you're much more likely to live a lot longer.[19]

Essentially, the human body functions in accord with Mayer's First Law of Thermodynamics: Energy cannot be created or destroyed—only changed.[20] In terms of weight control, this means that if your total food calories exceed your daily energy use, excess calories will accumulate and be stored as fat. On the other hand, when your caloric intake equals your caloric expenditure, your body weight will remain constant. Very simple.

Working within Mayer's Law, there are only three ways we can tip the energy balance equation to produce weight loss.

1. Reduce calories below daily energy requirements (eat fewer calories).

2. Maintain normal calories and increase energy use through additional physical activity (eat as usual, but exercise more).

3. Decrease calories and increase energy use (eat fewer calories *and* exercise more).

Reducing calories alone (essentially, dieting) is tough going because the body actively defends against low caloric intake by lowering its basal metabolic rate (BMR). Your BMR is the number of calories that your body burns at rest. It's like your body's thermostat and is the major determinant of how quickly you burn calories.[21] It has a set point that goes up or down according to calorie intake. When you reduce calories alone, your BMR goes down and alerts your body to burn calories more slowly as a defense against perceived starvation. The two ways to get your BMR back up are to be physically active, as activity raises BMR and keeps it up hours after the activity stops, and to build muscle tissue, as muscle burns more calories at rest than fat. Physical activity simply increases the energy output side of the equation, and it's even more important as we get

Figure 2.3

AGING AND ENERGY BALANCE:
WHY DO WE GAIN WEIGHT WITH AGE?

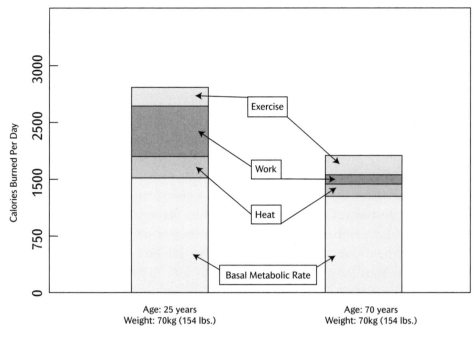

Note: Even if you weigh the same at age seventy as you did at age twenty-five, you will burn fewer calories at rest (BMR), you will burn less as heat, your workday is usually less strenuous, and you likely exercise less. Thus, the energy balance equation (output) is working against you. The solution is to exercise more (more calories out) and eat lower on the CD Pyramid (fewer calories in), thereby balancing the energy equation.

older, as BMR naturally slows down with aging. That means as we get older, if we don't expend more energy or cut back on calories, we'll almost certainly gain weight (see figure 2.3).

Obviously, working both sides of the energy equation—decreasing energy input *and* increasing energy output—is the ideal plan, a twofer in terms of weight control, and it is what the Okinawan elders do.

A DELICATE BALANCE

Your body's energy balance is more sensitive than you may think. Recent studies published in the leading medical journal *Science* suggest weight problems can be created by overshooting our calorie count by as little as 15 calories a day—that's less than a carrot's worth.[22] A daily energy imbalance of only 1 percent more input than output would increase your body weight by forty to fifty pounds during your adulthood—a common occurrence in Americans. If caloric intake exceeds output by only 100 calories per day (equivalent to one-quarter of a typical piece of cream pie), the surplus calories consumed in a year would add up to 36,500. Because 1 pound of body fat contains 3,500 calories, this caloric excess would cause a yearly gain of about ten pounds of body fat. Even Yuletide binges can upset the balance. One study reported that the average American gains one to two pounds during the yearly holiday season alone.[23] Over ten years, that amounts to a ten- to twenty-pound weight gain. Merry Christmas!

Before you get totally depressed, here's the good news: If your daily food intake decreased by just 100 calories and your energy expenditure increased by 100 calories, say by walking an extra mile, then your yearly fat loss would be twenty-one pounds! This means that just by making small changes in your eating habits and including a few extra activities in your day, such as taking the stairs instead of the elevator, you can effect a very different outcome in your body weight and health over the long term.

This is an exceptionally important point. Let's say you knocked off those 100 calories per day so that you were slightly under your body's set point on a regular basis. You'd not only be well on your way to lifelong healthy weight maintenance but also positioned to cash in on a valuable bonus. When your body's energy balance is tuned just below its set point (i.e., you eat slightly less than you require), your body has to defend that set point against being underweight rather than overweight. This allows you to tap into those tremendous calorie restriction benefits we mentioned earlier— slower aging and much lower disease risk.[24] This is partly because the lower set point leads your body to believe that a famine (or other bodily stress) is on the way, which causes it to shift its priorities from reproduction to maintenance. In other words, it fine-tunes your machine so it will be able to last a very long time under "harsh" conditions.

This fine-tuning may be the work of recently discovered uncoupling proteins (UCPs).[24] These proteins decide what percent of your calorie intake goes into making usable energy and what percent gets burned off as excess heat. If you take in more calories than you need, your energy efficiency could be as low as 25 percent. That may cause you to feel more sluggish and less sharp, and to tend to gain weight. You'd be like an old gas-guzzling car chugging along. But, on the other hand, if you take in slightly fewer calories than you need—say that magic 100 calories per day (just a handful of potato chips or a half of a chocolate bar) or you simply walk a mile, your body will turn the energy efficiency up as high as 50 percent.[22] Then your body would remodel itself along the lines of a new fuel-efficient car. You'd not only get yourself a sleeker chassis out of the

Figure 2.4

EFFECT OF CALORIC RESTRICTION AND EXERCISE ON GROUPS OF MICE

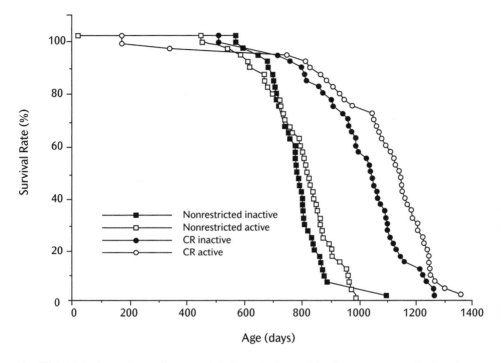

Note: While it is hard to put humans in a cage, calorically restrict them, and then have one group exercise, these data illustrate an important point—eating fewer calories and staying active (exercising) has strong additive benefits on life span in mammals. The mice that were calorically restricted (CR) *and* exercised survived the longest of all the groups. Adapted from Kim, et al.[25]

deal, but you'd likely feel sharper and look younger. Not a bad trade-off for half a chocolate bar (see figure 2.4).

HARA HACHI BU

One simple eating habit that helps the Okinawan elders stay energy efficient, and will be a boon to you too, is *hara hachi bu*. Loosely translated, it means "stop filling your stomach when you're eighty percent full," and it's something the elders have done all their lives. They simply stop eating before they feel they have to loosen their belt. It's a great habit to get into—you could easily knock 100 calories off a meal this way. Physiologically, *hara hachi bu* makes a lot of sense. The stomach takes about twenty minutes to signal the brain that it has filled to capacity, so by the time you feel full, you've actually overeaten a bit. If you eat until you're 100 percent full, you're essentially eating about 20 percent over capacity. On the other hand, if you stop *before* you feel full—if you just leave a little room in your stomach at the end of each meal—you could be eating 20 percent less—a real energy balance coup.

Bottom line: Input, output. Body fat depends on the balance between calories eaten and calories burned. When more calories are consumed than expended, the excess calories are stored as fat (in the form of cells called *adipocytes*). We've already seen how the prevalence of supersize portions and increased food availability in our culture make it easy to consume excess calories. Well, pair that with our penchant for inactivity, and you've got a classic energy imbalance. Studies show that only about 20 percent of Americans achieve the minimum public health goal of thirty minutes of moderate-intensity physical activity most days of the week, whereas about twice that number of Okinawans and three times that number of Okinawan elders meet that goal (see figure 2.5). This percentage of active Americans has essentially been the same for nearly three decades, but the population has increased by almost 60 million during that time. The result: 48 million more sedentary persons.[26] Physical activity has been all but engineered out of our workday and our leisure time.

Figure 2.5

ENERGY BALANCE IN OKINAWANS VERSUS AMERICANS

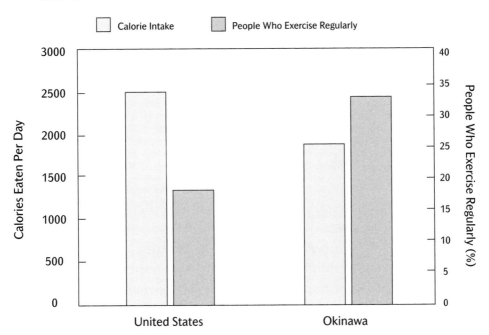

Note: Current diet of Okinawans and Americans. See chapter 1, note 26 for more information.

Computers, television, and video games may be enjoyable pastimes, but they also are big-time contributors to America's collective weight problem. Technology has done more than its share to shift the energy balance in the wrong direction. It's time to reverse the tide.

KEY FINDING #3
Macronutrient Balance Is Key to Healthy Weight Management and Loss

Food essentially contains two kinds of nutrients: *macronutrients,* which provide energy, and *micronutrients,* such as vitamins and minerals, that help the body use the energy. Carbohydrates, protein, fats, and alcohol are the main macronutrients. We'll disregard alcohol, for now, as we're concentrating on food. Water can also be considered a macronutrient because it's essential to processing the energy. To function properly, the body needs water and a certain amount of energy from carbohydrates, protein, and fats every day. That energy is measured in calories. Fat provides more than twice the calories per weight than carbohydrates or protein do, which is why reducing dietary fat is such an effective way to trim calories. Fat is the most concentrated source of energy, packing a whopping 9 calories per gram as opposed to carbohydrates and protein, which both weigh in at 4 calories per gram.

Nutrient	Calories per gram (caloric density)
Fat	9
Alcohol	7
Carbohydrate	4
Protein	4
Water	0

A diet that promotes health and helps you reach and maintain your ideal weight is based on a well-balanced combination of carbohydrates, protein, fats, and other nutrients—which perfectly describes the Okinawa diet. Our study has found that the elders have always had a healthy macronutrient balance in their diet— neither overly restrictive in one area nor overly permissive in another. But before we get into the specifics of the Okinawa diet, let's take a close individual look at the macronutrients to see what they're made of and what it takes to keep them in balance—and you out of trouble.

Fat

You've probably heard a lot of conflicting reports about fat over the years. At one point, it was considered a nutritional bogeyman, and for pretty good reasons. It's high in calories, it raises our cholesterol, and it was an omnipresent staple in our diets as we morphed into a fast-food nation. But then researchers came up with findings that turned the tide and took the pressure off fats. They reported that the Greeks and other Mediterranean populations who eat relatively high amounts of healthy monounsaturated fat, mostly olive oil, suffer no ill effects.[27] They also found that fat itself is essential to brain development, children's nervous systems, and, indeed, our overall health, and that the *right fat* could even help lower our cholesterol levels, decrease inflammation in the body, and possibly lower our risk for cardiovascular diseases and cancer.[28] So fat got a reprieve—it wasn't all bad, it was just misunderstood. And then fat became an overnight sensation. Thanks to weight-loss gurus like Dr. Atkins, whose mantra is "Eat fat to lose fat," it was hailed as a nutritional hero—although a dubious one. There are still quite a few of us in the vanguard of nutritional research—including, not coincidentally, the American Heart Association—who heartily disagree with Dr. Atkins and his followers, and we'll tell you why.[29] First, the facts.

FAT—THE LARGEST CONTRIBUTOR TO EXCESS ENERGY

Fat is a large food molecule that acts as a building block for cell walls, cholesterol, hormones, and other important components of the body. Its main role is to provide a dense source of stored energy, and it plays that role well. As we noted, it has more than twice the calories per gram than protein or carbohydrate, which makes it a potent energy source—and a macronutrient that has to be kept in proper balance for long-term weight management.

Fat metabolism research has revealed interesting facts. One of the most intriguing is that high-fat diets seem to bring on certain physiological changes that lead to weight gain. Dr. David York of the Pennington Biomedical Research Center, Baton Rouge, Louisiana, found that leptin, a hormone that rises in our bloodstream when we gain weight and helps shift metabolism into high fat-burning gear, loses its effectiveness in overweight people.[30] In other words, heavy people become resistant to leptin, just as diabetics become resistant to insulin. Dr. York found that high-fat diets could decrease the ability of leptin receptors to pick up the signal to burn fat. If the body doesn't receive the signal, it fails to crank up the metabolism, no fat is burned, and it gains weight. This is an excellent reason to watch the fat in your foods.

From a purely caloric perspective, the high caloric density of fat (not to mention its appealing taste) makes it all too easy to inadvertently slip into high-calorie territory. You don't feel you're eating much, but when you start counting the calories, you're way up there. So some fat limitation is critical to weight management. If your fat intake stays within 5 to 25 percent of your total calories, chances are you won't get in any serious trouble. But if you go beyond that, the percentage of your carbohydrates must be reduced, as they constitute over half of our usual calories. So if you eat much more than 25 percent fat, you can forget about ever having another bagel, but you can eat all the butter and cream cheese you want. Welcome to the Atkins Diet. (Actually, even Dr. Atkins wisely modified his original diet to exclude the worst of the fats and include healthy carbohydrates.)[29]

Your other option in terms of achieving energy balance on a fat-heavy diet is to run a couple of marathons per week. With all that energy input, you'd need to expend a *lot* of energy to stay balanced. Remember, the main reason Okinawan youths have lost their energy balance is excessive fat intake. Carbs have also contributed, as we discuss later, but keep the 25 percent fat rule in mind (see figure 2.6).

Figure 2.6

DAILY ENERGY BALANCE AND FAT INTAKE

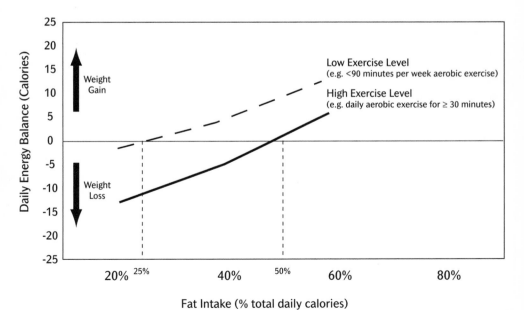

Note: If you eat more than 25 percent of your diet as fat and you don't exercise, you will tend to slip into positive energy balance territory and gain weight. If you eat a lot of fat (e.g., 50 percent of diet), you will have to be extremely active or severely restrict carbohydrate intake to stay in energy balance.

DIETARY FAT IS PREFERENTIALLY
STORED AS BODY FAT

Another reason to cut back on dietary fat is that it is more easily stored as body fat than either carbs or protein. Yes, this *is* true, despite all the misinformation being disseminated.[31] When you think about it, that the fat you eat is easily stored as body fat makes sense. The body is simply more efficient at converting fat to fat because it doesn't have to rearrange molecules to create an entirely new substance, which is the case when it converts proteins or carbs.[32] Fat to fat—it's easy. Only about 3 percent of the fat calories are used up during the conversion process, whereas the energy expended in making body fat from carbs is 25 percent, almost ten times as much![19] Changing one substance to another takes time and energy.

If you're in perfect energy balance, and your energy input exactly equals your output, you will burn off all the protein, carbs, and fat beyond what you need for energy replacement. On the other hand, the minute you slip into energy excess (positive balance) where you take in more calories than you expend, you start converting dietary fat to body fat. For practical purposes, this process mainly affects weight *gain,* not weight *loss.* When you lower calories enough to dip into negative energy balance (expending more calories than you take in) you will lose weight, no matter what the fat content of your diet, because you have to make up the energy from somewhere. Remember Mayer's Law?

Here's the interesting thing. If you eat too many calories from any source, be it fat, carbs, protein, or alcohol, you'll gain weight; but if those calories are from fat you'll gain *more* weight for the same number of calories.[33] This may seem counterintuitive, as we're often told a calorie is a calorie no matter what the source. But, alas, this is not quite true. The bottom line: An unfortunate property of fat is that the body absorbs it quickly and easily, and if we're in excess energy balance, most goes directly to the waistline—or whatever your body's favorite storage site is.[34] So if you eat an extra 500 calories per day from fat as opposed to carbs, you will gain an extra four pounds per year. Not much, but over a few years it could be responsible for that unwanted potbelly or those not-so-lovable love handles.

Carbohydrates

Like fats, carbohydrates have been in and out of favor with respect to weight management. They're currently coming up short in terms of popularity because they've been targeted as a weight-gain factor—which is not necessarily true. Like fat, not all carbs are alike. Certain carbs affect blood sugar and insulin (the hormone that signals the body to store fat) differently than others.[35] Here's how it works.

The main job of carbs is to provide immediate energy use and short-term energy storage (glycogen) in the liver and muscles. Carbs are the first place your body goes when it needs energy. Excess carbs you eat—those not needed for energy or glycogen replenishment—are simply burned off as heat.[36] Technically, all carbs are collections of carbon, hydrogen, and oxygen atoms (hence the name.) Depending on molecular structure, they can take the shape of simple sugars (one or two sugars joined together) like fructose (fruit sugar) and sucrose (table sugar). Some of these sugars, like sucrose, are rapidly converted to blood sugar (glucose); others, like fructose, convert very slowly. When three or more simple sugars are strung together, you get more complex collections of sugar molecules called *starches.*

Starch comes in two forms: amylopectin, which quickly converts to blood sugar, and amylose, which converts more slowly.[37] These are two important carbs to consider in weight control. A third key carb is fiber. Fiber comes in many forms: the most common type is cellulose, an indigestible stringy protective coating found in plant walls. Because fiber is indigestible, it slows the conversion of other carbs to blood sugar.

Generally, more than one of these three carbs (sugar, starch, fiber) is contained in any particular food. Fruit, for instance, has one simple carb (fructose) and two types of complex carbs (starch and fiber). This is what makes the carb story a little complicated. How a carb affects your weight is not just a matter of whether it is simple or complex, as many people think. It's the particular mix of carbohydrate types in a food that makes the difference, because that's what determines how rapidly that food is converted to blood sugar. For example, let's look at the complex carb wheat (starch and fiber). When it's made into white bread it's still complex because it has starch, but the fiber has been "refined" out during its processing into white flour. Often it has sucrose (table sugar) added to it when baked into bread. Before it was processed, the wheat was a high-fiber whole grain and would have been slowly converted to blood sugar. But as white bread without the fiber, it is rapidly converted to blood sugar. So processing is an important factor when it comes to carbs—and your weight.[35–38]

The rate of conversion from carb to blood sugar is called the *Glycemic Index* (GI). Very simply, the Glycemic Index tells us how much our blood sugar rises after we eat a particular kind of carb food.[35,37–38] Rapidly converted carbs cause a large rise in blood sugar levels—which is not a good thing. Increases in blood sugar lead to increases in insulin levels, which have been linked to a host of problems, including obesity, diabetes, cardiovascular disease, certain cancers, and even aging itself.[35,39] Bottom line: Any food that gets your insulin levels too high is bad news.

The good news is that, contrary to popular belief, not all carbs cause a large increase in your insulin levels. That misconception took root because all carbs were lumped together regardless of whether they were good carbs—unrefined, high-fiber, high-amylose carbs—or bad carbs—refined, low-fiber, high-amylopectin carbs. It doesn't quite work that way. Aside from the fact that many carbs have a low GI and don't cause large insulin reactions, certain protein-heavy and fat-heavy foods can also cause large insulin spikes.[40] Insulin scores for cheese, beef, and fish, for instance, are higher than porridge and other amylose-rich foods,

Figure 2.7

INSULIN SCORES OF SELECTED FOODS

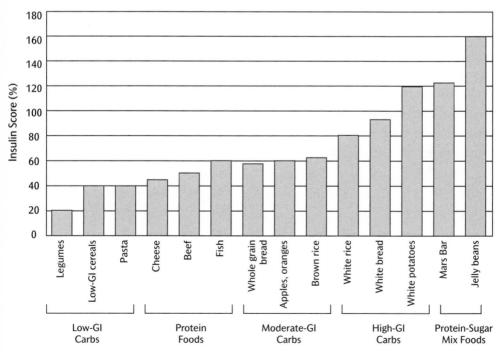

Adapted from Holt, S.H.A., et al. *American Journal of Clinical Nutrition* 1997, 66:1264.

and significantly higher than pasta. So it's the food itself, not the macronutrient group it belongs to, that determines insulin response.

While it helps to understand all this science, the most important point to remember is that Western staples that are highly processed or high in amylopectin (bad starch) such as white bread, white potatoes, bakery goods (cookies, pies, cakes), and fat- or protein-rich sweets (jelly beans, chocolate bars) are the biggest insulin culprits. Whole foods, or foods in their natural state, such as vegetables, fruits, whole grains, and other unprocessed foods, tend to have low GI scores and induce low insulin levels (see figure 2.7). They are low in caloric density and are your biggest allies in your struggle to control your weight.[40,41]

CARBOHYDRATE—NOT AN IMPORTANT SOURCE OF BODY FAT

Let's set the record straight on carbs before we move on to our next macronutrient. Many studies have shown that eating too many high-GI carbs—cookies, waffles, white bread, and the like—raises triglyceride levels in the blood.[42] Because triglyceride is a major component of body fat, people thought that the body turns carbohydrates into body fat. That's not the case. In reality, when you eat too much of *any* kind of calories you turn on the fat switch in your body's adipocytes (fat cells). That switch says "Store fat," so the body begins to convert dietary fat to body fat rather than burning it off. We've seen in tightly controlled metabolic studies that when subjects were fed many more calories than they needed, but these calories were all from carbohydrates, pushing them into highly positive energy balance—sumo wrestler territory—they nonetheless stored only a maximum of 12 carbohydrate grams per day as fat.[36,43] That's 108 calories. The rest of the body fat came from dietary fat.

While the distinction is subtle, it's nonetheless important because the belief that carbs make us fat has led a lot of us to avoid healthy, low-GI carbs such as vegetables, fruit, and high-fiber whole grains, which are antioxidant-rich and the mainstay of any low-cal diet. It is extremely hard to keep your calorie intake low if you're eating a lot of fat. Also, remember that some carbohydrate foods have a lot of fiber in them, which is entirely free of calories. Some of the carbohydrate foods in the Okinawan diet, such as *konyakku* (e.g. sukiyaki noodles), have been used specifically as weight-loss foods in Japan.[44] They're filling, tasty, and almost calorie-free. Bottom line: Eat like the Okinawan elders and you won't have to worry about getting fat from carbs (see table).

Americans Who Eat the Fewest Carbs Tend to Be the Most Overweight

Variable	≤30% of energy from carbohydrate	30–50% of energy from carbohydrate	>55% of energy from carbohydrate
Energy (kcal)	2,026	2,166	1,895
Total fat (% kcal)	46	37	25
Saturated fatty acids (% kcal)	16	12	8
Carbohydrate (% kcal)	25	45	62
Protein (% kcal)	22	17	14
Mean BMI—men	26.9	26.6	26.1
Mean BMI—women	26.8	25.9	25.4

Note: This study of what average Americans are eating shows that those who eat fewer carbs tend to be the most over-weight and those who eat more carbs are less overweight. A body mass index (BMI) >25 is overweight. The Okinawan elders most resemble the group on the right (>55% carbs). From *Clinical Diabetes* 2001;19:108.

Protein

At the moment, protein is the most popular of the macronutrients—and there's some justification for that. We all need it. Protein is an essential component of the body. The organs, muscles, brain, nerves, and immune system are all, to some degree, composed of protein; just name a body structure, and it probably has some protein in it. Because protein is one of the fundamental building blocks of the body, it's crucial that you get enough of it in your diet—but not too much. Too *little* can lead to protein malnutrition; too *much* can set us on the path to high blood pressure, kidney stones, and arterial aging, just to name a few related health concerns.[45] So proper balance is once again the name of the game.

We humans do very well when our protein intake is from 10 to 20 percent of our total calories.[45] If that includes a good variety of protein foods, we get plenty of the amino acids we need to rebuild our body's cells and tissues, and the kidney does a pretty good job of getting rid of the excess protein. If you're eating a wide range of healthy foods it is, in fact, difficult to eat more than about 20 percent of your diet as protein. You'd have to severely restrict carbs in order to do so.

PROTEIN AND WEIGHT CONTROL
You need to know four essential facts about protein in respect to weight control:

1. Protein helps with satiety.[46] It dulls the appetite and makes you feel fuller. So when cutting calories, it's important to eat enough protein to meet your daily needs. We'll show you the best ways to do that in the next chapter.

2. When cutting calories, getting enough protein is essential for preserving your muscle tissue.[47] Your body has to make up the energy loss from somewhere. The first thing it does is get more efficient at using whatever nutrients you do give it. Then it looks to energy storage sites within the body for extra calories. When you eat adequate amounts of protein and carbs, your body prefers to get the rest of the calories it needs for energy from stored fat—exactly what you want to get rid of. But if you're on a low-carb diet, your body tends to break down muscle tissue for usable energy—and muscle is *not* what you want to lose.

3. Getting protein from vegetable sources is important. Overconsumption of the amino acid methionine, a byproduct of animal sources—mostly meat—can result in high levels of the artery-toxic substance homocysteine, which is strongly linked to coronary heart disease, stroke, dementia, and even aging itself.[48] Plant proteins have very low levels of this amino acid. So if you eat mostly low-methionine plant proteins and plenty of vegetables that contain folate and vitamin B_6, which processes homocysteine into cysteine or other harmless substances, you'll have a lower homocysteine level.[49] Loading up on healthy plant proteins and folate- and B-vitamin–rich foods has given Okinawans extremely low homocysteine levels—among the lowest of any human population.[50] The kicker: Keeping levels of methionine extremely low leads to slower aging, lower body weight, and a much longer life in animals.[48] That's likely to hold true for humans too. Stay tuned.

4. Protein is the least energy-efficient nutrient.[32–34,51] Your body loses about 40 percent of protein calories in the conversion to energy, and only 3 percent of fat calories and 26 percent of carb calories. Simply put, your body prefers protein for growth and repair, carbs for fuel (immediate use and short-term storage in the liver), and fat to make body fat (long-term energy storage).[32–34,51] Most excess protein is burned off as heat in a process called the *thermogenic response*.

Because your body doesn't like to use protein for energy unless forced to (when no carbs are available), many weight-loss gurus recommend eating lots of protein when trying to lose weight. Some people do lose weight on high-protein diets over the short term, but you can't stay on these kind of diets too long—if you want to stay healthy, that is. They can cause kidney stones and heart rhythm disturbances in certain people, and most people regain any lost weight as soon as they go off the diet.[52,53]

Moreover, the excess heat—the thermogenic response—indicates that the body's energy efficiency is being turned down, which unfortunately may lead to a shorter life.[19] Studies of the long-term effects of high-protein diets on rodents showed that the higher their protein intake, the higher their risk for coronary heart disease, cancer, and prostate and kidney disease.[54] When they ate 30 to 40 percent of their diets as protein (commonly recommended by low-carb advocates) it tripled their risk for coronary heart disease, mildly increased their risk for cancer, and doubled their risk of kidney failure and prostate disease.

The American Diabetes Association recommends that people with diabetes consume no more than 20 percent of their calories from protein.[55] Yet protein makes up about 35 percent of the calories in the Atkins and Protein Power diets and 30 percent in Sugar Busters and The Zone.[56] In the short term, this might be fine for the average person. If when dieting you cut your total calories in half but maintain the same protein intake, then 30 percent of your diet as protein is just about the same total amount in grams as in a typical protein-rich American diet (15 percent of the usual U.S. diet comes from protein—about 75 grams per day).[45] The real danger comes when you try to stick to the same pattern (35 percent or more) once your calorie count crawls back up to normal. Then high levels of protein can increase the risk of kidney damage. It certainly does for people with diabetes and existing kidney disease.[53] And recent studies of non-diabetic people on high-protein, low-carb diets, who have stronger kidneys than diabetics, showed they too risked kidney damage under certain circumstances.[57] Ouch! Vegetables are sounding better and better.

KEY FINDING #4
Biomarkers Show Health Benefits of the Okinawa Diet

One of the most exciting recent scientific advances is the discovery of biological markers of healthy weight and healthy aging.[58] Biomarkers are biological or physiological factors in our bodies that can be measured to help predict our risk for certain diseases, how long we will live, and how many of those years will be vital ones (given relatively healthy lifestyles). They give us clues as to why some people are in excellent physical and mental condition at one hundred years old, while others have extensive physical or cognitive difficulties by the time they reach seventy. In short, biomarkers help gauge our biological age (also referred to as *functional age, real age,* and *physiological age*), which is a far more important indicator of our health and potential life span than our chronological age. An eighty-year-old may be physiologically younger than a sixty-five-year-old; the aging process catches up with individuals at different times. Biomarkers estimate how far along we are in the aging process. The better our biomarkers, the younger our biological age and the better chance we have at a long, healthy life.

The science is still in its infancy, but our research group has measured several of the more promising biomarkers in Okinawan elders. Predictably, they were significantly better than those in Americans of the same age, reflecting better health and a much slower rate of aging. The Okinawans' cardiovascular biomarkers showed better cholesterol profiles, lower homocysteine levels, lower blood pressure, and lower pulse wave velocity;[59] their hormonal biomarkers show a slower decline in DHEA levels;[60] and their biochemical biomarkers reflect lower free radical production.[61] There's no question that the major factor in these healthy biomarkers is diet.

Our study shows that one of the best ways we can improve our biomarkers of aging is by eating fewer calories, choosing the right foods, and losing excess weight. Let's take a look at some individual biomarkers and see the bonus health benefits you can look forward to when you follow the Okinawa Diet.

Bonus Benefits of the Okinawa Diet

YOUNGER ARTERIES IN THE HEART, BRAIN, AND BODY

Cardiovascular (from *cardio,* for "heart," and *vascular,* for "blood vessels") refers to the arteries of our heart, brain, and indeed our entire body. The health of our arteries—the pipes that carry the blood from the heart throughout the body— is critical to how long we live and how well we age. So biomarkers that reflect the health of the arteries, such as cholesterol levels, homocysteine levels, blood pressure, and pulse wave velocity (the speed of blood flow in the aorta, our biggest blood vessel) are important.

Cardiovascular disease, mainly coronary heart disease and stroke, is the most common cause of death among the elderly.[62] Stiffening of the arteries, also known as *arteriosclerosis,* is a big problem as we get older because it leads to higher blood pressure, which increases our risk of heart attacks, stroke (brain attacks), and a host of other arterial problems. Arterial stiffening increases at different rates during aging, so it's a key biomarker of your health and longevity.

Between the ages of thirty and eighty, systolic blood pressure (the top number on your blood pressure reading, which reflects how hard the heart has to pump to get blood to the far reaches of your body) generally shoots up about 40 points. It shouldn't. The pressure increases because the walls of the arteries get plugged with cholesterol and eventually calcify like an old garden hose. That pressure leads to tiny cracks in the artery wall; these need to be repaired with still more cholesterol, the body's cement. Constant high pressure means constant buildup of cement, which cracks again under more pressure. Eventually, the whole thing starts breaking apart, sending chunks into the arteries, which plug up at narrowed spots in the heart or brain. That's a heart attack or brain attack (stroke).

Until recently, this kind of stiffening was considered normal because it is so common in America.[63] Fifty percent of older Americans (age sixty-five and beyond) experience arterial stiffening to the degree that it leads to the development of isolated systolic hypertension (when the top number in your blood pressure reading rises above 140 mm Hg). That kind of high blood pressure is a serious risk factor for stroke, coronary artery disease, heart attack, heart failure, and even dementia in older Americans.[63] But it doesn't have to be that way. Diet, as the Okinawans have shown us, has a big influence on the health of arteries.

LOW PULSE WAVE VELOCITY

In our study of the Okinawa elders, we measured not only blood pressure but also pulse wave velocity (PWV).[59] This is an excellent measure of how stiff your arteries are—and, in the case of Okinawans, it reflects how diet and maintaining a healthy weight, among other factors, can keep our hearts healthy.

Pulse wave velocity is the speed of the blood through the arteries. If the arteries are stiff, they don't absorb the strong pulse of blood coming from the heart. The blood rushes through the arteries as if they were made of steel instead of flexible rubber. The stiffer the arteries, the higher the PWV score. PWV is among the best ways to gauge biological age because the score tends to increase at a steady clip the older you get and at an even faster rate if you are aging too quickly. As Dr. William Osler, a famous nineteenth-century physician, used to say, "You are as old as your arteries."[64] When Osler died in 1919, all our Okinawan centenarian subjects were already adults—and aging rather slowly. Osler would have been amazed at how young their arteries are, and thrilled at their equally healthy cholesterol and homocysteine levels as well.

Some of the foods that contribute to their young and healthy cardiovascular biomarkers are antioxidant-rich vegetables, fruit, and legumes, which all contain phytonutrients especially important to heart health, including vitamin E, carotenoids, and flavonoids.[65] Vitamin E, a fat-soluble antioxidant, is incorporated into the cholesterol particle, forming a last line of defense against corruption by free radicals. Carotenoids, plant compounds found mostly in brightly colored vegetables, are plentiful in Okinawa. The beta-carotene in carrots and orange sweet potatoes and the lycopene in tomatoes, watermelon, and purple sweet potatoes are the best known of the more than six hundred carotenoids.

Flavonoids are antioxidant and hormone-like plant compounds (there are some four thousand of them) found in, among other sources, soy foods, onions, broccoli, red wine, and green, black, and oolong teas. Healthy omega-3 fats, found in canola, soy, and fish oils, are also an important part of the elders' diet, and like the other components mentioned, have been shown in well-conducted studies to play an important role in our cardiovascular health.

IMPROVING YOUR CARDIOVASCULAR BIOMARKERS

Researchers have known for years that small dietary changes—a scoop of fiber here, a splash of canola oil there—can improve cardiovascular biomarkers. But there are still those in the medical community ready to pooh-pooh the whole idea. They complain that you get only a 4 to 7 percent improvement in cholesterol levels by making one of these changes, and that no one knows if the effects are additive or even might cancel each other out when more than one change is made. Hardly worth the bother, they say. We heartily disagree with that line of reasoning. If you eat a healthier overall diet, like the Okinawans, you can make whole-scale changes to your biomarkers, and small changes do add up.

This was clearly shown in experiments by two of our colleagues. In the first, Dr. David Jenkins of the University of Toronto recruited several dozen people and put them on a diet strikingly similar to the Okinawan elders' diet. He dubbed it the "Garden of Eden Diet."[66] It looked, in fact, very much like the East-West Fusion Track we provide for you in chapter 7. It followed a seven-day plan, which people remained on for up to a month, and consisted of foods available in regular supermarkets, including Okinawan veggie winners such as broccoli, carrots, red peppers, tomato, onions, cauliflower, okra, and eggplant. Other foods included were whole grains such as oats and barley; vegetable-based low-trans margarine; soy protein from products such as soymilk and soy sausages, soy cold cuts, and soy burgers; and almonds, among other ingredients.

Dr. Jenkins found that when these antioxidant-rich high-fiber foods, healthier fats, and soy were mixed into the diet, after a week the subjects' levels of LDL cholesterol (the so-called bad cholesterol believed to clog coronary arteries) were reduced by a dramatic 29 percent. The finding suggests that this combination diet may be as effective as the class of drugs known as statins, which have been the standard drug therapy for high cholesterol for the last fifteen years. A host of other benefits became apparent too—weight loss, markedly less inflammation, and likely lower insulin levels too.

A similar study was conducted by Dr. Roy Walford, another physician renowned for his work involving low-cal diets, healthy weight, and aging. On a recent visit, Dr. Walford told us that over the first six months of his Biosphere 2 study, in which subjects ate a diet that he likened to the traditional Okinawan diet, his male subjects lost an average of 18 percent of their body weight, the women 10 percent.[67] Dr. Walford also reported that their blood pressure fell 20 percent on average. Indicators for diabetes, such as blood sugar and insulin levels, decreased by 30 percent on average; and cholesterol levels fell from an average of 195 (considered good) to 125, considered extremely healthy. A remarkable biomarker improvement all around—and it was accomplished by diet alone.

Let's take a look at the remarkable cardiovascular biomarkers of the Okinawan elders versus those of similarly aged Americans. The comparison should definitely wipe away any lingering doubts about the cardiovascular benefits of eating the Okinawa way (see table).

Cardiovascular Biomarkers in Okinawans Versus Americans

Traditional Biomarkers

Group	HTN (%)	Cholesterol	Overweight (BMI > 25)	Diabetes (prevalence)
Okinawan centenarians	1.5	Total: 152 HDL: 49.8 Ratio: 3.1	<1%	<1%
Okinawan elders	37.0	Total: 212 HDL: 57.5 Ratio: 3.7	26%	8%
U.S. elders	61.0	Total: 221 HDL: 37.0 Ratio: 6.0	64%	12%

From Willcox, B.J., Willcox, D.C., and Suzuki, M. *Circulation* 2003; Japan National Nutrition Survey, 1990–2000; NHANES III. HTN = Hypertension.

Emerging Biomarkers

Elders	Homocysteine (μmol/L)	Flavonoids (mg/day)	Vitamin E (μg/ml)	Omega-3 (DHA) (% CE fraction)
Okinawa	8	100.9	16.8	1.6
U.S.	10	12.9	12.6	0.6

From Willcox, B.J., Willcox, D.C., Todoriki, H., and Suzuki, M. *JAGS* 2001.

Note: Elders are standardized to ages 65–74 for comparative purposes. Centenarians are aged 101 on average. While a quarter of Okinawan elders are now overweight, this was virtually unheard of when they were eating a more traditional diet a generation ago. Note that virtually no centenarians are overweight. As you can see, eating the Okinawa way helps keep you lean, keep your blood pressure within normal limits and your total cholesterol low (with high good cholesterol), and gives you excellent cardiovascular and nutritional biomarkers. All of these factors are associated with a longer, leaner, and healthier life.

YOUNGER HORMONAL BIOMARKERS

Hormones are compounds that are released into your bloodstream from glands or organs to regulate many of your body's functions (the endocrine system). They bind to the surface of cells and exert an effect on the cells' function. Obese people tend to have higher levels of key hormones linked to aging, including insulin and insulin-like growth factors, estrogen, and leptin. Many hormones decline with advancing age and seem to decline faster in those who weigh more and eat more calories.[68, 69]

The most interesting point is that by eating fewer calories, choosing the right foods, and maintaining a healthy weight, you may be able to slow the inevitable decline of your hormones.[39] One of the most promising of these hormonal biomarkers is DHEA (dihydroepiandrostenedione). DHEA is produced by the adrenal gland, which sits on top of the kidneys and produces hormones such as cortisol that help us respond to stress. DHEA, which also helps make testosterone and estrogen, tends to naturally decline as we age, so theoretically, it's a good barometer of how quickly we're aging.

A recent study showed that people with slower age-related DHEA declines had a better chance of living longer than those with a rapid decline.[39] Preserving a high DHEA level has been associated with better cardiovascular health as well as better overall health. This doesn't mean we should all rush out and get DHEA shots. Supplemental forms have *not* been shown to be helpful in either reversing or preventing disease. DHEA may simply be a biomarker of age, not a miracle age-erasing hormone. In other words, lower DHEA levels may be an *effect* of aging, not a *cause* of it.[70]

But while the effect of supplements is questionable, the effects of diet aren't; it seems to have a real effect on DHEA levels. What we eat makes a difference. In recent studies on rhesus monkeys (who share over 98 percent of our genes), the DHEA levels of the monkeys whose calories were carefully apportioned (equivalent to the difference between Okinawans and Americans) declined at a much slower rate than those of their fully fed counterparts.[70] Although no similar study has been done in humans, we compared DHEA levels in older Okinawans and Americans as part of our centenarian study and found the Okinawan level of decline appeared to be much slower (see figure 2.8).[71] This provides tantalizing evidence that the Okinawan diet not only keeps you lean but also keeps you hormonally young.

Figure 2.8

SLOWER PHYSIOLOGICAL AGING IN OKINAWANS THAN IN AMERICANS?

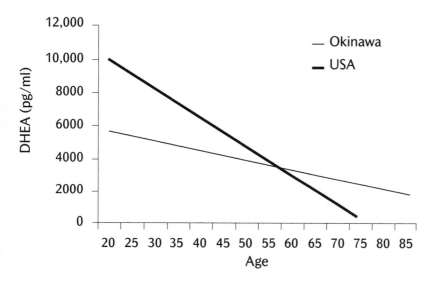

Note: Americans appear to start out with higher DHEA levels when younger, consistent with their larger size and higher body weight, but these levels appear to decline more rapidly than in Okinawans, suggesting a more rapid physiological aging in Americans.[71]

YOUNGER BIOCHEMICAL BIOMARKERS

On a biochemical level, we humans, and every other living thing, are composed of protons, neutrons, and electrons. The stability of those electrons, which whirl around the other cell components and bind them together electrically, appears key to holding our delicate cells together. Cumulative damage to our body's cells caused by free radicals—tiny, electrically charged particles created during energy production in our cells—may be at the root of health and aging.[72] What and how much we eat profoundly influences free radicals.[73]

The biggest source of cell-damaging free radicals is the body's production of energy from food.[74] Our mitochondria, the little nuclear reactors in every cell, produce large amounts of free radicals, and the more you feed them the more energy (and free radicals) they produce. Unfortunately, they damage the body's genes, its cells, and even themselves, more or less rusting the entire system over time. The oxidative process is essentially the same as the one that causes a car to rust when exposed to sunshine for extended periods.

On the other hand, free radicals are not all bad. They are an essential part of our body's immune system. Secreted by white blood cells in the face of "attack," their job is to defend against invading viruses, bacteria, and anything else the body recognizes as foreign. They set up their defense at a molecular level by stealing electrons from the invading cell's wall, DNA, or other essential component. Because electrons are the nano-size building blocks of cells, the cells eventually fall apart and die as their components disintegrate under free radical attack. This is great when you have an infection, but less so as you age when your body tends to lose its ability to recognize what's foreign and what's not.[75] Inevitable identity mistakes, if you will, can lead to your free radicals attacking your own cells and tissues (groups of specialized cells), causing pain and inflammation and fostering a wide variety of diseases.

The Okinawa diet helps counter free radicals on two fronts. First, because it's low in calories, fewer free radicals are produced. Second, it's rich in antioxidants that neutralize free radicals (see figure 2.9). About 90 percent of the traditional Okinawan diet consists of sweet potatoes, other vegetables, soy-based foods, and whole grains and fruits. These foods are supplemented by small amounts of fish and lean pork on special occasions as well as plenty of antioxidant-rich tea. The antioxidant intake is impressive. The elders' diet supplies some 3,500 percent of the recommended daily intake (RDI) for carotenoids and 700 percent of the RDI for vitamin C! Because most of this food is lightweight CD fare, and because Okinawans tend not to overeat, even now the modern diet tallies only about 1,800 calories a day compared with about 2,500 calories for Americans.[76] That's about a 30 percent calorie reduction—without even trying.

Although at this stage biomarkers are far from 100 percent in their predictive reliability, we are learning more every day and hope soon to use them not only to reliably establish our biological age but also to precisely track the effects of healthy living, predict our remaining life expectancy, and estimate our resistance to the major killer diseases. An exciting time lies ahead for us all.

KEY FINDING #5

The Okinawa Diet Fights Stress and Inflammation

A particularly provocative finding of our centenarian study is that when calorie intake is kept low, the level of stress hormones paradoxically increases—albeit mildly.[77] This turns out to be a very good thing. These slightly increased levels have been shown to bolster resistance to brain cell toxins and injury and to produce a marked decrease in many deleterious changes that normally appear in the aging brain.[78] The lower dementia rate in Okinawa compared to the rest of Japan and the United States suggests that the Okinawans may be at lower risk

Figure 2.9

FREE RADICALS

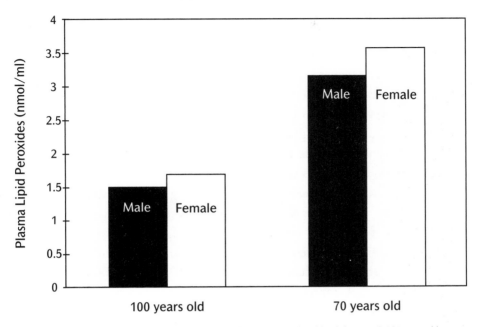

Note: Okinawan centenarians have less than half the level of free radicals in their blood than usual Okinawan elders. This is likely due to the centenarian habits of eating fewer calories, eating food that is richer in antioxidants, and possibly to better genes.

for brain-related illnesses, consistent with a protective effect of their low–caloric density diet.[79] So reducing your calories now may put you at reduced risk for age-related dementia and a host of other chronic diseases later.

Here's how it works. Stress hormones help us in acute and dangerous situations when our fight-or-flight response is triggered and we need instant energy to either stay and fight or run away. Whichever route we take, a stress hormone primer is fired off from the adrenal glands in the form of glucocorticoids. These hormones cause a high-energy surge of glucose (blood sugar) to be released into the bloodstream from the liver, where there's a backup supply of quick-access carbohydrate for just such a purpose. (It's the same supply of carbohydrate, by the way, that low-carb diets burn off, giving you a false sense of early weight loss.)

The interesting thing about glucocorticoids is that they have a dual effect. For the short term, they improve memory and physical performance, but over the long term, high elevations of glucocorticoids cause decreased ability in both areas; they break down our stored carbohydrate, raise our blood sugar levels, and cause many of the age-related changes we see in overweight people.[80] Consuming fewer calories helps produce the consistently right amount of glucocorticoids—

just enough to keep us sharp, but much less than we'd experience in a stressful situation. It also mildly elevates our level of corticosterone, a key stress hormone that protects against age-related brain disease.

So there seems to be an interesting paradox: Low-calorie diets increase stress hormone levels, which leads to decreased risk for stress-associated injury to the brain and other tissues. More research is needed, but chances are good that the explanation lies in either an anti-inflammatory response to the stress hormones or a longer-term reduction of cell-damaging free radicals.

ANTI-INFLAMMATION

Inflammation plays a key role in the chronic diseases of aging, such as coronary heart disease, stroke, and cancer, as well as in aging itself.[81] Reducing inflammation decreases damage to cells and tissues. And here again, cutting back on dietary calories seems to be extremely beneficial. The increase in glucocorticoid hormones produced by lower calorie consumption exerts powerful anti-inflammatory effects.[78,82] The hormones stop the production of unhealthy cytokines—proteins that function as immune system messengers—and can rev your anti-inflammatory response, much the same way as anti-inflammatory drugs such as aspirin and Cox-2 inhibitors (Vioxx, Celebrex) and cortisone do.

Inflammatory proteins have been implicated in a wide array of human diseases, such as coronary heart disease, cancer, stroke, diabetes, and rheumatoid arthritis. Our HLA genes, which we discussed a little earlier, help control the level of immune surveillance of our body. Our immune system can either be geared up and attacking invaders or broken down and unable to prevent pathogens from entering our body (as in AIDS or auto-immune deficiency syndrome). Usually it's somewhere in between—on guard yet not bulletproof; some pathogens slip in under the radar. But as we age, the whole system tends to fall apart; our white blood cells attack inappropriate targets and fail to attack appropriate ones.

The good news is that certain substances we eat can reduce inflammation and have been linked to lower risk for inflammation-related disease—and they are all important facets of the Okinawa diet. These include omega-3 fats (from certain plants and fish oils), plant-derived antioxidants, and anti-inflammatory substances such as the curcumin found in spices like turmeric.[83] We'll talk about them more in detail in the next few chapters. The important thing to keep in mind here is that eating the Okinawa way can help you lose weight *and* improve your overall health. Even modest reductions in weight—5 percent to 10 percent —have been shown to reduce the risk of many illnesses.[84] That said, we think the tools in the next chapter will help you do much better than that.

Chapter 3

MAKING CALORIC DENSITY WORK FOR YOU

Kamuru ussaa mii nayun.
The more you eat, the more you gain.

Now that you're more knowledgeable about how the body works, we're ready to get down to the real business at hand—how you can lose weight and keep it off. We want to help you get on track with the lean, long-lived, robust Okinawan elders. They've enjoyed great food while keeping weight gain at bay all their lives, and you can too. Let's see how to incorporate the principles of eating the Okinawa way into your life.

The major concept behind the Okinawans' healthy weight management is the principle of caloric density. While it may sound complex, it's really quite down to earth in practice. We all have to eat a certain amount of food to feel comfortably full—usually between two and three pounds a day.[1] If we eat less than that, we tend to feel those gnawing hunger pangs often associated with dieting. So cutting back too much on the amount of food we eat is the wrong approach to weight loss. If you feel hungry all the time, sooner or later your willpower will crumble; then there goes the diet, and back come the lost pounds. A much better approach is to eat the same amount of food but to reduce your caloric intake by reducing the caloric density of each mouthful of food. On the most basic level, that's really what the caloric density of your diet is—the amount of calories you put in your mouth. Not the amount of food; the amount of calories.

Caloric density (CD) is measured by the gram, so a food's CD number tells you how many calories are in 1 gram of that food. So, for example, if you see that a particular food has a CD of 2.5, it means that 1 gram of that food contains 2.5 calories. There are 28 grams in an ounce, so 1 gram of food is a pretty small amount. Obviously we're not going to go around calculating the gram weight of every morsel of food we eat, but because food is always listed in grams on the food label, CD is a good thing to know—and it makes it very easy to figure out the caloric density of various foods.

Obviously, the lower the CD of a food, the better it is for weight control, because you can eat a good deal more of it without greatly increasing your calorie intake. The result: more food, fewer calories, no hunger. Which do you think would help you feel fuller longer: a doughnut or a bowl of oatmeal with fruit? If you answered oatmeal and fruit, you're right. Both oatmeal and fruit are high-satisfaction foods—you can eat a good amount of them and feel fully satisfied without getting a lot of calories. While the oatmeal-fruit combo is low-cal, it actually weighs more per calorie than the doughnut because both cooked oatmeal and fruit are packed with fiber and water and are lower in fat, which means they have a low caloric density. Low-CD foods include broth-based soups and stews, vegetables, fruits, legumes like soy, some whole grains (especially those cooked with water), fat-free dairy products, and very lean meats. The bonus is that these very same foods are recommended for good health. By choosing foods with low caloric density, you'll eat fewer calories, feel fuller, get excellent nutrition—and in all probability, feel a great deal better too.

Calculating Caloric Density from Food Labels

We've listed the caloric density of the most common foods in our Caloric Density Index for Selected Foods (page 59) and illustrated the concept in our Caloric Density Pyramid (page 58), which will make it easy for you to determine a food's caloric density. After a very short time, differentiating between high- and low-CD foods will become second nature. When it comes to packaged foods, all you have to do is check the label. Although the CD isn't listed per se, it's extremely easy to calculate. Just divide the number of calories per serving (which is always listed on the food label) by the serving size (weight in grams). So, for example, if the label tells you that prunes are 110 calories per serving and the serving size is "5 prunes (weight 42 grams.)" You simply divide 110 by 42, which gives you a CD of 2.6. Remember, the CD is the number of calories per gram, so the lower the CD number, the better—ratings run from a CD of 0.0 for water (0 calories per gram) to vegetable oils with a CD of 8.8 (almost 9 calories per gram). Foods that are low in fat and high in water or fiber tend to have a low caloric density. *This is the secret that could save you from a lifetime of excess weight and possibly even an early grave.* Burn this caloric density measurement into your consciousness: *calories per gram.* Understand this concept, and you will have mastered one of the most important concepts for weight control.

Here's another label calculation example: In the breakfast cereal label in figure 3.1 you can see that the serving size is ¾ cup, which weighs 32 grams. Pay attention to those grams first. The next line tells you the number of calories per serving—110 in this case, and the same calories per serving, in fact, as the prunes. Now divide the calories by the weight in grams. So, 110 calories divided by 32 grams equals a caloric density of 3.4. The CD of that breakfast cereal is 3.4—higher than the prunes. Even though the prunes and the cereal are both 110 calories per serving, the cereal is actually higher in caloric density. Pretty interesting!

This cereal, by the way, is actually one of the healthier packaged cereals on

Figure 3.1

CALCULATING CALORIC DENSITY

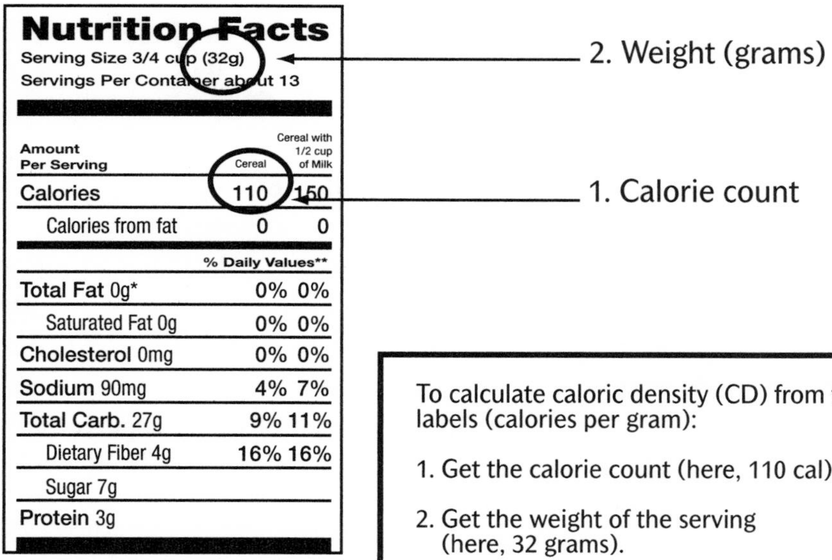

To calculate caloric density (CD) from food labels (calories per gram):

1. Get the calorie count (here, 110 cal).
2. Get the weight of the serving (here, 32 grams).
3. Divide the calorie count by the weight.

   110 cal/32g = 3.4 cal/g

   So there you have it. The caloric density, or calories per gram, of this food is 3.4—so watch out, it's a heavyweight!

the market, but like most packaged cereals it has added sugar (in the form of fruit juice) and is a processed grain, both of which raise caloric density. It still has about 5 grams of fiber and lots of vitamins and minerals, so as far as breakfast cereals go it's rather healthy. But eating this stuff by the handful—and especially the bowlful—will give you a big wallop of unwanted calories.

There *is* a way you can have your cake (or cereal) and eat it too. Here's how: Have a smaller serving than that recommended on the box—say, ½ cup instead of the recommended ¾ cup. Then fill your cereal bowl with low-CD fruit—say, ½ cup strawberries (CD 0.3) and add ½ cup low-fat soymilk (CD 0.3) or skim or 1% milk (both CD 0.4) (Our favorite is vanilla-flavored soymilk.) Now you have a breakfast with an average CD of 1.3 (equal portions of cereal CD 3.4, fruit CD 0.3, soymilk CD 0.3; divided by 3). You have dropped the CD of this meal into sensible low-CD territory—and enjoyed a large serving of healthy antioxidant, fiber-rich, tasty food. Now you are on your way to a healthy weight!

You could add more low-CD fruit and a cup of tea, or experiment with other healthy combinations. For example, by eating cooked oatmeal (CD 0.6) instead of that packaged cereal (CD 3.4) you could eat even more food, but that is entirely up to you. So find the calories, divide by the grams, and try to stay in the low-CD range overall. We give you an easy way to do just that with our Caloric Density Pyramid (page 58) and Caloric Density Index for Selected Foods (page 59) and plenty of delicious and healthy recipes.

BEWARE OF THE "SERVING SIZE"

Keep in mind that serving sizes are based on the amount people generally eat according to standards set by the USDA.[2] So they are not necessarily *recommended* amounts but rather the most *common* amounts—and we all know that most of us eat too much. All of the nutritional information on the package label is based on one serving size; the package may contain several servings. A small bag of chips might contain three servings. If you eat the whole package, you will have eaten three times the amount of calories and other nutrients listed on the package for one serving! Sort of takes the fun out of it, doesn't it?

RANKING THE CALORIES

A calorie is a measure of the energy food provides to your body. The number given on the food label indicates how many calories are in one serving. Although calorie requirements vary for each person, depending on age, weight, gender, and activity level, food labels are based on a diet of 2,000 calories a day. That's likely more than you need to stay slim and healthy, unless you are a very active woman or a fairly active man (see chapter 6 for more details on your calorie needs).

Take a look at the Caloric Density Pyramid again. You'll see that we've ranked foods according to their caloric density *and* the quantity we suggest for healthy weight loss and weight management. We've done it this way to give you a good idea of the foods you can eat freely and the kinds you really have to watch out for. The names of each category are fairly self-explanatory—heavyweights will make you heavy, middleweights could add a little weight to your middle; lightweights keep you light; and featherweights keep you light as a feather. Easy! Here's the CD category breakdown.

- **Featherweights** are foods with a CD of *less than 0.7*. You can eat as much of these foods as you want to—guilt-free. This group includes foods like water-based vegetable soup (0.3); apples, berries, peaches, and most other fruit (~0.7); broccoli, squash, green peas, and most other veggies (~0.5); low-fat plain yogurt (0.6); and tofu (0.5).

- **Lightweights** have a CD *between 0.8 and 1.5*. They can be eaten in moderation—that is, normal medium-size portions a few times a day. These are foods like white flaky fish (1.0); cooked whole grains such as rice and pasta (1.4); sushi (1.4); and cooked beans (1.5).

- **Middleweights** have a caloric density of *1.6 to 3.0*. You want to have relatively small portions of these foods. Middleweights are items like hummus (1.7); red fatty fish (1.8); whole-wheat bagels (2.0); soy cheese (2.5); and raisins (3.0.)

- **Heavyweights,** as the name suggests, are the most dangerous. They have a caloric density of *more than 3.0* and, like Mike Tyson, they pack a wallop. You have to eat these sparingly—infrequently or in very limited amounts. This group includes foods such as full-fat cheddar cheese (4.0); graham crackers (4.2); plain rice cakes (3.8); bacon (5.0); smooth peanut butter, (5.9); butter (7.2); and vegetable oil (8.8). All these foods are either high in fat and sugar or low in water content or fiber. Many of them are processed foods like doughnuts (4.3) and corn chips (5.4)—both processed grains—and French fries (3.2), which are processed potatoes. Processing removes the fiber (nondigestible carbohydrate), often removes water, and frequently adds sugar or fat, making these foods the most calorically dense of all and the most detrimental to your waistline. In small amounts, some can be quite beneficial, such as nuts and omega-3-rich cooking oils, but remember—good things come in small packages.

Interestingly, the higher you climb on the CD scale, the more likely you are to encounter foods that trigger the highest insulin response. Insulin and its associated growth factors (such as IGF-1) are lower in animals and in humans who eat fewer calories.[3] Those humans also are leaner, suffer less heart disease and cancer, and age a lot more slowly. So eating low-CD fare promises a host of benefits in addition to a slimmer body.

Once you realize that water, fiber, and fat content are the keys that separate dangerous heavyweights from healthy featherweights, it's easy to figure out which is which. Think of grapes versus raisins. Grapes are high in water, while raisins are dry and compact and have had all the water squeezed out of them. Grapes are a featherweight and have a CD of 0.7; raisins are a middleweight with a CD of 3.0.

Most salads (with low-fat dressing), vegetables, fresh fruits, tofu, and broth-based soups and stews fit in the featherweight or lightweight category. You can—and should—eat a lot of them. If you are vegetarian, this will be a cinch—just stick to your fruit, veggies, legumes, and cooked whole grains, and go easy on the processed, high-CD grains.

The Three-to-One Rule

If you enjoy animal foods, healthy eating is still possible. Simply eat *mainly* veggies and fruits, legumes, and whole grains, but add low-fat animal foods in limited quantities. Ideally, less than a quarter of your diet should be animal foods. We think of this as the three-to-one rule. Fill your plate with three parts plant foods to one part animal foods. That's three-quarters veggies and unprocessed grains and one-quarter lean versions of meat or poultry or fish or dairy products—not the other way around, as is often the norm here in the West.

Clearly, the best way to make the energy equation work in your favor is to replace high-CD foods in your diet with low-CD foods. Switching to low-fat foods may seem like a sensible way to achieve that goal, but you have to be careful. The low-fat replacement foods many people choose are often high in sugar, low in water and fiber, and all too easy to eat in large amounts—think of tubs of low-fat ice cream, jumbo low-fat muffins, and economy-size packets of low-fat pretzels. Although these foods may be up to 99 percent fat-free, they can be extremely calorically dense. You have to read the labels and do a quick CD calculation. Foods made with lots of oil and butter or that contain big amounts of processed grains or sugar have the highest caloric density; they pack a lot of calories into a small serving. You cannot eat a lot of this fare without gaining weight.

High-Fiber Carbs

Eating moderate to high amounts of good carbohydrates is an important part of a healthy diet. High-fiber carbohydrates, such as whole-grain breakfast cereals and whole-grain varieties of bread, rice, and pasta, can be included in meals and snacks, but watch the CD. Low Glycemic Index versions of carbohydrate-rich foods, such as porridge and low-fat muesli, also improve the satiety value of meals. You leave the table feeling full and satisfied. For breakfast, you could even go all-out Okinawan and try low-CD miso soup and brown rice. (Don't knock it 'til you try it.) Legumes such as soy and other beans and al dente pasta are good options for other meals. All these strategies should be underpinned by eating plenty of fruits and vegetables and by meeting your fluid needs with low-CD choices, especially healthy teas, water, and broth-based soups.

Why Dieting Fails:
Breaking the Caloric Density Principles

To many people, dieting means eating things like meat and mashed potatoes, beef lasagna, or macaroni and cheese in small microwaved portions, and attempting to limit each meal to a few hundred calories or less. But when you look at the average caloric density of these kinds of meals, they usually have a CD of 2.0 or higher. Eating them sets you firmly in middleweight territory. Where you want to be is in with the featherweights and lightweights—meals with a CD less than 1.5.

If you stick to a high-CD diet and just try to eat less, *you will often feel hungry* because a satisfying amount of 2.0 CD food is more than a few hundred calories. If you eat only a few hundred calories of your "diet" food, your stomach won't be very full. Remember, most of us need to eat two to three pounds of food per day, or we start feeling those hunger pangs. Once the hunger sets in, food becomes your obsession, and you fall into the classic pattern of guilty binging—and before you know it, you've gained back all the weight you lost with such difficulty, and then some. Sound familiar? The reason your diet failed wasn't lack of resolve; it was eating foods with high caloric density.

Trendy high-protein/low-carb diets have their problems too. They emphasize foods high in animal protein and fat, such as meats, eggs, and dairy, and "work" by inducing ketosis in the body, which dulls hunger.[4] Normally, the cells in the body run on glucose from carbohydrates. Without carbs, your body taps its stored carbs (glycogen) in your liver and muscles. These stored carbs carry six times their weight in water, so it's like emptying a bucket of water. It looks great on the scale, but since it's essential water it will come back when you eat carbs again. When this runs out, your body metabolizes fat and protein from your muscles and forces the cells of the body to run on ketones—a type of alternative fuel. This process causes you to lose weight, much of it water, but the diet is unsustainable. Because it's excessively high in animal protein and fat, it eventually becomes unpalatable and dull—you'll kill for a bagel or even a piece of fruit. Thus, sooner or later, you'll drop the diet. Then you'll attempt to restrict calories again, which leads to chronic hunger, which leads to binges, and the whole tedious cycle starts all over again. So while you can lose weight here and there on high-CD diets, it's virtually impossible to keep it off permanently—and that's what we all want; that's the universal goal.[5]

The typical American diet of meat, processed grains like white bread, and full-fat dairy with added oils and fats is a natural heavyweight diet—just the ticket for pro wrestlers but a washout for the rest of us. In contrast, a diet composed mostly of plant foods is a natural lightweight diet, low in caloric density. When put together healthfully, lightweight diets center on vegetables, fruits, legumes (such as soy), and whole grains (such as brown rice), plus smaller amounts of lean seafood, meat, or dairy. A typical meal might be brown rice, vegetables, and fish, or oatmeal with fruit. But you have to be smart here too, because a diet based on cheese pizza, corn chips, French fries, white bread, sodas, white rice, sugared cereals, and cookies could technically be considered a plant-based diet, even though these refined and processed foods contain mostly empty calories and are deficient in vitamins, minerals, fiber, phytochemicals, and everything else that's good for you. They're also very high in caloric density. You'd not only gain weight in a New York minute eating those kinds of foods, but your health would take a nosedive while you were at it.

PROCESSING AND REFINING

Here's the problem with refined and processed grains. As soon as whole grains, which are relatively low in caloric density, are milled into flour, their caloric density shoots way up. So while wheat berries have a low caloric density of 0.5, once the berries become whole-wheat flour, their calorie density is 3.3; refine them again into white flour, and the CD is 3.6—more than seven times as much! Thus products made from that flour, such as cracked-wheat bread (2.6), English muffins (2.5), and apple muffins (2.7), tend to have a high caloric density. And this is why even though whole-grain breads (3.0) and bagels (2.0) are a healthy addition to one's diet, they should be eaten judiciously. Go for the mini bagel, not the jumbo!

And then there's the fat. All too often, we greatly increase the caloric density of foods by adding fat. A raw potato, for example, has a caloric density of 0.3—a real featherweight—but that same potato, when processed into French fries, has a caloric density of 3.2, which is ten times higher. A salad has a caloric density of about 0.3. That same salad with French dressing and pieces of ham and cheese has a caloric density of 2.4, which is 8 times higher. You can save yourself a lot of extra pounds by paying attention to food preparation and optional extras.

The Traditional Okinawan Diet

The traditional diet of the Okinawan elders remained mainly intact from the 1600s to the 1960s. It was both low-fat and free of processed grains. It was composed principally of sweet potatoes; other unrefined, unprocessed starches such as brown rice as well as beans, cabbage, soy, and winter squash; other green and yellow vegetables; some fresh fruits; some whole grains (e.g., millet); and limited amounts of fish and lean meats. It was (and still is) the epitome of a natural, healthy low-CD diet. You can see why Okinawans could eat virtually as much as they wanted without gaining weight and why it was so rare to find obese or overweight people in Okinawa—until the local diet became more Westernized, of course. Unlike our typical Western diet, with its overemphasis on animal proteins, fats, and processed and refined foods, the Okinawan diet was filled with unprocessed plant foods that are high in fiber, phytonutrients, vitamins, and minerals and are naturally low in fat. This diet provides more than adequate protein, has little cholesterol, and has been shown to dramatically improve health.

The Caloric Density Pyramid

A quick look at the Caloric Density Pyramid in figure 3.2 will help you visualize just where various kinds of foods stand in terms of caloric density. It presents a complete picture when paired with the more comprehensive and precise calculations in the Caloric Density Index for Selected Foods that follows the pyramid (see page 59). When you study the pyramid, you'll see general patterns emerge in the foods on the different tiers. Unprocessed whole foods such as vegetables and fruits, water-rich foods like soups, and low-fat foods like lean proteins form the base of the pyramid. Those are the featherweights you can eat freely. As you go up the pyramid, the caloric density of the foods gradually increases, and you should eat progressively less and less of them, as their calories

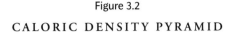

Figure 3.2

CALORIC DENSITY PYRAMID

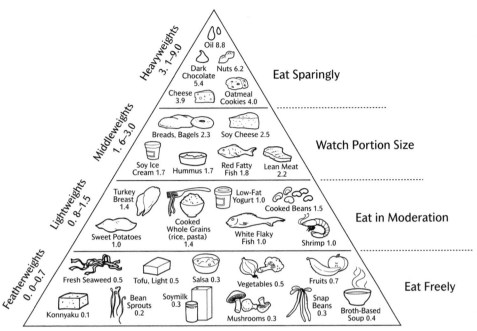

quickly add up. At the very top of the pyramid you'll find sweets, oils, meat, full-fat dairy foods, and other foods that are either very high in fat or very low in water. Some of those foods—nuts, healthy cooking oils (olive or canola oil), and chocolate (or other favorite sweets)—can and should be incorporated into your diet, but sparingly. Carnivores can still have steaks, of course; just have smaller portions and eat them less frequently. Save them for the Sunday barbecue and remember to have an extra-big serving of salad beforehand.

If you chose all your foods from the featherweight tier, you can eat with total impunity. Eat as much as you want; you'll never be hungry and you'll never get fat. But for more variety, take three-fourths of your food from the featherweight category and then add small amounts of other foods. You'd end up in solid light-weight territory. That's where the lean Okinawan elders have always been. Remember, it's the balance that counts. If you choose too many foods from the top tiers and eat them too often—have too many American steak-and-egg breakfasts, for instance—you'll tip the scale into heavyweight, high-CD territory. Even if you added a featherweight bowl of soup or a piece of fruit now and then, you'd still be in the land of the middleweights. And remember, a middleweight diet means fat around your middle—not to mention the thighs, tummy, and derriere. It will have you waging a continual battle with extra pounds over your lifetime—and the pounds will eventually prove victorious.

Unless you are a marathon runner, you'll find it very difficult to win the battle of the bulge without eating a mostly plant-based diet. Eating very few carbs and lots of meat à la Atkins can help dull the appetite and lead to short-term weight loss, but it's not a sensible long-term strategy. Watching your CD enables you to eat plenty of food without getting plenty of calories. As the Okinawans have shown us, it is the most effective and healthiest lifelong weight management strategy going—and, as you will soon find out, it's a delicious way to go.

Caloric Density Index for Selected Foods

Featherweights (0.0–0.7)

Water	0.0	Soup, vegetarian vegetable, prepared with water	0.3
Tea, jasmine/green/black	0.0	Soymilk	0.3
Cucumber	0.1	Strawberries	0.3
Lettuce, romaine	0.1	Cantaloupe	0.4
Konnyaku yam cake	0.1	Carrots	0.4
Summer squash	0.2	Milk, nonfat	0.4
Asparagus	0.2	Papaya	0.4
Bitter melon	0.2	Peach	0.4
Bean sprouts, boiled	0.2	Shiitake mushrooms	0.4
Celery	0.2	Soup, tomato, prepared with water	0.4
Daikon Japanese white radish	0.2	Winter squash	0.4
Hechima loofa gourd	0.2	Apricots	0.5
Spinach, boiled	0.2	Dandelion greens	0.5
Swiss chard, boiled	0.2	Orange	0.5
Tomato	0.2	Orange juice	0.5
Bamboo shoots	0.3	Soup, black bean and vegetable, fat-free	0.5
Bell pepper, red	0.3	Tofu, firm light	0.5
Broccoli	0.3	Wakame seaweed, rehydrated	0.5
Grapefruit, pink/red	0.3	Apple	0.6
Mushrooms	0.3	Blueberries	0.6
Salsa	0.3	Cheese, cottage, fat-free	0.6
Snap beans	0.3	Cranberry juice cocktail	0.6
Soup, chicken with rice, prepared with water	0.3	Milk, whole	0.6

Pear	0.6	Soy dressing	2.0
Yogurt, low-fat, plain	0.6	Soy sour cream	2.1
Grapes	0.7	Beef rib steak, lean, broiled	2.2
Light tuna, canned in water, drained	0.7	Cheese, mozzarella, part skim	2.5
		Cheese, soy	2.5
Mango	0.7	Pork chop, center cut with fat, braised	2.5
Tofu, regular, firm	0.7		
Yogurt, soy, plain	0.7	Ice cream, Häagen-Dazs, vanilla	2.6
		Bread, pita, whole-wheat	2.7
Lightweights (0.8–1.5)		Bagel, white	2.8
Banana	0.9	Muffin, wheat bran, low-fat	2.8
Red snapper	0.9	Beef rib steak, with fat, broiled	3.0
Cheese, cottage, 4% fat	1.0	Bread, whole-wheat	3.0
Cod, baked or broiled	1.0	**Heavyweights (3.1–9.0)**	
Shrimp, cooked	1.0	Cheesecake	3.2
Soba buckwheat noodle, cooked	1.0	Crackers, fat-free, whole-wheat	3.6
Sweet potato, boiled	1.0	Cheese, Swiss	3.7
Yogurt, low-fat, with fruit	1.0	Popcorn, air-popped	3.8
Potatoes, baked	1.1	Cheese, cheddar	4.0
Rice, brown, cooked	1.1	Doughnut, glazed	4.0
Scallops, steamed	1.1	Oatmeal cookies	4.0
Pasta, whole-wheat, cooked	1.2	Soybeans, dry-roasted	4.5
Pasta, enriched, cooked	1.4	Chocolate-chip cookies	4.6
Soybeans, green, boiled	1.4	Slim-Fast Peanut Crunch Snack Bar	4.6
Turkey breast, skinless, roasted	1.4		
		Sweet chocolate candy	5.1
Middleweights (1.6-3.0)		Corn chips, plain	5.4
Chicken breast, skinless, roasted	1.7	Dark chocolate	5.4
Ground beef, 5% fat extra-lean, broiled	1.7	Potato chips	5.4
		Cashew nuts	5.7
Hummus	1.7	Pistachio nuts	5.7
Soybeans, boiled	1.7	Pork bacon, broiled	5.8
Soy ice cream	1.7	Peanuts, dry roasted	5.9
Trout, baked or broiled	1.7	Peanut butter, smooth	5.9
Salmon, cooked, dry heat	1.8	Almonds	6.0
Tuna, cooked, dry heat	1.8	Pecans	7.1
Ice cream, Häagen Dazs, low-fat, vanilla	1.9	Macadamia nuts	7.2
		Butter	7.2
Bagel, whole-wheat	2.0	Mayonnaise, full-fat	7.2
Pork chop, center cut, lean, braised	2.0	Oil, vegetable	8.8

Chapter 4

THE TEN OKINAWA DIET PRINCIPLES FOR LIFELONG HEALTHY WEIGHT

Shinzi gusui.
It is important to get the right balance.

Now that you're familiar with the concept of caloric density, let's talk about how to put it to work for you. These ten principles will help you stay on target and add interest and punch to your diet. They are the meat and potatoes—or, should we say, the veggies and tofu—of the Okinawa diet.

PRINCIPLE #1
Build Meals on a Featherweight Foundation

The mini-list of featherweight foods in our Just the Facts box (page 62) should give you ideas about how to construct a low-CD meal, or even how to grab a quick and healthy low-CD snack. Many of these foods form the cornerstone of the Okinawa diet. The most important thing to remember here is that filling your plate with CD featherweights and lightweights will lower the caloric density of the entire meal. If you are eating a diet with an overall CD of close to 1.0, as the Okinawans have traditionally done, you can even break the *hara hachi bu* rule and still remain quite trim—although laying down your chopsticks when you feel that first twinge of fullness is always a smart move.

Because low-CD foods will help you feel satiated, eating mainly lightweights or featherweights will ensure that you reduce the portion of middleweight and

Just the Facts

- Make featherweight or lightweight foods the bulk of every meal.

- Follow the three-to-one rule: at least 3 parts featherweights or light-weights to 1 part middleweights or heavyweights on any plate. Typically, this means 3 parts plant food per 1 part animal food, as plant food is usually lower on the CD scale.

- Featherweights are eat-as-much-as-you-want foods. Prime examples are strawberries (CD 0.3); grapefruit (CD 0.3); cantaloupe (CD 0.4); papaya, apple sauce (CD 0.5); *konnyaku* (CD 0.1); lettuce (CD 0.1); tomato (CD 0.2); cooked broccoli (CD 0.3); gazpacho soup (CD 0.2); miso soup (CD 0.1); veggie soup (CD 0.3); chicken, rice, and veggie soup (CD 0.5); salsa (CD 0.3); carrot sticks (CD 0.4) . . . and lots more. Please refer to the list on pages 59 to 60 for a more extensive offering of featherweight and light-weight foods.

heavyweight foods like cheese, bread, beef, and chicken. It also will guarantee that you get your daily recommended servings of cancer-fighting vegetables and fruits. If you love fatty beef (a big heavyweight), you don't have to give it up completely; just reduce your portions and limit your big steak dinner to once a week—and the leaner the beef, the better. And always remember the three-to-one rule: a plate with at least three parts plant food and one part animal food is a healthier plate than the other way around.

MUST-KNOW EASY HERBAL VEGGIE BASICS

As you'll see when you get to the recipes, lots of delicious dishes contain light-weight and featherweight veggies. But we want you to embrace two basic ways to prepare vegetables that you can use over and over again. They should absolutely be part of your Okinawa way cooking repertoire, as they turn all and any vegetables into side-dish sensations that can be served with almost any meal. The techniques are *oven roasting* and *marinating* (the marinade doubles as a salad dressing). Make them part of your cuisine vocabulary, and you'll never be at a loss for what to do with veggies again. Examples of each of these techniques from two of our Okinawan gourmet friends appear on pages 313 and 320.

Tips For Incorporating Featherweights and Lightweights into Your Diet

• **Go for the veggie juice.** It's healthy and filling. In a study published in the journal *Appetite,* men who drank a 14-ounce, 88-calorie glass of vegetable juice before lunch took in an average of 136 fewer calories at the meal than men who didn't get the drink.[1]

• **If you are a milk-drinker, switch to nonfat or low-fat milk**—or, better yet, our favorite, soymilk. Drinking milk or soymilk before or with a meal helps you feel full sooner and eat less at the meal.[2] The lighter the milk, the greater the effect. Fat-free milk works better than 1% milk, and both work better than 2% milk. Going low-fat also takes a load of calories out of your diet.

• **Color your rice brown.** Brown rice has been a staple in societies full of thin people for millennia. It used to be considered the food of the poor, as milling rice to make it white (which removes the B-vitamins and fiber) was an expensive process. Long-grain brown rice and wild rice score the lowest on the CD scale and still have their B-vitamins and fiber intact. The same goes for bread—brown is better than white.

• **Add extra veggies to *everything*!** That means pizza, sandwiches, salads, soups (canned and homemade), casseroles, pasta, take-out Chinese, omelets—any dish that can handle it. This is one of the single best CD-lowering strategies around. Adding a handful of veggies to a meat dish is a friendly, subtle way of making sure your carnivore mate or children get their veggies. And for vegetable fans, it's just more of your favorite thing. Adding lovely florets of broccoli to a pepperoni pizza, for instance, will lower its CD and transform it from a heavyweight to a middleweight.

• **Eat fruit at every meal and for snacks.** Add fruit to breakfast cereals, salads, desserts, snacks—any place that works.

• **Drink low-CD beverages**—water; low-calorie or calorie-free beverages such as green tea, jasmine tea, and herbal tea; fruit juice diluted with seltzer; and diet soft drinks (if you absolutely must have a soft drink).

• **Avoid sugared beverages of any sort.** Read those labels! Even some seemingly healthy bottled green and herbal teas contain so many calories they can tip your delicate energy balance into dangerous territory with the first swallow. Super-size herbal teas and juices can contain 300 or more calories in a single bottle. While calories per serving may be listed at 100, the bottle could contain two or more servings—the old multiple-servings-in-the-innocuous-container trick. Make sure you don't fall for it and wind up getting double or triple the calories you bargained for.

• **Choose healthy liquid snacks.** For snacks, try "liquid foods" such as vegetable cocktails. Soy protein drinks are also good choices and leave you feeling full longer because of the hunger-supressing effects of protein.

PRINCIPLE #2

Anchor Main Meals on Low-CD Protein

Proteins are the chemical building blocks from which our cells, organs, muscles, and other tissues are made. They also serve double duty as hormones, enzymes, and antibodies, which help our body fight off invading germs. So it's important that we get enough proteins in our diet. Proteins are made of long chains of smaller building blocks, called *amino acids,* that determine the size, shape, and length of protein molecules. They also give protein molecules the odd ability to coil and uncoil like tiny cellular snakes, which is important for structural integrity when building cell walls and body tissues.

Experts aren't entirely sure of the exact amount of protein we need to eat; estimates have been revised often in recent years. The international organizations that advise us on nutrient requirements have calculated the standards to meet or exceed the requirements of practically everyone, explicitly taking into account individual variation. So the levels they recommend have a wide safety margin built in. In the United States it's recommended that we get at least 0.4 grams of protein a day per pound of body weight.[3] That means an adult who weighs 150 pounds should have about 60 grams of protein a day (0.4 grams multiplied by 150 pounds equals 60 grams of protein). A simple way to calculate this in your head is to multiply your weight by four and divide the result by ten (e.g., $150 \times 4 = 600 \div 10 = 60$ grams of protein). That's about as much as you'd find in three card-deck-size servings of tofu or meat. Under certain circumstances, such as pregnancy or severe stress, the body requires more. Most of us could probably get by on far less.

A typical U.S. diet provides 60 to 100 grams of protein per day; women usually eat about 65 grams; while men take in about 90. So a 120-pound woman who requires only 48 grams per day ($0.4 \times 120 = 48$ grams of protein) is getting almost 40 percent more protein than she really needs—and this for a

---

Just the Facts

- Protein is an essential part of any healthy eating plan—especially when you're trying to lose or maintain a healthy weight.

- High-protein foods can help decrease hunger and prolong satiety more than high-carb or fatty foods.

- Be sure to get 0.4 grams of protein daily for every pound you weigh, particularly when losing weight, so you preserve as much muscle mass as possible and burn fat rather than muscle.

- Choose lean, healthy, low-CD proteins. Eating mostly plant sources of protein, such as tofu, vegetable-protein meat replacements, cooked beans, and whole grains, will help you meet this goal. White flaky fish, low-fat dairy, and lean meat are other good sources.

---

requirement that has already been set on the high side. The kidneys are pretty good at getting rid of the stuff, but excessively high intakes of protein in people who don't get enough calcium and vitamin D can increase osteoporosis risk and lead to the accumulation of waste products, such as uric acid, that increase risk for gout and kidney stones. These are frequently mentioned side effects of low-carb diets such as the Atkins Diet.[4-6]

PROTEIN HELPS YOU FEEL FULLER LONGER

One aspect of protein that shouldn't be overlooked is its satiety factor—it helps you feel full better than carbs and fat do. So including a high-protein food in your main meals is always a good idea. Obviously, the fewer calories you consume, the higher the percentage of protein should be in your diet if you want to get your 0.4 grams per pound daily allowance. That means the percentage of protein in your diet will naturally increase when you're keeping calories at a relative minimum to lose weight, and decrease as you up your calorie intake to maintenance level after you've reached your healthy weight goal. Say, for example, you were the same 120-pound woman who requires 48 grams of protein per day, and you were on a 1,200-calorie-a-day diet. Eating only 10 percent of your calories as protein, you'd be getting only 30 grams of protein—not enough to support your fat-burning lean muscle tissue. In that case, you'd have to go to the upper ranges of the protein recommendations (closer to 20 percent). It's not rocket science, but it does require a little thought. As we mentioned, healthy plant foods can provide plenty of protein—tofu is 40 percent protein. The traditional Okinawan diet contained only 8 to 10 percent protein in the old days, and although it's now closer to 15 to 20 percent, the protein is still mostly from plants. Ten to 20 percent protein is considered very healthy by most experts, and far below the 50-plus percent recommended by some popular diet books.[5]

HOW MUCH IS TOO MUCH?

Millions of people around the world don't get enough protein. This leads to the condition known as kwashiorkor, which can cause growth failure, loss of muscle mass, decreased immunity, weakening of the heart and respiratory system, and, ultimately, death. It's very rare in the United States and other developed countries, where it's easy to get the minimum daily requirement of protein. A cereal and milk breakfast, peanut butter and jelly sandwich lunch, and a dinner featuring a piece of fish with a side of beans adds up to about 70 grams of protein—and remember, you need only 0.4 grams per pound of body weight daily. So getting enough is not the problem for most of us. The real question is, How much is too much?

The digestion of protein releases acids the body usually neutralizes with calcium and other buffering agents in the blood. Eating lots of protein, like the excessive amounts recommended in high-protein/low-carb diets, requires lots of calcium. Some of it may be pulled from bone.[6] Consuming a high-protein diet for a few weeks won't have much effect on the strength of your bones, but over the long term, it could weaken them. In the well-known Nurses' Health Study, for example, women who ate more than 95 grams of protein a day were 20 percent more likely to have broken a wrist over a twelve-year period than those who ate an average amount of protein (less than 68 grams a day).[7]

And, as we mentioned, high-protein diets can also adversely affect the kidneys because of the stress required to process proteins. Increased protein consumption leads to hyperfiltration—a state in which the kidney faces increased pressure to filter and remove waste from the body. Over the long term, hyperfiltration can lead to kidney damage, as was reported in a recent Harvard study.[4] (Deeper analysis in this study showed that the risk was significant only for animal protein, not plant protein. That strongly suggests that the source of protein is an important factor.) For most of us, too much protein intake should not be an issue—unless it makes up more than 35 percent of our diet for an extended period of time.

CHOOSE VEGETABLE PROTEIN OVER ANIMAL— AT LEAST SOME OF THE TIME

Animal protein and vegetable protein both break down into amino acids after digestion, but animal proteins give you some extras that you don't want. They have more methionine (which makes artery-clogging homocysteine) and more saturated fat (which packs a high CD punch), are devoid of healthy antioxidants, and are associated with increased risk for cardiovascular disease and certain cancers.[8] So while the amount of protein is important, the whole "protein package" has the greatest influence on your health. Consider a 6-ounce broiled porterhouse steak. It's a great source of complete protein—38 grams' worth. But it also delivers 44 grams of fat, 16 of them the saturated kind that raises your LDL, or bad cholesterol. (Think of the *L* in LDL as "lethal" and you'll never be confused again.) Sixteen grams of saturated fat is almost three-fourths of the daily cap on saturated fat. Add sour cream to your baked potato and you're over the limit. The same amount of salmon, on the other hand, gives you 34 grams of protein and a mere 18 grams of fat, only 4 of them saturated. A cup of cooked lentils also has 34 grams of protein, but less than 1 gram of fat—and that fat is all the healthy kind. Getting the picture?

GO NUTS

One particularly healthful source of plant protein is nuts. While many people think of nuts as just another junk food snack, they are, in fact, an excellent source of protein and other healthful nutrients. One surprising finding from nutrition research is that people who regularly eat nuts are less likely to have heart attacks or die from heart disease than those who rarely eat them. Several of the largest cohort studies (the Adventist Study,[9] the Iowa Women's Health Study,[10] the Nurses' Health Study,[11] and the Honolulu Heart Program[12]) have shown a consistent 30 to 50 percent lower risk of heart attack, stroke, and diabetes associated with eating nuts several times a week. Finally—a snack food we can feel good about eating!

Several factors contribute to the heart-healthy effect of nuts. The unsaturated (good) fats they contain help lower bad LDL cholesterol and raise good HDL cholesterol (think of the *H* as "healthy"). One group of unsaturated fats, the omega-3 fatty acids, found in certain nuts and seeds, including walnuts and flaxseed, prevent the development of erratic heart rhythms.[13] Omega-3 fatty acids (which are also found in most fish) may also prevent blood clots, partly by decreasing inflammation, much like aspirin.[14] Nuts are also rich in arginine, an amino acid needed to make a molecule called nitric oxide that relaxes constricted blood vessels and eases blood flow. And they contain vitamin E, folic acid, potassium, fiber, and other healthful nutrients.

On the downside, eating nuts will definitely expand your waistline if you gobble them down *in addition* to your usual snacks and meals. At 185 calories per ounce and a CD of ~6.2, they are a real CD heavyweight. A handful of walnuts a day could add 10 pounds or more in a year if you don't cut back on something else. This weight gain would tip the scales toward heart disease, not away from it. So eat nuts *instead of* chips or other less healthy snacks. Or try using them instead of meat in main dishes, or to replace croutons in salads. Go nuts, but don't go crazy!

Tips for Balancing Protein Intake

- **Get a good mix of proteins.** Almost any reasonable diet (including vegetarian) will give you enough protein each day if you eat a variety of healthy foods.

- **Maintain the minimum.** If you are cutting calories, try to keep your protein intake to at least 0.4 grams per pound body weight daily. This is rarely a problem unless you are on a very low calorie diet (less than 1,000 cal/day), which we do not recommend. Typically, most of us get about 50 percent more protein than we need, so as long as you don't drastically cut protein foods, you'll still get enough. Cut down on high-CD fats and processed carbs instead of protein foods and eat a variety of lean protein foods, and you should do just fine.

- **Pay attention to the "protein package."** You rarely eat straight protein. Some comes packaged with lots of unhealthy fat, like when you eat marbled beef or drink whole milk. If you eat meat, steer yourself toward the leanest cuts, such as pork tenderloin, chicken and turkey breast, shellfish, fish, and egg-white omelets. If you like dairy products, nonfat or low-fat versions are healthier choices. Plant sources, such as beans, soy, nuts, and whole grains, offer protein with healthy fats, fiber, antioxidants, and micronutrients.

- **Balance carbohydrates and protein.** Cutting back on highly processed carbohydrates and increasing plant protein over the short term lowers levels of blood triglycerides (bad fat) and raises HDL (healthy cholesterol), and so reduces your risk of heart attack, stroke, and other forms of cardiovascular disease.[15] The protein will also make you feel full longer and stave off hunger pangs.

• **Eat soy.** Soybeans, tofu, tempeh, miso, and other soy-based foods are an excellent alternative to red meat. Larger amounts of soy may also soothe hot flashes and other menopause-associated problems.

• **Eat nuts.** Try nuts instead of chips or other less healthy snacks. Use them instead of meat in main dishes, or as a healthful crouton replacement in salad.

Dietary Sources of Protein and Caloric Density

Vegetable Protein	Serving Size	Protein (g)	CD
Soybean and Soy Products			
Soymilk	1 cup	6.6	0.3
Tofu, silken	3 ounces	4.7	0.6
Tofu, firm	3 ounces	7.0	0.7
Soy yogurt, with fruit	1 6-ounce container	4.0	1.0
Soybean sprouts	½ cup	4.6	1.2
Soy hamburgers	one, 71 grams	13.0	1.3
Soy sausage, wiener	one, 57 grams	11.0	1.4
Soybeans, green, or *edamame*	½ cup	10.6	1.4
Soybeans, boiled	½ cup	14.3	1.7
Tempeh	½ cup	15.4	1.9
Soy cheese, cheddar	1 ounce	6.0	2.5
Soy cheese, mozzarella	1 ounce	3.0	2.5
Soy cream cheese	2 tablespoons	1.0	2.7
Soy flour, defatted	¼ cup	11.8	3.3
Soybeans, roasted	¼ cup	17.0	4.5
Other Legumes and Bean Products			
Chili, vegetarian	1 cup	13.0	0.7
Refried beans, low-fat, canned	¾ cup	4.5	0.9
Fava beans, boiled	½ cup	6.5	1.1
Lima beans, boiled	½ cup	5.8	1.2
Green or yellow peas, boiled	½ cup	8.2	1.2
Kidney beans, boiled	½ cup	7.7	1.3
Lentils, boiled	½ cup	8.9	1.2
Adzuki, or azuki, beans, boiled	½ cup	8.6	1.3
Pinto beans, boiled	½ cup	7.0	1.4
Garbanzo beans, or chickpeas, boiled	½ cup	7.3	1.6

Other Protein	Serving Size	Protein (g)	CD
Animal Proteins			
Milk, nonfat	8 fluid ounces	8.4	0.4
Egg white, raw	1	3.5	0.5
Yogurt, plain, low-fat	1 6-ounce container	7.0	0.6
Cottage cheese, low-fat, 1% fat	½ cup	14.0	0.7
Cream cheese, fat-free	2 tablespoons	4.3	1.0
Egg substitute, cooked	¼ cup	6.9	1.2
White fish	3 ounces	16.2	1.3
Egg, hard-boiled	1	6.3	1.6
Chicken breast, meat only, cooked	3 ounces	26.4	1.7
Extra lean beef (5% fat)	3 ounces	22.3	1.7
Turkey, meat only, cooked	3 ounces	24.9	1.7
Salmon, cooked	3 ounces	21.6	1.8
Tuna, cooked	3 ounces	25.4	1.8
Cheese, cheddar	1 ounce	7.1	4.0
Grains, Nuts			
Oat bran	½ cup	8.1	2.5
Whole wheat flour	½ cup	8.2	3.3
Rolled oats	½ cup	4.9	3.7
Almond butter	2 tablespoons	4.8	6.3

PRINCIPLE #3

Make Soy a Principal Protein

The soybean, a member of the legume family, is the basis of a remarkably varied number of foods and ingredients. Many foods are made from the soybean itself; others are made from specially formulated soy-based ingredients, so soy comes in all kinds of textures, shapes, forms, and caloric density levels. Soy nuts, which are very concentrated, for example, are rated at 4.5, rather high on our Caloric Density Index, while tempeh is 1.9 and silken tofu is only 0.6.

Soybeans contain all the amino acids essential to human nutrition that cannot be synthesized by the body—the ones that must be supplied by our diet.[17] Animal-based foods have complete proteins too, but, as we discussed, they also contain more fat, including harmful saturated fats. So we highly recommend replacing animal foods with soy protein products—at least some of the time. It's easy to do, even without any other major adjustments to your diet—and our recipes guarantee you'll thoroughly enjoy the process.

A POWERFUL CONTRIBUTOR TO HEALTH

Other cultures, especially Asian cultures, and Okinawan in particular, have used soy extensively for centuries. While soy is a huge cash crop in the United States, it's used largely as livestock feed. Mainstream America has been slow to move dietary soy beyond a niche market status, but that's changing as its health benefits are becoming better known—and there are many. Soy may lower your risk for several common chronic diseases, heart disease and breast, prostate, and colon cancers among them.[17–20] Although cardiovascular disease is a major cause of death in the United States and most developed countries, it's comparatively rare in Okinawa.[19] The death rates from cardiovascular diseases such as heart disease, including heart attack, stroke, and high blood pressure, in the United States are three times higher than in Okinawa. And death rates for breast and prostate cancers are more than four times higher in Americans than Okinawans. Our studies show that soy is likely an important contributor to this statistical discrepancy (see figure 4.1).[16–17]

Americans typically eat only 1 to 3 grams of soy protein a day. In Asia, on the other hand, the average soy protein intake ranges from about 10 grams a day in China to between 30 and 50 grams a day in Japan and 60 to 120 grams in Okinawa.[16,18,21] But when Okinawans and other Japanese migrate to the West and have less soy in their diets, their cancer risk rises. The same holds true for heart disease.[22] Studies by our colleagues at the Pacific Health Research Institute

---

Just the Facts

- Soy is a very important part of the Okinawa diet and is an extremely nutritious low-CD food.

- Soy is the highest-quality plant protein and is equivalent in quality to animal proteins.

- Soy comes in a variety of caloric densities, depending on processing.

- Miso soup is a mainstay of the Japanese and Okinawan diets and has an exceptionally low CD—only 0.1.

- Older Okinawans have among the highest consumption of soy in the world, between 60 and 120 grams per day, which may play a role in their very low death rates from cardiovascular disease and cancer as well as their healthy weight.[16–19]

Figure 4.1

HIGH ISOFLAVONE INTAKE IN OKINAWAN JAPANESE
VERSUS JAPANESE CANADIANS

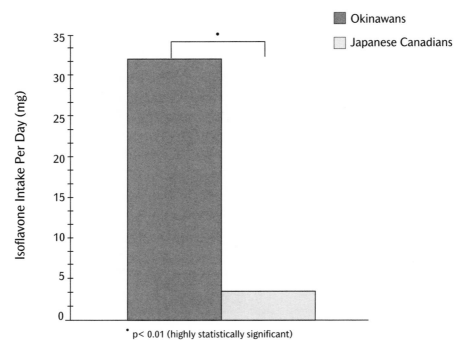

Note: Isoflavones come mainly from soy foods, such as tofu and miso, and may play a role in the markedly low risk for cardiovascular disease and cancer in Okinawans.[16–18]

and Hawaii Cancer Institute show that dietary westernization, including reduced soy food intake, plays a role in the increased risk of heart disease. Soy is, in fact, one of the few foods allowed an official USDA health claim for lowering heart disease risk.[23]

Exceptionally high consumption of soy protein has helped Okinawans easily meet their protein requirements while keeping their intake of high-CD animal protein low. That, of course, lowers the overall caloric density of their diet. The soy "protein package" also comes with cholesterol-lowering saponins, antioxidant flavonoids, and many other healthful phytonutrients. So soy has helped Okinawans stay lean as it's added many other healthy nutrients to their diet. That makes it an A-number-one food in our book. Let's take a look at some ways you can take advantage of this amazing food.

LOW-CD SOY WINNERS

SOYMILK (CD 0.3) Soymilk is made by cooking dehulled ground soybeans in water. Once the solid matter is filtered out, the liquid remaining is the soymilk. Soymilk has several important health advantages. Plain, unfortified soymilk provides high-quality protein, B-vitamins, and iron; contains no cholesterol or lactose; and is naturally low in saturated fat. Some brands of soymilk are fortified with calcium, vitamin D, or vitamin B_{12}.

How to use: Soymilk is extremely versatile. You can drink it as a cold beverage, stir it in your coffee, pour it over your cereal, and use it in lieu of evaporated milk in desserts and all other cooking and baking. Try a frosty soy smoothie—cold soymilk blended with your favorite fruits. Be careful mixing soymilk with acidic ingredients, such as lemon juice and wine, as it tends to curdle.

Availability: Soymilk is available in regular and low-fat varieties and in several flavors. It can be found in containers on regular grocery store shelves and in cartons in the refrigerated dairy case. You can also find powdered soymilk, which you mix with water—a great pantry staple because it has a long shelf life. Our favorite for breakfast cereal is low-fat vanilla-flavored soymilk, as we find some of the plain soymilk brands taste a little beany; plain, however, works better in baking and cooking. All brands taste a little different, so experiment with several until you find one you like.

Storage: Refrigerated soymilk must be kept cold, and nonrefrigerated types of soymilk require refrigeration after they are opened. Once opened, a container of soymilk should stay fresh for about five days in the fridge. Always be sure to check the expiration date.

TOFU (CD 0.5) Tofu, or soybean curd, is the best known and most widely hailed traditional soy food. It's made much like regular cheese. First, hot soymilk is curdled by the addition of a calcium-based coagulant. The curds are subsequently drained and pressed to remove excess liquid. Removing more liquid results in firmer tofu, which is what the Okinawans use. In the United States, you'll find firm tofu with a texture like compressed cottage cheese; silken tofu with a custardlike texture; and soft tofu, with a texture that falls in between. They all have a bland, slightly nutty flavor, which makes them adept at absorbing the flavors of other foods and ingredients when cooked. Tofu is an excellent source of B-vitamins in addition to protein. It contains some healthy fat in the form of soybean oil but, unlike dairy products, doesn't contain cholesterol. Tofu also provides a good source of calcium, especially when a coagulant containing this mineral is used to make it. In Okinawa, tofu is traditionally made with seawater, which adds to its taste and mineral-rich health properties.

How to use: Firm tofu is dense and solid. Cut it into cubes and grill or stir-fry. Or use cubed firm tofu to increase the protein power of soups, stews, and casseroles. (For a meatier texture, press the water out and freeze. Then thaw the frozen tofu before using it.) Firm tofu works great in recipes calling for cottage cheese, ricotta, or cream cheese. Try mixing firm tofu with lemon, garlic, vinegar, and honey to make a protein-powerful mayonnaise substitute. Blended firm tofu can replace eggs or dairy products in some pies and other desserts. Soft tofu is ideal for blending into other foods; it gives a thick, creamy texture to dressings and sauces. Try substituting it for sour cream or yogurt. Use creamy silken tofu instead of sour cream in dips and recipes, or mix it with fruits and juices to make a delicious smoothie.

Availability: Most grocery stores now carry tofu. You may find it in the produce section, dairy area, deli, or Asian or health food sections. If you get chilled water-packed tofu, be sure to keep it refrigerated and check the expiration date to ensure its freshness. Water-packed tofu tastes better if you drain away excess water before using it. Press the tofu between two flat surfaces (cutting boards, cookie sheets, or plates) and tilt it to let the water run off.

Storage: Some types of tofu, unlike water-packed, don't require refrigeration until the package is opened. Read labels. After tofu is opened, it should be stored in fresh water (changed daily) and refrigerated. If tofu is properly stored, it keeps for about a week. You can also freeze tofu for up to six months.

GREEN SOYBEANS (*EDAMAME*) (CD 1.4) Green vegetable soybeans, or *edamame,* are harvested when they are still immature. They're high in protein and fiber, and they provide all the nutritional benefits of soybeans. Sweeter than mature beans, they can be served with or without the pod. We like them in the pod, because it is fun to hull them.

How to use: Edamame can be served in any number of ways—as a main vegetable dish, a snack, and as a healthy addition to soups, stews, and salads. Boil them in lightly salted water for 10 minutes; remove from the pods to use in soups, stews, and salads, or eat the beans out of the pods for a snack.

Availability: Edamame, with or without pods, are commonly available in many supermarkets, Asian grocery stores, and health food stores.

Storage: Edamame keep for several months when frozen.

SOYBEANS, BOILED (CD 1.7) Soybeans ripen in the pod into hard, dry beans about the size of a pencil eraser. The most common variety is yellow, but you'll also find brown and black soybeans. The black ones have the mildest taste. Soybeans can be cooked or baked like other beans and added to stews, soups, and sauces to increase the protein content. Make your own soynuts by soaking and then roasting soybeans.

How to use: To prepare and cook soybeans, first pick out any shriveled beans and other debris, then wash and drain. Soaking the soybeans shortens the cooking time and improves flavor and texture. Soak soybeans for 8 hours (or overnight), using 4 cups of water for each cup of beans. If time is short, soak the soybeans in boiling water for 2 to 5 minutes, allowing 6 to 8 cups of water for 1 pound of soybeans. After soaking, drain off the water and rinse the beans. In a large pot, add 4 cups of water for each cup of beans you originally had and bring to a boil. Reduce the heat and skim off the excess foam. Simmer for about 3 hours, adding more water as needed. Cook until the soybeans are tender but still somewhat firm. Black soybeans take less cooking time—about 1½ hours.

A pound of raw soybeans (about 2 cups) yields 4 to 6 cups of cooked soybeans. You may want to season your soybeans with onion, garlic, and bay leaf while they're cooking. Don't add salt or acidic ingredients (tomatoes, lemon juice, vinegar, etc.) to yellow soybeans until after they're cooked, or they'll take extra time to soften. But it's perfectly fine to add any of these ingredients to black soybeans while they're cooking, as salt and acids actually help them retain their shape.

Availability: Try looking for soybeans where bulk beans are sold in your grocery store. You can also look where other bagged dried beans are located. Frozen and canned soybeans are also readily available in most markets.

Storage: Stored in an airtight container, uncooked soybeans last months.

TEMPEH (CD 1.9) Tempeh is a soybean cake made by fermenting whole soybeans, sometimes mixed with a grain such as rice or millet. This traditional Indonesian food has a smoky or nutty flavor, provides high-quality soy protein, is low in saturated fat, and contains no cholesterol.

How to use: Tempeh's chunky, tender, chewy texture makes it an excellent choice for a meat extender or alternative. It can be prepared in many ways: steamed, baked, sautéed, deep-fried, grated, microwaved. Try adding chunks of tempeh to spaghetti sauce, Sloppy Joe mix, soups, chili, and casseroles. To grill: Steam first, marinate in barbecue sauce, then grill until brown.

Availability: Tempeh is growing in popularity, so there's a good chance you'll find it in the refrigerated case in the produce section of your regular grocery store. If you don't, try an Asian or natural food store. When you buy tempeh, look for grains that are bound tightly together.

Storage: Frozen and packaged tempeh lasts at least a year.

MISO PASTE (CD 2.0) If you've ever enjoyed a steaming bowl of miso soup (CD 0.1), you've tasted this popular soy food. Miso is a rich, full-bodied, salty paste made by fermentation. Cooked soybeans are mixed with salt and a fermenting agent that has been cultivated in a barley, rice, or soybean base. Traditionally, this mixture is aged for one to three years. The quick types of miso now commonly on the market are fermented for only five to thirty days, and they tend to have less flavor. Miso is easily digested and contains high-quality protein and B-complex vitamins. It's a basic condiment in Japanese cuisine and is popular in many other Asian countries as well. Miso soup is an important contributor to the Okinawan elders' low-CD diet.

How to use: In addition to its use as a base for soup, miso can be used to flavor other foods, such as spaghetti and barbecue sauces, stews, marinades, dips, and toppings. You can also substitute miso for salt in some recipes. Miso ranges in color from a creamy shade, often used in soups and sauces, to a deep brown. As a rule, darker-colored miso has a stronger flavor, which makes it preferable for heavier dishes.

Availability: Miso comes in two forms: paste and dehydrated. We prefer the paste. It is readily available in health food stores, Asian markets, and possibly the international section of your grocery store.

Storage: Miso paste has a refrigerator life of six months (store in a tightly sealed container). Dehydrated miso should last up to a year when stored in cool, dry surroundings.

EASY EVERYDAY SOY SUBSTITUTES

SOY BEVERAGES (CD 0.3) Soy beverages and shakes made with isolated soy protein come in a variety of delicious flavors. Some formulas are even higher in protein than soymilk. Read labels to find out the amount of soy protein in one serving. Some soy beverages are on grocery shelves; others are refrigerated. Convenient soy beverage mixes are also readily available in health food stores and may be carried by your regular grocery store.

SOY YOGURT (CD 0.9) Soy yogurt is a creamy product made from soymilk. It's similar to dairy yogurt and comes in the same wide variety of flavors. Use plain soy yogurt as a substitute for sour cream or cream cheese

MEAT ALTERNATIVES (CD 1.3–1.8) Meat alternatives (also called *meat analogs*) are soy-based foods made to resemble various types of meat—burgers, hot dogs, turkey, bacon, bologna, and so on. While some meat alternatives contain tofu, most are based on textured vegetable protein, usually made from soy flour, soy protein concentrate, isolated soy protein, or a combination of these ingredients.

How to use: Soy-based meat alternatives can be used in place of meat in most any recipe. A 12-ounce package of soy burger–style crumbles, for example, can replace a pound of ground beef in dishes like spaghetti, chili, Sloppy Joes, and casseroles.

Availability: Soy-based meat alternatives are easily found in all natural food stores and most supermarkets. They're sold in several forms—frozen, refrigerated, canned, and dried. They're often stocked near the product they resemble—look for soy-based veggie burgers near the hamburger patties in the frozen foods section. Remember to read labels carefully; meat alternatives vary in nutritional content, and not all soy-based meat alternatives are low in fat.

Storage: Store frozen and refrigerated products accordingly. Canned and boxed products can be kept on your pantry shelves if indicated.

SOY CHEESE (CD 2.5) A creamy food made from soymilk, soy cheese is available in many flavors—American, Swiss, pepper jack, provolone, cheddar, and mozzarella, just to name a few. Use soy cheese as a replacement for most cheeses, sour cream, or cream cheese, alone or in recipes. They're all healthy alternatives and taste almost like the real thing. You'll be happier with the calorie count too. Here, for example, is a quick nutrient comparison of regular cheese and soy cheese:

Calories	Regular: 110 cal	Soy: 40 cal
Saturated fat	Regular: 6 g	Soy: 1.6 g
Monounsaturated fat	Regular: 1.5 g	Soy: 2.7 g
Flavonoids	Regular: 0 mg	Soy: 1.7 mg

NON-DAIRY FROZEN DESSERTS (CD 1.7) Nondairy frozen desserts are typically made from soymilk, soy yogurt, or tofu, and they can truly satisfy your yearning for ice cream and conventional frozen yogurt. Be sure to read labels to find out the protein and fat content of these foods, as they can vary greatly.

SOY FLOUR (CD 3.3) Grinding roasted dehulled soybeans into a fine powder makes soy flour. Soy flour ground so that it still contains soybean oil is known as *natural* or *full-fat soy flour;* when it's processed to remove the soybean oil, it's called *defatted soy flour.* We recommend defatted for weight-loss purposes. Soy flour is 50 percent protein (based on dry weight), making it an excellent source of soy protein. It also contains iron, B-vitamins, calcium, and fiber.

How to use: When using soy flour to replace wheat flour in baking, be sure to add a little more water than the recipe calls for. Also, slightly reduce either the baking time or the oven temperature to prevent your baked goods from becoming too brown. Adding soy flour gives bread a slightly nutty flavor and a dense, moist texture in addition to increasing its protein content. Soy flour doesn't contain gluten, so if you try to make yeast-raised bread with just soy flour, the dough won't rise. The solution is to combine flours. For best results in yeast-raised baked products, put 2 tablespoons of soy flour in a measuring cup before filling it with all-purpose, whole-wheat, or another gluten-containing flour. When making quick breads that are not yeast-raised, you can replace up to one-fourth of the all-purpose or whole-wheat flour called for in a recipe.

Because soy flour retains more moisture than other flours, it helps prevent your baked goods from becoming stale. You can increase the nutty flavor soy flour gives to foods by lightly toasting it in a dry skillet. Use the toasted flour to thicken gravies and sauces or for baking. Be sure to fluff soy flour before measuring it, as it tends to become packed.

Availability: Soy flour is stocked in all heath food stores and may be found in your conventional supermarket on the shelf with other flours or in the health food section.

Storage: Refrigerate or freeze full-fat soy flour in a tightly covered container. Defatted soy flour doesn't need to be refrigerated and, properly stored, should keep for about a year.

PRINCIPLE #4

Balance Your Fats and Choose the Right Ones

FATS AND CHOLESTEROL: THE GOOD, THE BAD, AND THE BALANCE

How often has your doctor told you, "Your cholesterol's a bit high. You really ought to consider a low-fat, low-cholesterol diet"? For some of us, these words are so familiar we can recite them in our sleep. Lowering cholesterol has been prescribed for some time now as a way to lose weight and prevent heart disease, stroke, cancer, and even gallstones. But unfortunately, the message is way too simplistic. Detailed research—particularly that done by our former colleagues at the University of Toronto, at Harvard, and by our present colleagues at the Pacific Health Research Institute—shows that the *total amount* of fat in the diet, whether high or low, has less impact on disease than the *type* of fat in the

---

Just the Facts

- Any diet that leads to an energy (calorie) deficit, no matter what the fat content, will induce weight loss.

- Fats (CD 9) have more than double the CD of either carbs (CD 4) or protein (CD 4), so cutting fat makes it easier to cut calories, lose weight, and prevent weight regain.

- Fats are not as satiating as protein and low-GI, high-fiber carbohydrates, and are easy to overeat.[24]

- A low to moderate fat intake (10–25 percent of calories) allows you to eat bigger portions of other foods and stay satisfied longer.

- It's not a good idea to cut fats out altogether because they enhance food flavor, and some of them are actually good for you.

- Substituting low-fat foods for high-fat foods may not reduce calories if the low-fat food is too high on the CD scale (e.g., sugar-laden fat-free cookies).

- The overall solution is moderate fat intake, portion control for weight management, and choosing the right fats for good health—like the Okinawan elders have done.

diet.[22,25] There are bad fats that increase the risk for certain diseases and good fats that lower that risk. There are even fats called *essential fats,* without which we would die. The key to good health and weight management is to substitute good fats for bad fats.

The cholesterol in food—all that tasty fat in shrimp, eggs, and other foods—isn't quite the food villain it's been made out to be. While dietary cholesterol plays a small role in heart disease, it isn't enough to kill you.[22,25–27] Much more important is your blood cholesterol. High blood cholesterol levels greatly increase the risk for heart disease, stroke, and other cardiovascular diseases and may even accelerate aging itself. The connection between blood cholesterol and heart disease is a given—there's no debate; it's not up for question. What gets people mixed up is the fact that the amount of cholesterol in food is not very strongly linked to cholesterol levels in the blood. *The biggest determinant of your blood cholesterol levels is the type of fat you eat—whether it's good fat or bad fat.*

THE CHOLESTEROL–HEART DISEASE CONNECTION

Cholesterol is a waxlike substance made by the liver. It sticks to carrier proteins called *lipoproteins* that dissolve in the blood and are transported to all parts of the body. And it's important stuff. Cholesterol plays essential roles in the formation of cell membranes, some hormones, and vitamin D, and it plugs cracks in artery walls, where high blood pressure can cause damage. So it's a vital material, but too much of it in the blood can lead to a slew of problems. Again, it's all about balance.

Scientists established a link between high blood cholesterol levels and heart disease in the 1960s, when they found that deposits of cholesterol could build up inside arteries.[27] These deposits, called *plaque,* can narrow an artery enough to slow or block blood flow. This narrowing process, called *atherosclerosis,* commonly occurs in arteries that nourish the heart (the coronary arteries). When one or more sections of heart muscle fail to get enough blood, chest pain, known as *angina,* may result. Worse, the plaque can rupture, causing blood clots that may lead to heart attack, stroke, and sudden death. Fortunately, the buildup of cholesterol can be slowed, and even reversed, by medication—or, better yet, diet, which we'll talk about in a minute.[28]

But first, it's important to understand that while cholesterol-carrying lipoproteins play a key role in the development of atherosclerotic plaque and cardiovascular disease, there are two main types of cholesterol that basically work in opposite directions. Low-density lipoproteins, or LDL (remember the *L* for "lethal"), carry cholesterol from the liver to the rest of the body. When

Dietary Fats

Type of Fat	Main Source	State at Room Temperature	Effect on Cholesterol Levels	Good?
Monounsaturated	Almonds; Avocados; Canola oil; Flaxseeds/oil; Margarine;* Olives/oil; Peanuts/oil	Liquid	• Lowers LDL • Raises HDL	☺
Polyunsaturated (Omega-3)	Borage oil; Canola oil; Fish oil; Flaxseeds/oil; Grapeseed oil; Hemp oil; Mackerel; Margarine;* Omega-3 eggs; Other fish;‡ Pumpkin seeds; Salmon; Sardines; Soybean oil;† Tuna; Walnuts	Liquid	• Lowers LDL • Raises HDL	☺
Polyunsaturated (Omega-6)	Corn oil; Cottonseed oil; Grapeseed oil; Margarine;* Poultry; Safflower oil; Sesame oil; Soybean oil;† Sunflower oil	Liquid	• Lowers LDL • Raises HDL	☺
Saturated	Animal fat; Butter; Cocoa butters;§ Coconut oil; Margarine;* Palm oil; Red meat; Whole dairy products	Solid	• Raises LDL • Raises HDL	☹
Trans	Cookies; Deep-fried foods (e.g., French fries); Hydrogenated and partially hydrogenated oils; Margarine;* Pastries; Pies	Solid or semisolid	• Raises LDL • Lowers HDL	☹

* Varies widely; read labels

† More omega-6 than omega-3

‡ Most cold-water fish

§ The best of the bad fats, doesn't raise cholesterol much

there is too much LDL cholesterol in the blood, it can be deposited on the walls of coronary arteries. LDL is referred to as "garbage" or "bad" cholesterol. High-density lipoproteins, or HDL (remember the *H* for "healthy"), carry cholesterol from the blood back to the liver, which eliminates it from the body. HDL makes it less likely that excess cholesterol in the blood will be deposited in the coronary arteries, which is why HDL cholesterol is often referred to as the "good" cholesterol, or the "garbage truck."

The higher your LDL and the lower your HDL, the greater your risk for coronary heart disease and other cardiovascular diseases. For adults aged twenty years or over, the most recent federal guidelines from the National Cholesterol Education Program recommend that you aim for these target levels:[29]

• Total cholesterol less than 200 milligrams per deciliter (mg/dl). (*Note:* Twenty-five percent of all heart attacks in Americans occur in people with cholesterol levels of 150–200 mg/dl; very few occur in people under 150, so it's best to aim for the lower limits. Most Okinawan elders are under 180 mg/dl.)[30]

• HDL cholesterol levels greater than 40 mg/dl. Levels above 60 are considered a protective factor. Most Okinawan elders are near 55 mg/dl.[30]

• LDL cholesterol levels less than 100 mg/dl.

• Total:HDL ratio less than 4.5. (Most Okinawan elders are less than 3.3.)[30]

BAD FATS

Trans Fats—The Baddest of the Bad. Trans fatty acids are fats produced by heating liquid vegetable oils to very high temperatures under great pressure in a process is known as *hydrogenation.* Basically, hydrogenation turns unsaturated fat into saturated fat. The more hydrogenated an oil is, the harder it is at room temperature and the more trans fatty acids it contains. For example, spreadable tub margarine is less hydrogenated (and less hard) than stick margarine and so has fewer trans fats.

Most of the trans fats in the American diet are found in commercially prepared baked goods, margarines, snack foods, and processed foods. Commercially prepared fried foods, like French fries and onion rings, also contain a good deal of trans fat. Trans fats are worse for cholesterol levels than saturated fats because they not only raise LDL (lethal) cholesterol but also lower HDL (healthy) cholesterol—a real double whammy.[31]

Saturated Fats—Just Plain Bad. Saturated fats (SFAs) are mainly animal fats. They're found in meat, seafood, whole-milk dairy products (cheese, milk, and ice cream), poultry skin, and egg yolks. Full-fat dairy products and meat appear to raise blood cholesterol the most.[32] Some plant foods are also high in saturated fats, such as coconut and coconut oils, palm oil, and palm kernel oil, although they usually have much less effect on cholesterol than the animal fats.

Some Trans-Heavy Foods

	SFA (%)	MUFA (%)	PUFA (%) Omega-3	PUFA (%) Omega-6	TRANS (%)
Vanilla frosting, ready-to-eat	21	46	<1	11	20
Potato chips	13	40	<1	21	21
Doughnuts, glazed	20	44	1	9	21
Saltine crackers	17	45	<1	14	22
Taco shells	14	49	<1	8	23
Popcorn, oil-popped	16	47	<1	6	24
Shortening	21	44	<1	12	22
French fries, fast food restaurant	19	47	<1	7	25
Biscuit dough, frozen, high fat	17	46	<1	5	25
Vanilla cream-filled cookies	15	48	0	4	25
Imperial 70% Soybean Stick®	18	2	<1	29	23
Chocolate-coated cookies with caramel	32	45	0	3	24

GOOD FATS

Unsaturated Fats—Polyunsaturated and Monounsaturated. These are good fats because they lower cholesterol levels.[33] Unsaturated fats are found in products derived from plant sources, such as vegetable oils, nuts, and seeds. There are two main categories: polyunsaturated fats (PUFAs), found in high concentrations in sunflower, corn, and soybean oils; and monounsaturated fats (MUFAs), found in high concentrations in canola, peanut, and olive oils. In studies in which polyunsaturated and monounsaturated fats were eaten in place of saturated fats or processed carbohydrates, these good fats decreased LDL levels and increased HDL levels.[34] The table on page 81 will help you separate the good from the bad in your pantry.

Types of Fat in Common Oils and Fats

	SFA	MUFA	PUFA		TRANS
			Omega-3	Omega-6	
Oils					
Canola	7	59	9	21	0
Coconut	87	6	0	2	0
Corn	13	24	0	59	0
Olive	13	74	1	7	0
Palm	49	37	0	9	0
Peanut	17	46	0	32	0
Safflower	9	12	<1	75	0
Sunflower	10	20	0	66	0
Soybean	15	43	3	35	0
Cooking Fats					
Butter	60	26	0	5	5
Lard	38	43	<1	13	2
Shortening	21	44	<1	12	22
Margarine/Spreads					
Benecol®	11	44	<1	33	11
Fleischmann 67% Spread, Corn & Soybean Tub®	16	27	<1	44	11
Imperial 70% Soybean Stick®	18	2	<1	29	23
Promise 60% Tub, Sunflower, Soybean and Canola®	18	22	<1	54	5
Shedd's Country Crock 48% Spread, Soybean Tub®	17	24	<1	49	8
Take Control®	13	56	<1	25	6

Note: All values are given as percentages. Not all values add up to 100 percent due to rounding.

DIETARY FATS AND HEART DISEASE

Many health authorities, including the American Heart Association, recommend limiting fat intake to 30 percent or less of total daily calories as a preventive strategy.[35] But in truth, there is no "perfect" amount of total fat for a healthy diet. Several large studies, including the Nurses' Health Study and the Health Professionals Follow-up Study, have not found strong links between the overall percentage of calories from fat and heart disease.[36] What they *have* found to be most important is again the *type* of fat in the diet—and that's what we want you to pay strict attention to. There are strong links between the types of fat you eat and the effects they have on your blood cholesterol and thus your risk of heart disease—the number-one killer in America.

Of the bad fats, trans fats are the worst for heart disease. The Nurses' Health Study found that replacing only 30 calories (7 grams) of carbohydrates every day with 30 calories (4 grams) of trans fats nearly doubled the risk for heart disease. Saturated fats increased the risk as well, but not nearly as much. For the good fats, there is consistent evidence that high intake of either monounsaturated or polyunsaturated fat *lowers* the risk for heart disease. Replacing only 80 calories of carbohydrates with 80 calories of either polyunsaturated or monounsaturated fats lowered the risk for heart disease by 30 to 40 percent![37]

Fish, an important source of the polyunsaturated fat omega-3, has received a lot of attention for its potential to lower heart disease risk,[38] and many studies back this up (although not all have shown consistent benefits). One recent large trial found that by getting 1 gram per day of omega-3 fatty acids over a 3.5-year period, patients who had previously suffered heart attacks could lower their risk of dying from heart disease by 15 percent—that's equivalent to one daily serving of fatty fish, such as mackerel, salmon, sardines, or swordfish.[39] The American Heart Association currently recommends that everyone eat at least two servings of fish per week.[40]

Best Omega-3 Sources

Animal Sources	EPA/DHA: g/3 oz.	Plant Sources	α Linolenic Acid: g/1 tbsp.
Halibut	0.7	Walnuts, English	0.7
Oyster	0.7	Soybean oil	0.9
Tuna, white, canned in water	0.7	Canola oil	1.3
Tuna, fresh	0.8	Walnut oil	1.4
Trout, rainbow	0.9	Flaxseeds	2.2
Mackerel	1.0	Flaxseed oil	8.5
Salmon	1.1		
Sardines	1.3	**Alternatives**	EPA/DHA: g/g
Herring	1.8	O-3 concentrate	0.5

Data from USDA Nutrient Data Laboratory.

CHOOSE A HEALTHY COOKING OIL

Aside from fish, one of the main sources of healthy oils in the Okinawan elders' diet comes from their cooking oil, which supplies about a third of their total fat calories.[41] The main cooking oil in Okinawa is a canola–soy oil blend—one of the healthiest oils on the market. (Cold-pressed canola oil, which is produced without heat, is the best kind.) It comes out on top when compared head to head with any other oil—even olive oil—because it is very low in saturated fat (which produces cholesterol in the body) but high in monounsaturates (which helps reduce LDL while boosting HDL.) Canola oil also has heart-healthy omega-3 fat and very little omega-6 fat, which is implicated in higher breast cancer rates in animals (most vegetable oils are primarily omega-6 fatty acids).[42] Because we already get plenty of omega-6 fat in our diet, we're better off replacing it with omega-3. But remember, oil is extremely calorie dense, so spray it *on* rather than pouring it *in*. The American Heart Association also recommends getting your omega-3 fatty acids from plant sources such as tofu, walnuts, and flaxseed.[40]

Heart disease is not the only condition linked with fat intake. Researchers have long known of a similar association of dietary fat with certain cancers.[42] And here, once again, the *type* of fat, not the total amount, seems to be most important factor. Good fats are generally protective; the bad fats increase risk. While dietary fat was once considered (and dismissed) as a possible cause of breast and colon cancer,[43] some European studies have reported lower breast cancer risk among women with a high intake of monounsaturated fats—mainly in the form of olive oil.[44] And while fat intake doesn't seem to increase colon cancer risk, it appears that high consumption of red meat does,[45] and there is also evidence that diets high in animal fat and saturated fat increase prostate cancer risk as well.[46]

THE BOTTOM LINE ON FATS

Although the types of fat have a varied and somewhat complex effect on health and disease, the basic message couldn't be simpler: Limit the bad fats and replace them with good fats. We, as well as other experts, recommend you get at least equal amounts of polyunsaturated fat to saturated fat—and double the monos. If you use mainly mono-rich cooking oils (canola oil and olive oil), eat according to the three-to-one rule (at least three-quarters of your diet as plant food), eat nuts on occasion, go for fish, and choose low-fat versions of dairy or lean meats (if you eat animal foods), you will automatically be in this healthy range.[40] As you'll see in the next chapter, that's a big part of eating the Okinawa way.

The trickiest part is limiting the stealthy trans fat; it lurks in many types of food and is seldom included on the food content label. Fortunately, as awareness about trans fats increases, more products like "trans-fat free" or "nonhydrogenated" margarines are becoming available.[47] Labeling is improving too. While listing the trans fat content in food labels has long been up to the manufacturer's discretion, a report from the Institute of Medicine, concluding that there is *no* safe level of trans fats in the diet, finally prompted the Food and Drug Administration to require that trans fats be listed as part of the Nutrition Facts food label.[48] This decision came after several years of negotiations. Until trans fats are labeled, which will be in the year 2006, it still takes a little detective work to uncover their presence. The simplest approach: Check the ingredient list for "hydrogenated oils." The higher up these are listed, the more trans fats the food contains.

EGGS—TO EAT OR NOT TO EAT?

Several studies have shown that moderate egg consumption—up to one a day—does not increase heart disease risk in healthy individuals.[49] While it's true that egg yolks have a lot of cholesterol and may slightly affect blood cholesterol levels, eggs also contain nutrients that may help lower the risk for heart disease, including protein, vitamins B_{12} and D, riboflavin, and folate. So it's a pretty even trade-off. Bottom line: When eaten in moderation, eggs can be part of a healthy diet. Individuals with diabetes should limit themselves to no more than two or three eggs a week, though, as the Nurses' Health Study found an egg a day might increase the risk for heart disease in diabetics.[49] And people who find it difficult to control their blood cholesterol should choose foods made with egg whites or try omega-3 eggs (available at most health food stores).[50]

Tips for Getting the Right Fat Balance

• **Clean the pantry.** Toss out all cooking oils that are not either monounsaturated fat-rich and/or omega-3 rich. Stick to canola oil and olive oil.

• **Reduce trans fats.** Eat less commercially prepared baked goods, snack foods, processed foods, and fast foods. Choose liquid vegetable or soft tub margarines that contains little or no trans fats. When foods containing hydrogenated or partially hydrogenated oil are unavoidable, choose those that list the hydrogenated oils near the end of the ingredient list.

• **Cut meat portions down to size.** Plan for no more than 3 ounces (90 grams) for each serving. That's about half a chicken breast, one loin pork chop, two loin lamb chops, a hamburger patty, or a plain fish fillet the size of a deck of cards.

- **Trim the fat.** Before cooking, trim all visible fat from meat and remove the skin from poultry.

- **Toss the frying pan.** Bake, broil, or grill instead of frying. To keep meat moist and add flavor, baste with broth, wine, or fresh lime juice. Braising and poaching are other good cooking techniques.

- **Invest in nonstick cookware.** No fat is needed, and cleaning the pots and pans is a cinch!

- **Go meatless.** Meatless dishes like vegetarian lasagna, pasta with chunky tomato-vegetable sauce, and old standbys like baked beans and pea soup are delicious alternatives to meat.

- **Add more veggies.** When making spaghetti sauce, use less ground meat and more vegetables. Good choices include mushrooms, eggplant, and green peppers. Add an extra can or two of kidney beans to chili to make the meat go farther.

- **Choose lean cuts.** There are higher and lower fat choices in all types of meat, fish, and poultry. Make your choices from among the leaner ones. Beef: Choose extra-lean ground beef, sirloin, round steak/roast, rump, strip sirloin, wing steak, stew beef, flank steak, tenderloin. Veal: All cuts are fairly lean. Pork: Go for leg or butt roast, picnic shoulder, tenderloin, center cut loin. Poultry: White meat has half the fat of dark meat. Fish: Have sole, halibut, haddock, cod, whitefish.

- **Reach for the tofu.** Replace some or all of the ground meat in sauces with extra-firm tofu: just drain first, then crumble or mash with a fork before adding it to your recipe.

- **Get saucy.** Serve meat, fish, and poultry with low-fat sauces like cranberry relish, chili sauce, salsa, chutney, and spicy mustard. When making gravy, skim the fat out of meat juices first, or thicken beef or chicken bouillon with cornstarch.

- **Spike the pizza.** Popular pizza toppings such as anchovies, bacon, pepperoni, salami, cheese, and sausage are loaded with fat. Lighten up with ham or sliced chicken and veggies like mushrooms, green peppers, broccoli, onions, and sliced tomatoes.

- **Be a limey.** Herb- or fruit-flavored vinegars can stand alone as simple salad dressings, or try a splash of fresh-squeezed lime juice. Go easy on high-fat salad ingredients like avocado, bacon bits, regular salad dressings, olives, nuts, and high-GI croutons.

- **Shop low-fat.** Check your supermarket for lower-fat and fat-free versions of salad dressings, mayonnaise, veggie dips, and other items that are traditionally high in fat.

PRINCIPLE #5
Eat Good Carbs/Avoid Bad Carbs

We've talked a lot about vegetables and fruits, so we want to concentrate on grains here. The main rule of thumb is that when it comes to grains, breads, pastas, and other carbohydrates, *brown is always better than white.* Brown usually indicates that a grain is whole and still has most of its fiber intact. Whole grains absorb water better and are less calorically dense than their overly refined white counterparts. So toss out doughy white breads and replace them with a loaf of thick, nutritious nine-grain bread—but don't eat too many slices. Most commercially available grains are middleweights or higher after they're processed into flour, but even so they are still a vast improvement over the refined white high-GI sorts, which are true CD heavies and offer far less nutrition.

The effect of carbohydrates on our health depends not just on how much of them we eat but what kind they are. Good carbs help us maintain a healthy weight; bad carbs actually increase the risk for obesity, diabetes, coronary heart disease, and cancer.[51]

WHAT ARE CARBOHYDRATES?

Carbohydrates are compounds that include sugars, starches, and fibers. They come from a range of foods, including vegetables, fruits, milk, beans, yogurt, bread, cookies, and pasta. But these foods contain very different types of carbohydrate. As with dietary fat, some are good for your health and some are hazardous to it. Traditionally, carbohydrates classified as complex carbohydrates—vegetables, fruits, bread, pasta, and other starches—were considered to be good, and simple carbohydrates or sugars—table sugar, candy, and honey—were thought of as bad. But the truth is more complicated than that.

Carbohydrates are necessary to a healthy diet because they provide the body with the energy it needs for physical activity and keep the body's organs running

Just the Facts

- Veggies and fruits are low-CD carbs; almost all are featherweights.

- Brown versions of rice and pasta tend to be lightweights (CD ~1.4), but they can be made even lighter when combined with sauces that contain lots of vegetables.

- Whole grains, such as wheat berries are lower CD, but after processing into flour or baked into bread, virtually all grains are middleweight or higher.

- Almost all breads, even brown bread (CD 2.5–3.0), weigh in as middleweight and border on heavyweight.

- Eat most grains in moderation, and stick to the brown kind.

smoothly. The brain even rewards you with serotonin, the "feel-good hormone," when you eat them, since it prefers glucose, a simple carb, for brain fuel.[52] Many foods rich in whole-grain carbohydrates are also good sources of essential vitamins and minerals. During digestion, all carbohydrates are broken down in the intestine into their simplest form—glucose, or blood sugar—which then enters the blood. As blood sugar levels rise, the body's normal response is to trigger the pancreas to release more of the hormone insulin into the bloodstream. Insulin helps the body's cells use the sugar for energy. This, in turn, helps return blood sugar levels to normal.

In some people, however, this response doesn't work well—in particular, in obese people, who are prone to type II diabetes.[53] This type is also known as *adult onset diabetes,* which is a bit of a misnomer, because as children and adolescents become heavier they're getting it too. Type II diabetics either don't have enough insulin, or their insulin doesn't work well; either way, the result is high blood sugar levels, or a condition known as *insulin resistance.* In this condition, both blood sugar and blood insulin levels stay high because the body's cells are so accustomed to high levels of insulin that they become resistant to its actions. Many factors can promote insulin resistance, including genetics, lack of physical activity, being overweight or obese, and eating high-CD foods like cake, candy, and cookies that cause big spikes in blood sugar.[54] The insulin index in chapter 2 identifies more of the usual suspects, as does the Glycemic Index.

Glycemic Index of Common Foods

Low: up to 55 • **Medium:** 56 to 70 • **High:** 71 to 80 • **Very high:** more than 81

Baked Foods	GI
Pumpernickel, whole grain	46
Sponge cake	46
Banana bread	47
Sourdough bread	52
Stoneground whole-wheat flour	53
Pita bread	57
Blueberry muffin	59
Whole-wheat bread	64
Croissant	67
White bread	70
White bagel	72
Waffles	76

Beverages	GI
Apple juice	40
Orange juice	46
Flavored syrup, diluted	66
Fanta	68
Gatorade	78

Dairy Products	GI
Whole milk	22
Skim milk	32
Yogurt, flavored, low fat	33
Chocolate-flavored milk	34
Ice cream, low fat	50
Ice cream, full fat	61

Fruit	GI
Cherries	22
Grapefruit	25
Peach, canned in juice	30
Apricot, dried	31
Apple	38
Pear	38
Plum	39
Peach, fresh	42
Orange	44
Grapes	46
Kiwi	52
Mango	55
Papaya	58
Banana	60
Raisins	64
Cantaloupe	65
Pineapple	66
Watermelon	72
Dates, dried	103

Grains	GI
Pasta, egg fettuccine	32
Pasta, ravioli	39
Spaghetti	42
Noodles, instant	46
Bulgur	48
Buckwheat groats	54
Rice, brown	55
Rice, white, long grain	56
Rice, basmati	58
Taco shells	68
Rice, white, short grain	72

Legumes	GI
Soybeans	18
Kidney beans	27
Lentils	30
Butter beans	31
Chickpeas	33
Navy beans	38
Baked beans	48
Broad beans	79

Snacks	GI		
Peanuts	14	Mars Almond Bar	68
Potato chips	54	Arrowroot cookies	69
Popcorn	55	Ryvita	69
Corn chips	72	Life Savers	70
Water cracker	78	Skittles Fruit Chews	70
Crispbread	81	Graham crackers	74
Pretzel	83	Vanilla wafers	77
		Jelly beans	80

Sugars	GI	Vegetables	GI
Fructose (fruit sugar)	23	Peas, green	48
Lactose (milk sugar)	46	Carrots	49
Honey	58	Yam	51
Sucrose (table sugar)	65	Sweet potato	54
Glucose (blood sugar)	100	Sweet corn	55
Maltose (malt sugar)	105	Potato, new	62
		Rutabaga	72
Sweets	GI	Potato, French-fries	75
Chocolate	49	Pumpkin	75
Snickers	41	Potato, red-skinned	88
Twix Cookie Bar	44	White (Russet) potato, baked	93
Oatmeal cookies	55	Parsnip	97
Shortbread	64		

Source: With permission, David J.A. Jenkins, M.D.

CARBOHYDRATES AND THE GLYCEMIC INDEX

The Glycemic Index (GI) is a relatively new system for classifying carbohydrates based on their blood sugar effects.[55] It's received a great deal of attention and has called into question many of the old assumptions about how carbohydrates relate to health. The index, created by our former research lab at the University of Toronto, measures how quickly and how strongly blood sugar rises after a person eats a food that contains carbohydrates. Diets filled with high–glycemic index foods, which cause quick, strong increases in blood sugar levels, have been linked to an increased risk for diabetes and heart disease.[56] Foods that raise glucose levels also tend to raise insulin levels, although the Glycemic Index predicts only about 30 percent of your insulin response.[57] Foods that are low in GI, such as certain proteins and fats, can also invoke a high insulin level, so some of the simplistic arguments made against avoiding all carbs because of their insulin-raising effects are off base.[56,57] There's no reason to avoid carbs; we just have to be discriminating and choose them wisely.

A number of factors determine a food's GI rating. One of the most important is how highly processed its carbohydrates are. In highly processed carbohydrates, the outer bran and inner germ layer are removed from the original kernel of grain; this causes bigger spikes in blood sugar levels than occurs with less-processed grains. Whole-grain foods tend to have a lower glycemic index than their more highly processed counterparts. Highly processed white rice, for instance, has a higher glycemic index than less processed brown rice.[58]

A number of other factors influence how quickly a food's carbohydrates raise blood sugar levels:

FIBER CONTENT Fiber helps shield the carbohydrates in food from immediate digestion, so the sugars in fiber-rich foods tend to be absorbed into the bloodstream more slowly.

RIPENESS A ripe fruit or vegetable has a higher sugar content than one that is still green or immature and therefore has a higher glycemic index.

TYPE OF STARCH The type of starch granules in a food influences how fast the carbohydrates are digested and absorbed into the bloodstream. For example, the main starch in white potatoes, known as amylopectin, is digested and absorbed into the bloodstream fairly quickly, whereas amylose, which is relatively higher in sweet potatoes, is not.

FAT CONTENT AND ACID CONTENT The higher a food's fat content or acid content, the slower its carbohydrates are converted to sugar and absorbed into the bloodstream.

PHYSICAL FORM Finely ground flour has a higher glycemic index than more coarsely ground flour.

Although the fine points of the Glycemic Index may seem complicated, the underlying message is fairly simple: Whenever possible, replace highly processed grains, cereals, and sugars with minimally processed whole-grain products. And white potatoes—once on the complex carbohydrate preferred list—should be eaten only occasionally because of their high glycemic index. Lower GI sweet potatoes, on the other hand, are highly recommended. The following table will give you a good idea of where foods fall in the index. Any rating over 70 is considered high; medium runs from 70 down to 56; and any foods under 55 are considered low. Like CD ratings, when it comes to the GI, lower is always better.

Carbohydrates and the Glycemic Index

Higher Glycemic	*Lower Glycemic*
Refined breakfast cereals (70s to 80s)	Whole-grain breakfast cereals, oats, bulgar, barley (50s to 60s)
Canned fruits (50s to 60s)	Whole fruits (apple, 39)
White bread (70)	Whole wheat (64), whole pumpernickel (46)
Instant white rice (80)	Cooked brown rice (55)
White spaghetti* (42)	Whole-wheat spaghetti (37)
French fries (70s)	Sliced, baked new potatoes with olive oil, sweet potatoes (50s)
Sugar-rich soft drinks (90s)	Fruit juice (40s)

Note: Virtually all pasta is low GI, but white is relatively higher than whole-grain pasta.

Tips for Getting Healthy Carbs

- **Eat your veggies.** Just like your mom told you to—especially more dark green, deep yellow and red vegetables like spinach, broccoli, green leafy lettuce, squash, and green and red peppers. Aside from their low CD, they are packed with health benefits: They improve blood pressure and digestive system health; decrease risk for diabetes and cardiovascular disease (heart attack and stroke); protect against a variety of cancers; and, possibly, slow aging.[59,60]

- **Eat brown instead of white.** Choose brown rice, whole-wheat or whole-grain bread, whole-grain pasta, buckwheat noodles, whole-wheat pitas and tortillas, etc. Whole grains are not only tastier but help protect us against a range of chronic diseases.[61]

  Processing, through refining or milling, removes a good part of the vitamins, minerals, healthy oils, and fiber found in the bran-rich outer layer of grains, thus diminishing their health properties. White bread, for example, has had the dark fibrous bran as well as the wheat embryo (wheat germ) removed, leaving little more than the starchy, carbohydrate-rich center. During the process, over 80 percent of the vitamin E, niacin, riboflavin, manganese, magnesium, vitamin B$_6$, and fiber are lost, as is over half the calcium, iron, thiamin, potassium, and most other vitamins and minerals. Little wonder law mandates that riboflavin, thiamin, niacin and a few other nutrients be added back in. But despite being "enriched," white bread has few of its original healthful properties and all or more of the calories. Worse yet, a diet high in this type of refined carbohydrate can lead to high levels of blood sugar, insulin, and triglycerides and low levels of HDL cholesterol—the pre-cursors to diabetes and cardiovascular disease.

• **Eat more legumes.** These include beans and tofu. They're among the lowest-GI and healthiest carbs around.[17,18]

• **Eat the right potatoes.** Replace white potatoes with sweet potatoes. If at all possible, get purple Okinawan sweet potatoes. If you live in a big city, they might be in your grocery store; if not, try an Asian market. But all sweet potatoes are low GI and full of vitamin C and healthy carotenoids—and considerably healthier than white potatoes. Despite being the most popular vegetable in America, white potatoes are made up mostly of easily digested starch, called *amylopectin,* which is turned into blood sugar very quickly. In fact, several studies have shown that eating this starch can lead to insulin resistance.[62] In terms of their insulin effects, high-amylopectin starches like potatoes are equivalent to table sugar. So if you are including white potatoes in your vegetable count, you're getting fewer benefits than you think. White potatoes just don't pack the health benefits of the antioxidant-rich green or yellow vegetables—or sweet potatoes.

PRINCIPLE #6
Keep Fiber in Mind

FIBER MADE SIMPLE

What Grandma called *roughage,* scientists know as *fiber*—and there's a lot more to it than crunch. Fiber is not a single food or substance; it is an indigestible complex carbohydrate found in plants. It has no calories in and of itself because the body can't absorb it. That's why high-fiber foods are low in fat and calories. Fiber can be divided into two categories according to physical characteristics and effects on the body: water-insoluble fiber and water-soluble fiber. Each form functions differently and provides different health benefits. Insoluble fibers, such as cellulose, hemicellulose, and lignin, don't dissolve in water and may help protect against cancer.[63] Soluble fibers, such as gum and pectin, dissolve in water and help lower cholesterol levels.[64]

Health experts are now advising people of all ages to include more of both kinds of fiber in their diets. A solid body of research shows that fiber and/or its associated phytonutrients help prevent cancer, diabetes, heart disease, and obesity. Fiber may owe its healthy protective qualities to several substances it contains, including lignans and folate, found in whole grains, and various other

---

Just the Facts

- Fiber is a complex carbohydrate that has no calories and usually has many phytonutrients that help protect against cancer and cardiovascular disease.

- Fiber (CD 0.0) not only reduces a food's caloric density but also helps you feel full on fewer calories.

- High-fiber foods give you a lot to eat for very few calories and take the edge off your appetite for longer than many other foods.

- Fiber adds a satisfying chewiness to food and aids in its digestion.

- Fiber is found in whole grains, vegetables, legumes, and fruit, but not in animal products.

---

phytochemicals, found in fruits and vegetables. Whatever the source, eating high-fiber foods definitely contributes to robust health, a leaner body, and better weight control.[60]

FIBER AND YOUR WEIGHT

Let's take a closer look at the two kinds of fiber and how they help with weight control. Insoluble fiber is found in fruits, vegetables, dried beans, wheat bran, seeds, popcorn, brown rice, and whole-grain products such as breads, cereals, and pasta. Soluble fiber is found in fruits such as apples, oranges, pears, peaches, and grapes; and vegetables, seeds, oat bran, dried beans, oatmeal, barley, and rye. So there's a lot of crossover; one food can contain one or both kinds of fiber. Insoluble fiber bulks up wastes and moves them through the colon more rapidly, preventing constipation and diverticular disease.[65] Soluble fiber, especially the stickiest kinds, called *gums* and *pectins,* help keep cholesterol under control by removing bile acids that digest fat, and help regulate blood sugar and obesity by coating the gut's lining and delaying stomach emptying.[66] As a result, they can slow sugar absorption after a meal and may reduce the amount of insulin needed.[67] Fiber, in fact, is a weight-watcher's dream, as certain fibers, namely cellulose and hemicellulose, take up space in the stomach, making us feel full and therefore reducing our food intake.

Another reason fiber makes you feel full is that the extra chewing required with fibrous foods signals the brain that a lot of food is coming, which causes the body to slow the passage of food through the intestines so hunger signals are delayed. A review of studies of the effects of a high-fiber diet on body weight showed that increasing dietary fiber of any type resulted in more body fat loss than usual weight loss interventions.[68] Over a four-month study period, when subjects ate more than 14 grams of fiber per day they lost between four and five extra pounds. When they both lowered their dietary fat and increased fiber, they experienced even greater weight loss.

BEST SOURCES OF FIBER

Although fiber is not considered an essential nutrient, the U.S. Surgeon General and many professional health organizations recommend a diet containing 20 to 35 grams of fiber a day.[69] The average American consumes half that—about 10 to 15 grams daily. The best way to up your fiber intake is to eat more complex low-GI carbohydrates, but go slowly. A large increase in fiber over a short period can result in bloating, diarrhea, gas, and general discomfort, so it's important to add fiber gradually over a period of three weeks or so to avoid abdominal problems.

Animal products like meat, cheese, and eggs contain zero fiber. Only plant foods—fruits, vegetables, whole grains, beans, nuts, and seeds—can provide the fiber essential to good health. Some are higher in fiber than others. For example, ½ cup cooked carrots has four times as much fiber as 1 cup raw spinach. A medium baked sweet potato contains more fiber than ½ cup cooked brown rice. Whole-wheat bread has twice as much fiber as white bread. But no matter what specific foods are selected, eating a variety of fruits, vegetables, grains, and beans can easily ensure the daily recommended intake of fiber. Five daily servings of fruits and vegetables plus several servings of whole grains and beans will provide not only essential fiber but also the nutrients and phytochemicals critical to lowering cancer risk.

Don't be intimidated by the numbers. It's not as hard to get your 20 to 35 grams of fiber as it may seem.

Try, for example adding to your

• *Breakfast:* 1 cup raisin bran cereal (7 grams) and 1 banana (3 grams)

• *Lunch:* a sandwich of 2 slices whole-wheat bread (4 grams) filled with ¼ cup hummus (4 grams), followed by 1 orange (3 grams)

• *Dinner:* 1 small baked sweet potato with skin (3 grams), ½ cup mixed vegetables (4 grams), and 1 cup strawberries (4 grams).

Total Fiber: 32 grams. Bingo! Each of our recipes lists fiber content, among other nutritional information, which will also help you keep track.

Tips for Increasing Dietary Fiber

• **Eat plant foods.** Only plant foods contain fiber, so load up on them.

• **Start early.** Start your day with a high-fiber breakfast cereal—one with 5 or more grams of fiber per serving. Opt for cereals with the word *bran* or *fiber* in the name. Or add a few tablespoons of unprocessed wheat bran to your favorite cereal.

• **Go the whole way.** Switch to whole-grain breads that list whole wheat, whole-wheat flour, or another whole grain as the first ingredient on the label.

• **Substitute whole-grain flour for white flour** when baking bread. Whole-grain flour is heavier than white flour. In yeast breads, use a bit more yeast, or let the dough rise longer. When using baking powder, increase it by 1 teaspoon for 3 three cups of whole-grain flour.

• **Eat brown.** Experiment with brown rice, barley, and whole-wheat pasta.

• **Reach for a carrot.** Take advantage of ready-to-use vegetables. Mix frozen broccoli into prepared spaghetti sauce. Snack on baby carrots.

• **Eat beans.** Eat more beans, peas, and lentils. Add kidney beans to canned soup or a green salad. Make nachos with black bean dip, baked tortilla chips, and salsa. A single 15-ounce (425-gram) can of baked beans has 30 grams of fiber. Beans on whole-grain toast gives you a full day's allotment!

• **Make snacks count.** Fresh fruit, raw vegetables, and air-popped popcorn are all good sources of fiber.

• **Eat fruit at every meal.** Apples, bananas, oranges, pears, and berries are good sources of fiber.

• **Go slow.** To avoid bloating and gas problems, increase your fiber intake gradually. Drink plenty of water (until your urine is clear) as you increase your fiber to promote regularity.

• **Read labels.** Check the fiber content, listed on product labels.

• **Eat oat bran.** It's one of the best sources of fiber. This grain contains a hefty dose of soluble fiber, as opposed to the nondigestible kind we often associate with fiber. Soluble fiber not only does everything a good low-CD food should, like fill you up on fewer calories, but also lowers your bad cholesterol.

• **Go for the berries.** With their appealing sweetness and juiciness, berries and other fruit may be the smartest high-fiber snack of all. Along with high water content, berries have lots of fiber, so they fill you up with few calories. Two cups of fresh strawberries is a satisfying snack, while other 100-calorie snacks, like ten jelly beans or eighteen fat-free pretzels, would not even put a dent in your appetite.

Some Healthy Sources of Fiber

Grains

100% bran cereal	⅓ cup	8 grams
Whole grain wheat flour	½ cup	8 grams
Oatmeal, cooked	1 cup	4 grams
Pearled barley, cooked	½ cup	3 grams
Whole wheat bread	1 slice	3 grams

Vegetables and Legumes

Baked beans, vegetarian	½ cup	6 grams
Kidney beans, boiled	½ cup	6 grams
Burdock root	⅔ cup	3 grams
Sweet potato	¾ cup	3 grams
Spinach	3 cups	2 grams
Sweet corn	½ cup	2 grams
Cabbage	1 cup	2 grams
Green beans	½ cup	2 grams
Tomato	1	1 gram
Konnyaku	2 oz.	1 gram

Fruits

Dried figs	¼ cup	6 grams
Apple	1	4 grams
Pear	1	4 grams
Apricots	½ cup	2 grams

PRINCIPLE #7

Go for Water-Rich Foods

One problem that makes weight control such a challenge is that our body's natural sensors don't tally our calories very well. We're designed to check food amount, not caloric content. It's this faulty feedback system that makes it so easy to overindulge in calorie-rich foods—like the carrot muffin that looks healthy but weighs in at 400 calories. But while this system is somewhat imperfect, it can also be your friend—when you take advantage of water-rich foods. Your body interprets the water in water-rich foods as actual calorie-bearing food, allowing you to fill up on fewer calories and not be hungry later.

A fascinating study by researchers at Pennsylvania State University clearly illustrates this point and demonstrates that it's the water in the food, not drinking water, that increases our feelings of satiety.[70] In the study, researchers served lunch to twenty-four hungry young women and measured how much they ate. The first course was a 270-calorie appetizer of chicken-rice casserole with varying amounts of water. Women who started with the casserole alone or drank a 10-ounce glass of water along with it went on to eat another 300 calories of food at the main course, whether they drank the water or not. But when the 10-ounce glass of water was added to the casserole—in effect, making it soup—each woman ate only 200 calories of food at the main course—about 30 percent less! These women did not feel hungrier later in the day or feel any need to make up those calories later. All women in the study ate about the same amount of calories at dinner, whether they had eaten less at lunch or not. The result? Same satisfaction for all, but fewer calories for the soup eaters.

Just the Facts

- In general, the more water a food contains, the less calorically dense it is—and the more of it you can eat.

- Broth-based soup decreases hunger and keeps you full far longer than water alone.

- Increased intake of water-rich fruits (up to CD 0.7), vegetables (up to CD 0.5), and broth-based soups (CD 0.1 to 0.8) will markedly lower the CD of your diet and help keep you lean.

These data reinforce the science that tells us that "eating" water and "drinking" water affect hunger and thirst through different mechanisms. You can use this science to your great advantage in managing your weight. When you drink water per se, it will quench your thirst but not quell that tiger in your belly— except perhaps momentarily. But when water is in soup, stews, vegetables and fruit, your body thinks of it as food, and it will help satisfy your hunger. So eating water-rich foods is one of the most important principles for healthy weight control. It has a huge impact on lowering caloric density, minimizing hunger, and, ultimately, helping you shed your unwanted pounds.

Most of the foods at the base of the CD pyramid are water-rich. They make up the majority of the featherweight and lightweight categories, which reflects the calorie density benefits of water. Water, in fact, has a far more powerful effect on caloric density of food than fat or fiber does because it's totally calorie-free, yet adds significant volume. Water-rich, weight-control wonder foods include vegetables and fruits, some even named for their high water content (e.g., watermelon), soups, stews, casseroles, and cooked water-rich cereals, such as oatmeal and cream of wheat. A little higher on the pyramid but still making the lightweight cut are cooked pasta (hooray, you can eat pasta!), steamed and boiled rice, steamed and poached fish, and low-fat frozen desserts such as sorbet and frozen yogurt. Many of these are Okinawan favorites, as you'll see in chapters 5 and 8. The table below quantifies this a bit better for you.

Water Content of Foods and Caloric Density

Food	Water Content	CD Range
Broth-based soups	90–97%	~0.1 to 0.8
Broth-based stews	85–95%	~0.3 to 0.9
Vegetables/Fruit	80–95%	~0.1 to 0.7
Cooked cereal	85%	~0.6
Seafood (including fish)	60–85%	~0.9 to 1.5
Boiled eggs	75%	~1.6
Pasta	65%	~1.3 to 1.5
Meat	45–65%	~1.2 to 5.0
Bread	35–40%	~0.9 to 5.0
Nuts	2–5%	~5.7 to 6.6
Cooking Oil	0%	~8.8

BROTH-BASED SOUPS

Not surprisingly, soup is the ultimate featherweight because its water content is so high. You can eat plenty of it. It's extremely difficult to overdose on soup calories. Soup makes you feel full by offering sensory stimulation at multiple levels, including smell, taste, and activation of the stomach's stretch receptors. Slow absorption by the stomach causes minimal increases in blood sugar with subsequent incremental increases in insulin.[57] Insulin then shuts off the hunger signal—which is exactly what you want. By the time you finish a bowl of soup, you are well on your way to feeling full and less likely to overeat higher-CD fare. Broth-based soups can get their flavor from almost any food—vegetable extract, mushrooms, kombu (kelp), bonito (tuna family), sardines, chicken, beef, and pork, among other possibilities; the sky's the limit.

We're definitely *not* saying to eat only soup—although that strategy has been proposed by others. Remember the cabbage soup diet? This was a trend diet that popped up some years back; it consisted of cabbage soup and little else, taking the low-CD principle to the extreme.[71] Some people, naturally, lost weight on the diet because it was so incredibly low-cal, but nobody stuck with it for long because it was so restrictive and boring. The all-soup-all-the-time strategy wasn't smart then and isn't smart now.

On the other hand, following the Okinawan example—where miso soup (CD 0.1) is eaten with almost every meal—is both smart and effective. The elders end up eating *less* at the main meal because they are partially full on featherweight fare when they start their main meal. Again, this doesn't mean you have to eat miso soup at every meal, but it *is* a good idea to fill up early on water-rich fare. Try soup, salad, and stew as appetizers, snacks, or even as a main course. Cold soups, like tomato-rich gazpacho, work just as well as hot soups. Chunky soups like chicken noodle soup work better than strained or clear soups because small chunks of low-CD veggies, tofu, seafood, rice, pasta, and spices help satiety by prolonging the digestion time in the stomach, ultimately making that feeling of fullness last longer.

STEW OVER IT

Stews are one-pot meals and lifesavers for busy cooks. Besides only having one pot to clean, there are no complicated steps, no fancy cooking techniques—nothing stressful to think about. Just heat up a big pot and throw in lots of goodies. One-pot stews, called *nabe,* are so important in Japanese cooking that each type has a special name. The best-known *nabe* are *yudofu,* a tofu-based stew;

dotenabe, a miso and oyster stew; and sukiyaki, a beef (or tofu) and *konnyaku* noodle stew.

It's easy to keep stews low-CD, and they can be readily adapted to fit vegetarian or carnivore preferences. Plus, you can easily include your entire day's allotment of low-CD vegetables in one meal—ten at a time, should you choose. Stews are also wonderfully compatible with other leftovers. If you cooked up one of the recipes in chapter 8, for instance, and had some left over, you could toss it into a stew pot the next day with a few fresh ingredients. It's already low-CD fare, and by adding water, miso, and a few more items, you'd have your next lightweight meal. It's hard to make a serious mistake, really—which gives you lots of room to be creative. And while you're cooking up one batch of stew, you can make extra to freeze for a quick, healthy lunch or dinner later in the week. Individual portions can be frozen and stored in plastic containers and are perfect to take to work or school. These make an instant healthy meal at about 300 calories apiece.

Bottom line: Stew doesn't have to be the boring high-CD meat-and-potatoes dish you may remember from your childhood. There are hundreds of superb, low-cal gourmet options now—meatless veggie stews, lean chicken stews, Okinawan sweet-potato stew, and on and on. You'll find some great recipes in this book to get you started. One thing is for sure, they'll help you get rid of that old image of stew as a dull, tasteless cold-weather staple and give you something wonderful to stew about.

WATER-RICH VEGGIES AND FRUITS

Most fruits and vegetables are water-rich, and most of them are featherweights. Lettuce, tomatoes, broccoli, winter squash, bitter melon, zucchini, cucumbers, celery, bamboo shoots, eggplant, strawberries, grapefruit, honeydew melon, apples, oranges, and many, many more have a CD of 0.7 or less—low even on the featherweight scale. The water-rich concept becomes clearer than ever when you consider dried fruit versus plump ripe fruit. Two cups of fresh apricots, for example, has about the same amount of calories as only ½ cup of the dried version you find in trail mix. You can eat four times as much fresh as dried. They're essentially the same food, only the trail mix type is lacking the water. So include more fresh fruit in your diet and less dried—grapes rather than raisins, plums rather than prunes—for more satiety and fewer calories.

Almost all fresh fruits and vegetables can be eaten in unlimited quantities. Find kinds you really enjoy and buy them in bulk so you have plenty around the house when you have a snack attack. Also use them liberally to lower the CD of common dishes. Pasta salads, for instance, can be jazzed up with zucchini, red peppers, carrots, green beans, and other veggies. Their high water content allows you to have a double portion for the same calories you'd get in one portion of the salad made without the veggies. Augment chili with lots of veggies and beans; add lots of sprouts, lettuce, and tomato to sandwiches.

Expand your horizons and try new foods. You might try shopping at new or different venues, such as farmers' markets and Asian food stores you may not have ventured into before. One of the most striking aspects of an Asian market is the dazzling array of native produce. The richness of their aroma, texture, color, and flavor is in extreme contrast to that of the rather limited selections in many American groceries. Some of the more exotic fruits are an acquired taste, so zero in on the ones you find most intriguing, try them a few times—and keep an open mind.

WATER-RICH OKINAWAN FOODS

It is no coincidence that water-rich featherweights form the bulk of the slim Okinawan elders' diet. Miso soup is eaten at breakfast, at lunch, *and* at dinner as an appetizer. Almost all vegetables are water-rich—some more than others, of course—but they are the single most frequently consumed food of the elders. All three major cooking styles used in Okinawa (stir-fry, simmered, and combo) are built around veggies. One of these styles, called *nbushi,* is based entirely on simmering the most water-rich veggies without cooking oil. The water drains out of the vegetables into the pan and then miso paste is added, along with the ingredients of choice. It's delicious, filling, and about as low-CD as you can go. (More on this in chapter 5.)

Although fruit is a smaller part of the Okinawan diet than vegetables, it's still an important aspect of the elders' lives and is surrounded by tradition and folklore. That's no more evident than on the Motobu peninsula at the northern tip of the main Okinawan island, which is like orchard heaven. There are miles and miles and miles of orange, pineapple, and papaya orchards. Watermelon (CD 0.3) is another Okinawan favorite. We give watermelons as gifts to thank the elders for participating in our studies, which is greatly appreciated; we're always invited back.

DON'T FORGET TO *DRINK* WATER, TOO

To start off the New Year in Okinawa, young boys haul water from a sacred spring in a tradition called *wakaubi.* It's said that drinking this water will chase away misfortune and help to keep you young. The sacred water is first offered to the Fire God in the kitchen and then brewed into jasmine tea, which is offered to the ancestors at the family altar. Then the family drinks the tea themselves.

While we're not suggesting that you engage in water-honoring rituals, we do want you to appreciate the value water has to your body—indeed, to your life. Water is a critical nutrient. It bathes our body's cells, is essential for energy production, and makes up two-thirds of our body mass. We lose water via breathing and sweating and in our urine and feces, so we need to replace it daily. Good hydration is essential to keep your body full of energy and performing at its best. Studies show that drinking plenty of water also is beneficial to the immune system and skin, helps alleviate constipation, and reduces the risk of kidney stones, and bladder and colon cancer. The U.S. National Research Council recommends you get 1 milliliter of water for every calorie you eat.[72–77] So if you eat 2,000 calories, you'll need 2,000 ml (2 liters), which equals 2 quarts (there's your eight-glasses-a-day rule.)

Your daily quota of water can come from both foods and drinks. You get about ½ quart from food if you eat a lot of water-rich foods. Drinks provide the rest. Caffeinated beverages count for only about half their volume, as they are also mild diuretics. Watch out for soft drinks, fruit juice, and sugared teas, as those calories quickly add up. The Okinawan elders love tea, and many studies support the health benefits of tea catechins (a class of flavonoid) in its ability to help metabolize fat, and for risk reduction in cardiovascular disease and cancer.[78]

In general, hard water, which is more mineral-rich than soft water (calcium and other metals removed and sodium added) is much better for you, so avoid drinking soft water if possible. We get enough salt in our diet! The hardness (mineral content) of drinking water has been associated with healthier hearts and lower risk for certain cancers in some studies.[79] However, don't be misled by fantastic claims being made about the coral calcium water of Okinawa. While Okinawan drinking water has higher calcium content than that in the rest of Japan, the actual amount of extra calcium Okinawans drink is only about 50 mg/day—a far cry from the 100,000 mg/day being claimed by some; it is unlikely to be much of a factor in their longevity.[80] The low calorie content of the diet is far more critical to Okinawan leanness, health, and longevity than their drinking water.[81]

We highly recommend spring water or filtered water as your main drinking water. Some studies have shown that up to 10 percent of gastroenteritis (inflammation of the digestive tract) hospital admissions come from microbes in tap water, particularly river water.[82] Some bottled water, however, is nothing more than tap water. If the label says "purified" water, not spring water, the water may have come from someone else's tap, as purification is the customary process used everywhere to remove the major contaminants. Check the source. Buyer beware!

Remember that dehydration can make you feel tired and lethargic and will decrease your capacity for exercise. Extra fluid is needed in hot weather and when you exercise. For each hour of exercise, you should drink an extra quart of fluid. If you have an illness that's causing diarrhea or sweating, you'll need to increase your fluid intake to make up for the loss. The color of your urine is a rough gauge of your water intake. If it's straw-colored (pale yellow or clear), you're probably getting enough. If it's dark yellow and/or has a strong odor, you probably need to drink more water. Another check: If you're urinating less than four times a day, you probably need more water. Proper hydration is an essential part of weight control and overall wellness—so bon appétit, and bottoms up!

Incorporating More Water-Rich Foods

- **Start meals with soup whenever possible.** Try to eat broth-based soups as an appetizer (and occasionally as a meal itself.) This is a major strategy employed by the Okinawans and other Japanese. In Japan, miso soup (CD 0.1) starts every breakfast, lunch, and dinner.

- **Eat more stew.** Water-rich stews should replace high-CD meats with vegetables, spices, brown rice, and whole-grain pasta.

- **Plan ahead and skim the fat.** Make soups or stews a day ahead and refrigerate. Skim off any fat that hardens on top. The meat itself will be leaner with a lower CD.

- **Go low-fat.** In cream soup recipes, use plain soymilk, low-fat or fat-free yogurt, buttermilk, or nonfat or 1% milk instead of cream.

- **Turn on the blender.** Use pureed, cooked vegetables (squash, sweet potato, carrots), whole-grain noodles, canned legumes, brown rice, or barley to make soups thick and hearty without added fat.

- **Take Manhattan.** If you like clam chowder, choose the water-rich, lycopene-rich tomato-based Manhattan style, rather than the creamed-based New England style. Smarter for calories; smarter for health.

- **Keep it right there.** Buy a small bottle of water and always keep it near you—on your work desk, kitchen counter, night table, and in your purse.

Whenever you see the bottle, have a sip. Soon you will get used to being well hydrated, so that when you have less water in your body it will be easier for you to notice that, too.

- **Don't throw away that bottle just yet.** Those little plastic bottles are great for carrying around your water. They never break and are light and refillable. Once you buy a bottle of water, refill it several times a day as you drink the water. You can use the same bottle for days—but keep it clean.

- **Go steamy.** When you cook vegetables that you can either steam or bake (or broil or grill), go for steaming. Steaming will keep a higher percentage of water in the vegetables, while baking, broiling, and grilling can evaporate most water. The water in the vegetables fills you up and is calorie-free.

- **No syrup.** Although real fruits are the best way of eating water-rich, low-calorie fruits, canned fruits are a convenient occasional alternative. But when you buy canned fruits, be conscious what liquid the fruits are stored in. There are four main types of liquid: heavy (or regular) syrup, light syrup, juice, and the fruit's own juice. The best is the fruit's own juice, then go for other juices. Never choose fruit stored in syrup—it's the triple whammy, high CD, heavy calories, and high GI!

- **Add vegetables and fruit to most dishes.** Add to pasta, pizza, chili, soups, and sandwiches in liberal quantities.

- **Plan ahead.** Cook a week's worth of soup, stew, casserole, etc., and store the food in plastic containers for later use.

- **Simmer your veggies.** Simmering veggies with miso paste is a delicious and healthy way to prepare them.

- **Buy smart.** If you go for commercial soups, make sure to choose low-salt versions, as many are exceedingly high in sodium.

PRINCIPLE #8

Herbs and Spices are Practically Calorie-Free

Many people avoid vegetables and other low-CD foods because they find them boring. But herbs and spices can make any food exciting—and they add up to so few calories that we don't even count them. The right blend of herbs and spices can transform the most featherweight veggie meal into a gourmet treat,

---

Just the Facts

- Herbs and spices give you a big bang for your calorie buck because they are dense in nutrients but almost calorie-free.

- Herbs and spices add wonderful taste and smell to foods and help make featherweight dishes highly palatable.

- Herbs and spices are among the most potent sources of antioxidants and may help with fat loss.

---

which is one of the reasons Okinawan cuisine is so sensational (as you'll see when you try our recipes).

And there's more good news. Herbs, which typically come from plant leaves, are also amazingly healthy. Recent studies at the USDA show that common herbs are a potent source of antioxidants—those free-radical fighters we need to protect our body from corrosive molecules produced during normal energy metabolism as well as from environmental hazards like smoking, pesticides, and exhaust fumes.[83] USDA researchers measured the antioxidant properties of numerous medicinal and culinary herbs, all of which were grown under the same experimental conditions, and found that the antioxidant activity of some herbs were actually higher than that of vitamin E. Most of the herbs they tested even surpassed foods long lauded for their antioxidant content, such as vegetables, fruits, and berries.

Of all the herbs, oregano was the clear winner. Three types of oregano—Greek, Italian, and Mexican—scored the highest in antioxidant activity. Oregano demonstrated forty-two times the antioxidant activity of apples, twelve times that of oranges, and four times that of blueberries, the most highly touted fruit. Oregano even had more antioxidant activity than the highly regarded garlic. That's a serious antioxidant! The most active component in most herbs is a phenol (similar to a flavonoid) called *rosmarinic acid*. Rosmarinic acid is also prominent in rosemary, as the name suggests.

But even the herbs that lost out to oregano are powerful antioxidants in their own right—and definite winners in terms of taste. We strongly recommend using herbs and spices for flavoring instead of salt and artificial chemical additives. Fresh herbs and spices usually contain higher antioxidant levels than their dried and/or processed counterparts. Fresh garlic cloves, for example, provide 1.5 times more antioxidant activity than garlic powder. We'll introduce you to some of the more impressive Okinawan herbs and spices in the next chapter; meanwhile, here are some you may already know. Some of our favorites, these are wonderfully versatile, flavorful, aromatic, and ready to let loose with a significant antioxidant punch on your behalf.

EIGHT HEALTHY HERBS

CILANTRO. Cilantro leaves are great for broth-based soups, salsa, and sauces, and also add a wonderful touch to fish and meat. Add near the end of cooking for peak taste. Cilantro looks similar to Italian parsley; make sure to tear a tiny piece off a leaf and sniff before buying. If you smell a distinctive, extremely pungent aroma, it's cilantro. Store a bunch in a cup with just enough water to keep one inch of the stems' end submerged and cover with plastic bags. You can use cilantro in many ways. Sprinkle chopped raw leaves into broth-based soups before serving. Add chopped raw leaves to salsa and sauces. Combine with whole-wheat flour or bread crumbs to coat fish or meat before cooking. It's also great for Asian broth-based soups such as Vietnamese *pho* and Thai *tom yum goong*, rolled into fresh spring rolls, and combined with breads, fish, meat, ratatouilles, and curries. To prepare cilantro, rinse before using, remove the leaves from the stems (the soft stems on the top part are also edible), and chop finely.

DILL (baby dill or dill weed). These feathery, light green leaves are best used fresh or added to food in the last few minutes of cooking so as not to lose the delicate flavor. Add dill to seafood dishes. Mix it with soy, yogurt, vinegar, and salt and toss with thinly sliced cucumbers. Include a few sprigs when making chicken soup. Add to vinaigrette dressing. Great for cooking with cabbage and onions, served with cheese, stir-fried with root vegetables, and folded into bread dough. To prepare dill, rinse just before using, remove the leaves from the coarse stems, and snip or chop the leaves.

MARJORAM. Marjoram has a flavor similar to oregano but is subtler and a little bit sweeter. The pretty pink flowers are an attractive garnish. Add marjoram to olive oil. Brush it on broiled or grilled fish or meat. Add it to salads. Stir it into creamy soy-based soups, tomato soup, pasta sauces, and lentils. Add it to chili near the end of cooking. To ready it for use, remove the leaves from the stems and chop leaves or use whole.

MINT. Peppermint and spearmint are the most popular varieties for cooking, although there are many other species. Both sprigs and flowers make a pretty garnish. Use mint to make a soothing tea: Crush the stems, add boiling water, and let it steep. Stir mint into fruit salads. Add it to citrus sorbets. Add it to liquid when poaching pears or other fruits. Sprinkle mint, finely chopped, over chilled cucumber or green pea soup. Garnish small appetizers. To prepare mint, pull the leaves from the stems. Use the small leaves whole, or chop or cut in strips.

OREGANO. Oregano is similar to marjoram, but the plant is tougher and more aromatic. Use it sparingly, or it will dominate other flavors. It's great in combination with basil. Sprinkle oregano on tomato halves before roasting or broiling. Add a sprig or two to pot roast. Add to tomato sauces for pasta, pizza, and so on. Add to salad dressings. Mince and add to soy cheese spreads. To use oregano, remove the leaves from the stems and chop leaves finely.

ROSEMARY. The strong, needlelike leaves of rosemary have a piney aroma. Although it has a strong flavor, it goes well with almost any dish. Coat new potatoes or sweet potatoes with olive oil and rosemary before roasting. Stir into bread dough. Stuff into slits in leg of lamb (with garlic slivers) or tofu before roasting. Sprinkle on rolled-out whole-wheat pizza dough for herbed focaccia. To prepare rosemary, remove the leaves by running two fingers down the tough stem from top to bottom. Chop leaves, or use whole.

TARRAGON. A delicate, sweet aroma distinguishes this flavorful herb. Add it to fish or chicken soups. Add it to beaten omega-3 eggs when making mushroom or cheese omelets. Add it to cream sauces for poultry and fish. Steep a few sprigs in a bottle of white wine vinegar and use in salad dressings or sprinkle over fish. Stir it into brown mustard for a delicious new flavor. Prepare tarragon by removing the leaves from the stems and chopping.

THYME. The longer you cook this herb, the stronger the flavor becomes in the pan. Use sparingly—only a tiny bit is needed for quick-prep dishes. Simmer thyme in stews. Add it to crumbled tofu to make tofu burgers. Sprinkle the leaves on fish or poultry before broiling or baking. Heat the leaves in apple jelly and use as a sauce with sautéed tofu and vegetables. To use thyme, remove the tiny leaves by running your fingers down the stem from top to bottom. Use the whole leaves.

TEN DELIGHTFUL SPICES

ALLSPICE (*Pimento officinalis*). A wonderful sweet spice that tastes like a mixture of cloves, cinnamon, ginger, and nutmeg. Allspice is great for stir-fries, sauces, soups, cooked meats, baked bananas, exotic sweets, mulled ciders, pies, and Christmas recipes. See the recipe for Spiced Cranberry Cider on page 355.

CARDAMOM (*Eletaria cardamomum*). One of India's most amazing spices. Store the delicate green but strong-flavored seeds in an airtight container. Grind whole cardamom with an herb grinder before cooking. Cardamom adds an exotic sweetness to cake dough, ice cream, milk tea, and fruity sweet dishes. See the recipe for Soy Masala Chai on page 353.

CHILI (*Capsicum frutescens*). As chilies mature, their spiciness increases. Okinawans like to place a handful of fresh chili in local rice wine. Makes a great flavoring for noodle dishes, vegetables, and fish dishes. (Chilies also get hotter the longer they're cooked.) Chilies are wonderful in stir-fries, guacamole, salsas, chili con carne, baked beans, deviled eggs, and curry spice mix. See the recipe for Cajun Hot Popcorn on page 360.

CUMIN (*Cuminum cyminum*). This spice, with its gentle flavor, is at its best when roasted over medium-low heat before adding other ingredients. Its seedy, caviar-like texture is a treat. Cumin is delicious in curries, sautéed and stuffed vegetables, cordials, liqueurs, roasts, and mixed with yogurt. See the recipe for Cumin-Chili Cauliflower on page 305.

FENNEL (*Foeniculum vulgare*). The leaves are called *I cho ba* in Okinawan, and its seeds are one of the most beloved spices in Okinawa—indeed, it's a favorite over the world. Store the seeds in a cool, dry place. To enhance fennel's great flavor, roast before use. Fennel adds distinction to fish soups, poached eggs, sauces, apple pies, custards, desserts, curries, breads, fish, roast pork, and served with cheese.

GINGER (*Zingiber officinale*). This multipurpose spice is great for almost everything. Slice the ginger bulb thinly when cooking with other ingredients and grate when using for dressing, soups, or tofu topping. Use ginger in stir-fries, tofu topping with green onions, hot curries, sweet dishes such as ice cream, ginger cookies and cakes, and desserts. Also, ginger is a traditional side with sushi and ideal for many Asian dishes. See the recipe for Soy-Sake Shiitake Mushroom Steak on page 303.

MUSTARD (*Brassica alba*). Another very popular spice in Okinawa and the rest of Japan. Simmered vegetables come to life with a splash of hot Japanese mustard. Stone-ground, Western-style mustard is also becoming popular in

Okinawa and Japan, especially to make sandwiches. Mustard is great for sandwiches, condiments for rice, served with simmered vegetables on the side, as dressing, dips, and sauces.

NUTMEG (*Myristica fragrans*). The amazingly aromatic nutmeg is not really a nut but rather the kernel of a small fruit. Buy ground, or grind fresh—our preference. Nutmeg is quite versatile—try it in stews, curries, custards, cakes, stewed fruit, biscuits, pumpkin pie, soups, breads, mashed potatoes, cabbage, rice, fish sauce, cheese dishes, and pickle chutney. See Veggieful Beef Stew recipe on page 277.

PEPPER (*Piper nigrum*). Use a pepper mill to grind fresh seeds for best flavor, as pepper quickly loses its flavor. White pepper is hotter than black, but black is more aromatic. You'll want to add pepper to vegetable soups, Caesar salad, stir-fries, vinaigrettes, soft cheeses, and almost any dishes calling for a bit of pizzazz.

TURMERIC (*Curcuma longa*). One of Okinawa's and India's essential spices. The ground powder is a beautiful yellow color and should be stored in airtight containers. Turmeric is good in curries, fish dishes, deviled eggs, rice dishes, coating for poultry and seafood, soups, folded into bread dough, and stir-fries. See the recipe for Turmeric and Rosemary Grissini on page 209.

Tips for Getting Herbs and Spice into Your Life

- **Spice up your veggies.** Try topping veggies with any of these winners, or add fresh chopped chives or vitamin C–rich parsley.

- **Replace butter with herbs and spices.** For a great low-CD treat, instead of using butter or margarine and brown sugar in mashed squash, try a mixture of cinnamon and nutmeg plus allspice or ginger. Orange juice and grated zest also add satisfying taste.

- **Mix a pinch or two of turmeric,** masala, or even a spoonful of mango chutney into your tuna salad. This gives an amazing hint of the exotic, and you can use much less mayonnaise—just a teaspoon of nonfat mayo is enough for a can of tuna.

- **Oatmeal takes on a whole new life with cinnamon**—makes it almost like a dessert. Sprinkle liberally.

• **Salsa, salsa, salsa.** Salsa often contains many tasty herbs and spices. Over two hundred varieties are available in stores. Try out a spoonful of salsa or fat-free yogurt or sour cream on your next baked sweet potato; top with a sprig of cilantro.

• **Get your colors.** Many herbs and spices have bright, beautiful colors. When you're missing a punchy color on your dish, sprinkle a bit of red paprika or chili powder on orange or purple mashed sweet potato; light-green cardamon seeds on yellow squash dishes; bright yellow turmeric on green spinach pasta. And so on—the only limit is your artistic imagination.

• **Sweet alternatives.** Spices are not only "hot"; there are also "sweet" spices, such as cloves, cardamon, allspice, anise, and cinnamon. Use them in lieu of sugar in tea and in cooking.

• **Get the best of both.** Whenever you can, try to combine both spices and herbs in your cooking.

PRINCIPLE #9

Graze Rather Than Gorge

While Mom may have had good intentions when she told you to finish everything on your plate, the strategy is questionable. Eating everything in front of you worked better when we were sleeping in caves and roaming the plains than it does now. Back then, it certainly would have helped to pack on the pounds and create significant fat storage for the lean times that were sure to come. Today, stuffing yourself at the dinner table not only leads to a bloated, uncomfortable feeling but is also bad for your health.

Just the Facts

• Replenish your energy supply regularly by having at least six small meals/snacks rather that three square meals in a day.

• Eating the same number of calories and same foods spread out over the course of the day in small meals instead of three large leads to lower blood sugar levels, lower insulin levels, and better health.

• Never skip breakfast. You will be hungry later in the day and make up the calories anyway.

This fact was beautifully illustrated in a study done at our alma mater, the University of Toronto. In this study funded by the National Institutes of Health (NIH), Dr. David Jenkins and colleagues fed two groups of volunteers the same food but in different increments throughout the day.[84] One group got three meals a day; the other got seventeen smaller meals spread out through the day. The results showed that the seventeen-small-meals-a-day group had an impressive decrease in blood sugar (4 percent), insulin (28 percent), and LDL cholesterol (13 percent). It was a beautifully simple experiment and had such important, long-term implications for insulin-related diseases such as obesity, diabetes, cardiovascular disease, cancer, and even aging itself, that it was published in the *New England Journal of Medicine*. Bottom line: It's better to have small meals throughout the day than to stuff yourself at two or three huge meals.

THE IMPORTANCE OF BREAKFAST

The percentage of us who skip breakfast is on the rise, from about 14 percent in 1965 to 25 percent in 1991.[85] If you're in this group, think about changing your ways. Eating breakfast is not just healthier; it will actually help you control your weight. A recent study of people who lost a significant amount of weight and were able to keep it off showed that breakfast was an very important meal and that those who ate breakfast consumed no more calories than those who skipped it.[86] The breakfast-skippers were making up the calories they omitted at breakfast at other points throughout the day—and messing up their insulin levels while they were at it. So eating a healthy breakfast not only keeps hunger at bay throughout the day but also positions you to better resist fatty and high-cal foods when they inevitably cross your path. The energy you get from breakfast nutrients also gives you the ability to be more physically active—and physical activity is an important part of overall weight management.

What you have for breakfast, of course, is a matter of individual choice. We've got suggestions for you in our menu track plans in chapter 7, and you'll find some terrific recipes in chapter 8 (don't miss the buckwheat pancakes!), but here are a few extra points to keep in mind.

• **Fiber up.** Choose a breakfast cereal that gives you at least 5 grams of fiber per serving. Use soymilk or nonfat milk instead of whole milk or 2% milk (2% milk is actually 35 percent fat; it's 2 percent butterfat).

• **Have fresh fruit.** Add strawberries, peaches, or apples to cereal; they're all very low CD. Eating half a pink grapefruit (CD 0.3) provides a big dose of prostate/breast cancer–fighting lycopene.

- **Frozen berries are fine.** They're convenient, relatively inexpensive, and amazingly good for you, as freezing doesn't destroy the acanthocyanid antioxidants. Frozen blueberries (CD 0.5) are our favorite. They can add a big antioxidant bang to your breakfast. Blueberries were even shown to help reverse some signs of memory decline in recent studies.

- **Go Okinawan.** Okinawans traditionally eat miso soup for breakfast, with sweet potatoes, a small piece of fish, and veggies. Switching your usual breakfast habits around from time to time will help you re-educate your palate. Try it a few times as an experiment.

KUTEN-GWA—SMALL PORTIONS

Another point to keep in mind at all meals and snacks is the size of your portions. You've heard the saying "all things in moderation." Well, the Okinawan elders may be among the few populations that actually practice moderation in the size of their food portions, and once again they can stand as a model for us. Okinawa's *kuten-gwa,* or "little portion," may be one of the best strategies for cutting calories. In Okinawa, serving sizes are half to two thirds the jumbo sizes we see in America. Here are a few simple strategies to help you keep your portion sizes under control.

Getting the *Kuten-gwa* Spirit— Tips to Decreasing Portion Size

- **Learn the measures.** If you are ever to get a handle on your calories without weighing everything you put in your mouth, you need to know how to assess portions at a glance. One 3-ounce serving of meat is the size of a deck of cards or a cassette tape. Half a cup of potatoes, rice, or pasta looks like a tennis ball cut in half.

- **Size up your servings.** Just how many servings are in that bottle of juice, can of soup, or box of cookies? How many potato chips make up a serving? Check the label and find out *before* you gobble them down; you may be shocked at how many servings you're actually eating. Assess what a portion of your favorite snack looks like by measuring it the next time you eat it. When you see what a serving really looks like, you'll be able to eyeball it from then on and avoid overeating.

- **Meet yourself halfway.** You don't have to give up all your favorite foods to lose weight. Try instead to cut your portion size by half. Eat just half of that deli

---

Picture This!
What Does a Serving Look Like?

One serving of . . .

Meat, poultry, fish	3 ounces	a deck of cards
Cheese	1 ounce	a pair of dice
Bread (pancake)	1 slice	a CD
Rice, pasta, cereal	½ cup	a tennis ball cut in half
Cooked vegetables	½ cup	a lightbulb
Salad greens	1 cup	a baseball
Fruit	1 medium	a tennis ball

---

sandwich. Cut the CD of your meal by supplementing it with raw veggies. Finish off with fresh fruit.

- **Take a rest and smell the tea.** After the first half of your sandwich, sip on a cup of green, jasmine, or black tea for a few minutes. Now wait and see if you're still hungry. By pausing after eating the first half and allowing yourself up to 20 minutes to feel full, you just may find you're too full to eat the other half.

- **Feed Fido.** Restaurant portions are mammoth—almost double the size they were two decades ago.[87] A strategy we've used with great success—although it admittedly turns a few heads—is to ask the waiter for a doggie-bag container as soon as he or she brings the main course. Put some of your food in the box before you even start eating. If you're still hungry, you can always take it back out to eat at the restaurant, but chances are you won't want to. Feed the leftovers to Fido, or eat them yourself for lunch the next day. Save time, money, and your waistline!

- **Downsize dinner.** Many restaurants offer lunch-size or child-size dishes. These are smaller than full-size dinner entrées and resemble more closely what you would get in Okinawa. Tell your server you're dieting, and he or she will probably sympathize with you.

- **Blow off the biggie size.** It's no secret that fast-food portions are oversize, so there's no need to add insult to injury by *super*sizing. No matter how much of a better deal upgrading your meal's size may be, don't be tempted! In fact, steering clear of meal deals altogether is wise. You're much better off ordering a chicken sandwich and a side salad. You could also order a kid's meal, which contains what used to be normal portions for us grown-ups (before there were value meals or combos, that is).

- **Good portions come in small packages.** In Okinawa, they say *kuu sa kana sa,* or "good things come in small packages." One of the biggest mistakes you can make is to buy large packs of potato chips or other snacks. You *will* overeat them. Either buy small, not at all, or, if you must buy big, portion the chips into single-serving snack bags as soon as you get them home.

- **Beware of buffets.** We often just skip all-you-can-eat restaurants. It is nearly impossible to practice portion control at these buffets. If you do end up at one, though, remembering the serving sizes we just discussed can be a lifesaver.

- **Share the wealth.** One of our favorite strategies is to order one meal at a restaurant but ask for two plates and split the meal. A great strategy for couples!

PRINCIPLE #10
Easy on the Alcohol and Sweets

Both alcohol and sweets can pack on pounds, and neither is essential for our survival or even our health. So theoretically, we'd do just fine without them. On the other hand, many of us have come to enjoy them. So a good strategy is not to cut them out altogether but rather to be smart about them.

ALCOHOL: THE BENEFITS AND RISKS

Alcohol is a compound of carbon, hydrogen, and oxygen produced when glucose is fermented by yeast—and humans have been making it for thousands of years. Fruits are used to make wines and ciders, and cereals such as barley and rye form the basis of beers and spirits. These substances provide the flavor associated with each individual spirit. During the brewing process, the alcohol content is controlled by the amount of yeast and the duration of fermentation. *Alcohol is a potent provider of calorically dense calories, with a CD of 7.*

Consumed in moderation, alcohol is thought to be beneficial in reducing the risk of coronary heart disease.[88] Indeed, alcohol or red wine consumption, in conjunction with high intake of fruit and vegetables, may partly explain the so-called French paradox. That's the unsolved mystery of how the French, with their traditionally high-fat diet (especially saturated fat), manage to have a lower death rate from coronary heart disease than any other Western country.[89] The answer may be the flavonoids in wine or the ability of alcohol to raise good cho-

---

Just the Facts

- It's not necessary to cut out either sweets or alcohol—just partake wisely.

- Alcohol is a heavyweight (CD 7.0—most distilled alcohols are CD 2.4–2.7), so moderation is advised.

- Moderate alcohol consumption is associated with longer life expectancy.

- More than 1 drink per day for women, 2 drinks per day for men, may increase risk for cardiovascular disease or cancer.

---

lesterol levels. So are we telling you to reach for your wineglass? Yes and no. The key word, once again, is *moderation.* The World Health Organization in 1997 concluded that coronary heart disease risk was lowered by the consumption of one drink every second day.[90] That's true moderation.

On the other hand, even when consumed in moderation, alcohol is linked to a wide range of other ailments and diseases, such as increased risk of mouth, pharyngeal, and esophageal cancers (and the risk is greatly increased if combined with smoking).[91] Furthermore, alcohol appears to increase the risk of colorectal and breast cancer, possibly through its association with higher levels of insulin or insulin-like growth factor or its tendency to destroy cancer-fighting folate.[92] The list doesn't stop here: High blood pressure; gastrointestinal complications such as gastritis, ulcers, and liver disease; and a depletion of certain vitamins and minerals are all caused by alcohol consumption.[93] Of course, excessive alcohol can have detrimental social and psychological consequences as well.

WHAT IS A DRINK?

Fourteen grams of alcohol is considered one drink. This is often taken to mean one 5-ounce (150-ml) glass of wine at 11 percent alcohol, one 12-ounce beer at 4 percent alcohol, or one 1.5-ounce shot of hard liquor at 40 percent alcohol. But the alcohol content of different products varies considerably. Some stronger beers and lagers may contain as much as 2.5 ounces of alcohol per half-pint. The size of drinks can also vary—home measures of spirits are usually more generous than pub measures. Cans of beer often contain about three-quarters of a pint rather than half a pint and so will contain 1.5 ounces of alcohol—and even more if the product is high-strength.

ALCOHOL ADDS POUNDS

Alcohol is a source of energy, providing 7 calories per gram of alcohol. Remember energy balance. Every pound of body fat is 3,500 calories, and so to lose one pound in a week, you need to cut out 500 calories per day through a combination of diet (reducing energy intake) and activity (increasing energy expenditure). Three glasses of wine each night provides about 300 calories. If you were to reduce the wine to two glasses on three nights per week, you would save an extra 1,500 calories in a week, which equals about ½ pound of body fat!

All this is to say that if you're serious about watching your waistline—not to mention your health— it's a good idea to cut down on the amount you drink and to monitor the type of drinks you choose. Alcohol pretty much lives up to its hype as a source of empty calories.[94] Some alcoholic drinks contain traces of vitamins and minerals, but certainly not in amounts that make any significant positive contribution to the diet. Because the calories provided by an alcoholic drink are dependent on the percentage of alcohol it contains, it's difficult to assess the calorie content for a particular alcoholic drink, but the following chart will give you a pretty good idea of the kind of caloric punch you're in for with various alcohol options.

Drink	Size	Typical calorie content
Beers, lager, and cider		
Brown ale	240 ml (½ pint)	80
Pale ale	240 ml (½ pint)	91
Stout, bottled	240 ml (½ pint)	105
Strong ale (barley wine type)	240 ml (½ pint)	205
Lager (ordinary strength)	240 ml (½ pint)	85
Light beer	240 ml (½ pint)	67
Nonalcoholic beer	240 ml (½ pint)	40
Sweet cider	240 ml (½ pint)	110
Dry cider	240 ml (½ pint)	95
Wines		
Red wine	125 ml (small glass)	85
Rose wine, medium	125 ml (small glass)	89
Sweet white wine	125 ml (small glass)	118
Dry white wine	125 ml (small glass)	83
Medium white wine	125 ml (small glass)	94

Drink	Size	Typical calorie content
Sparkling white wine	125 ml (small glass)	95
Nonalcoholic wine	125 ml (small glass)	8
Wine spritzer	230 ml (8 fl. oz.)	100
Fortified wine		
Port	60 ml (2 fl. oz.)	87
Sherry, dry	60 ml (2 fl. oz.)	64
Whisky and Spirits		
Whiskey, 45%	30 ml (1 fl. oz.)	74
Cognac	30 ml (1 fl. oz.)	73
Distilled alcohol, 80 proof (rum, vodka, gin)	30 ml (1 fl. oz.)	64
Sake rice wine	30 ml (1 fl. oz.)	73
Cocktails		
Alexander	90 ml (3 fl. oz.)	214
Bloody Mary	150 ml (5 fl. oz.)	116
Bourbon and soda	120 ml (4 fl. oz.)	105
Frozen daiquiri	120 ml (4 fl. oz.)	216
Gin and tonic	225 ml (7.5 fl. oz.)	171
Grasshopper	90 ml (3 fl. oz.)	247
Long Island iced tea	150 ml (5 fl. oz.)	142
Mai tai	120 ml (4 fl. oz.)	310
Martini	75 ml (2.5 fl. oz.)	157
Sangria	240 ml (8 fl. oz.)	159

Tips for Using Alcohol Wisely

- **If you drink, don't give it up entirely.** If you enjoy alcohol, it is probably better to have a drink from time to time. If you cut it out completely, you're more likely to feel deprived. Chances are you'll maintain dietary changes longer if you include foods and drinks you enjoy in your diet. (This obviously doesn't apply to alcoholics and other problem drinkers.)

- **Watch the calories.** Every gram of alcohol contains 7 calories, so its caloric density is high. Your body uses the calories from alcohol first because alcohol is a toxin.[95] This increases the tendency of dietary fat to be stored as body fat when you eat a meal containing fat together while drinking alcohol.

- **Alternate drinks.** Take measures to reduce your caloric intake from alcohol by alternating alcoholic drinks with nonalcoholic ones (not those high in sugar, though). Drink water between alcoholic drinks and use low-cal mixers.

- **Careful at the pub.** Watch out for the high-fat, salty snacks served at bars to encourage you to buy more drinks. Nuts, chips, and olives are all high in fat and calories.

- **Choose red wine.** Red wine contains flavonoids that act as antioxidants in the body and help to protect the heart, and possibly do much more than that. A recent study by a colleague of ours at Harvard showed that resveratrol, a flavonoid found in red wine, turned on the same biological switch thought to be in part responsible for the age-slowing effects of caloric restriction.[96,97] It is not advised that you start drinking to be healthy, but if you already drink, red wine is a comparatively healthy choice.

AND, FINALLY, SWEETS

Most of us crave sweets to some degree—some more than others. But don't feel bad about it; it's not your fault. It is thought that being able to identify sweet things played a critical role in human evolution.[98] Our love for calorie-rich sugary foods ensured we would choose them and thus be provided with the energy we needed to get through the next famine. The sweet taste also enabled our ancestors to distinguish between viable sustenances and bitter items like poisonous plants.

Two research teams fishing through the human and mouse genomes think they may have caught the sweet-tooth gene.[99] The difference between those of us who prefer two lumps of sugar in our tea and those of us who take it black (or green) could be the gene T1r3. According to Dr. Linda Buck and her team at Harvard Medical School, sugar turns on T1r3 in the cells of our taste buds. This gene makes a receptor protein that seems to stick to sugars that touch your tongue. This then triggers a biochemical and nerve-signaling cascade of sweetness signals to the brain.

In another recent study, scientists discovered that there are supertasters among us who are genetically more sensitive to both bitter and sweet tastes and don't much like them.[100] They consequently end up eating less of them. Knowing an individual's genetic taste preference profile may help us predict food preferences and more precisely tailor healthy and weight-friendly diets. In the meantime, those of us with a sweet tooth have to make do with other strategies. Here are a few that have worked for us.

- **Don't try to pull that sweet tooth.** It's too difficult to cut out sweets all together. When you feel the urge, try having just a hard candy or two. This strategy can very often satisfy your sweet tooth. One butterscotch candy has a high CD of 3.9, but it has only 24 calories and lasts a long time. Compare that to one chocolate chip cookie, eaten in a moment, at CD 4.6 and 140 calories.

- **Snack on fresh fruit** such as apples, oranges, and grapes. You can eat half a pound of grapes and still get fewer than 150 calories.

- **Lower-fat desserts can be delicious.** Fruit (even canned in juice) is great for any occasion. Pineapple is always a treat. When entertaining, try topping a small scoop of sorbet with an exotic fruit choice like papaya, mango, kiwi, pomegranate, or lychee.

- **Pass on the pastry.** Pastry is traditionally made with lots of high-CD and trans fat–laden shortening or lard. Try baking an apple, rhubarb, or berry crisp instead of a fruit pie—and don't forget the calorie-free cinnamon and nutmeg.

- **Be cool.** Serve fruit sherbet, low-fat frozen yogurt, or ice milk as cool alternatives to ice cream. You could even wedge a thin, crisp chocolate wafer alongside so it appears a more extravagant dessert.

- **Be angelic.** Angel food cake has only a trace of fat. The same is true of meringues. Serve either with sliced fruit or a sauce made from plain yogurt and berries.

- **Ban the butter.** Replace the butter, margarine, or oil called for in muffin, cookie, and cake recipes with prune puree or applesauce. To puree prunes, blend together about 1⅓ cups seedless prunes and 6 tablespoons hot water. Refrigerated, the puree keeps for up to a month.

- **Drink chocolate; don't eat it.** Crazy for chocolate? Next time, try a hot chocolate drink instead of a chocolate bar to curb those cravings. An 8-ounce mug of hot chocolate has only 140 calories and 3 grams of fat (only 1 gram of which is saturated). A typical chocolate bar, on the other hand, has 13 grams of fat (including 9 saturated) and 230 calories. The extra water in hot chocolate brings down the CD tremendously, so you can see the CD principle in action!

Chapter 5

THE POWER FOODS
OF OKINAWA

Nuchi gusui.
Eat as if your food had healing power.

Unlike Naha City (the capital) in southern Okinawa, which is quite Westernized, the northern village of Ogimi makes you feel like you've stepped back in time a half century or more. Ogimi is Okinawa's self-proclaimed "longevity village" because it is home to such a large number of healthy oldsters. That's where we met Ushi-san, one of the town's spry, slim elders. She was carrying a large garden hoe on her back as she walked home after a full day of working the clay-colored northern soil. Although less than five feet tall, she had a strong presence—and she was very curious to know what had brought two foreigners all the way to her country village. When we explained we were doing research on how the elders managed to stay so lean and healthy, this wiry, tanned old woman paused for a moment, as if drawing on some ancient well of sacred knowledge, and then said one word—*"imo"*—the Japanese word for "sweet potato." "Do you mean you ate lots of sweet potatoes when you were young?" we asked. At that, Ushi smiled as if indulging a not-so-bright child. *"Imo bakkari!"* she said. "Nothing but sweet potato."

We were still a bit befuddled, but over the next few days, Ushi-san took pity on us *shima gaicha* ("island adoptees," as she playfully called foreigners) and explained the immense value of the sweet potato and how it had proved to be a lifesaver to her community in times of floods and typhoons, when other crops were washed out. She gave us the full tour of her garden—and her kitchen. She nimbly guided us through rows of purple and orange sweet potatoes and showed us how the sweet potato is steamed to eat as a staple food, boiled and mashed to create desserts, and cooked in miso soup. We learned that its stems and leaves (called *kandaba*) are believed to possess medicinal properties and are used as a garnish or simply chewed when one has a fever or stomach ailment. Ushi-san, of course, had other vegetables and fruits in her garden, including rows of dark green leafy vegetables we had never laid eyes upon before, as well as familiar vegetables, legumes, and fruit, such as soybeans, carrots, green beans, Chinese cabbage, radishes, and papayas. But the sweet potato was the center of her traditional Okinawan diet, and it definitely held a special spot in her heart.

Tusui ya takara.
The elders are treasures to us.

On our last afternoon in Ogimi, we were invited to Ushi-san's house for turmeric tea and mugwort sake, the latter a favorite of Ushi-san's. As Ushi-san sipped her sake, she shared other lifestyle secrets with us. If we wanted to live as long as she has, she told us, we should always eat whole foods, always leave the table with a little room in our stomachs (*hara hachi bu*), and always think of food as a source of healing power (*nuchi gusui*). And then she sang us a song that her great-grandmother had taught her as a child. The song was called *"Nmu Ga Nashi"* ("Honored Sweet Potato"), and it expressed gratitude to the sweet potato for its sustenance in the days when people could afford little else. It was a poignant moment, for there was little doubt Ushi-san had greatly benefited from the sweet potato's nutritional qualities. As we watched her singing—her bright eyes still playful and a quick smile at the ready—we just couldn't believe she was over a hundred years old. Smart eating habits take you a long way.

The Traditional Okinawan Diet

In addition to Ushi's treasured sweet potato, the Okinawan elders' diet is filled with all kinds of antioxidant-rich vegetables, grains, flavonoid-rich soy products, fruit, omega-3-rich fish, and minimal meat and dairy products—exactly the type of diet that affords protection against most diseases associated with premature aging and gives us the best shot at remaining slim, healthy, and attractive for life.[1]

And their cooking methods are health-smart too. There are three main styles, all centering around vegetables. First is *chample,* which is essentially stir-frying vegetables and tofu with small amounts of fish, noodles, or lean meat with herbs, spices, and a little oil. Next is *nbushi,* in which water-rich vegetables such as daikon, Chinese okra, and pumpkin are seasoned with miso and simmered in their own juices. Small amounts of tofu, fish, or boiled pork and other flavor-enhancing vegetables and herbs like Asian chives are often added. Last is *irichi,* a combination of simmering and stir-frying. Less watery vegetables such as burdock, seaweed, dried daikon, and green papaya are used. Water, a hint of oil, bonito dashi broth (for flavor), and small amounts of chicken, fish, or boiled pork are added. Soy sauce and mirin (Japanese cooking sake) are optional.

	Okinawa, 1949	*Okinawa, 1993*	*USA, 1990–99*
Total Calories	1539	1927	2176
Total Weight (grams)	1557	1353	1321
Caloric Density (CD)	1.0	1.4	1.7
Food Group	*Weight in grams*		
Grains	111	248	302
Rice	108	176	23
Wheat and wheat products	3	64	87
Others (e.g., baked goods)	<1	8	192
Nuts, Seeds	<1	1	4
Sugars	2	6	25
Oils	3	19	14
Legumes (e.g., soy and other beans)	75	75	25
Fish	15	80	10
Meat (including poultry)	<1	98	187
Eggs	1	34	18
Dairy	<1	132	274
Vegetables	1348	308	189
Potatoes	1174	52	61
Sweet potatoes	1174	15	N/A
Other potatoes	<1	37	N/A
Fruits	<1	86	169
Seaweed	<1	4	<1
Beverages (including alcohol)	<1	262	104

Calculated based on CFSII, 1994–96; USDA Economic Research Service, 1990–99, 1990–94; U.S. National Archives Rural Okinawa data, 1949; Okinawa Prefectural Nutrition Survey, 1993, Government of Okinawa.

Note: The traditional diet of Okinawans contained little meat, dairy, or fruit on a daily basis, but these foods were eaten on festive occasions, along with awamori (Okinawan sake) several times a month. Notice the virtual absence of high glycemic index (GI) carbohydrates (e.g., sweet potato is low GI) and the healthy protein sources (e.g., fish, soy foods). For more information on the current elders' diet, see chapter 5, note 1.

A traditional Okinawan meal would start with miso soup (which may contain a small amount of seaweed and/or tofu, and sweet potatoes or rice). The main dish would be a *chample,* accompanied by the day's side dish, say *kubu irichi,* which is kombu seaweed and *konnyaku* cooked in *irichi* fashion. The meal would be served with freshly brewed jasmine or green tea. You can see how different Okinawan cuisine is from Japanese. Okinawan cooking is, in fact, heavily influenced by southern Chinese cooking and has stronger and spicier flavors than Japanese food. Vegetables, which made up about two-thirds of the traditional diet and about a third of the current elders' diet, are the most important food overall, followed by tofu and other legumes, grains (mostly whole), seafood, and fruits supplemented by lean meat and limited dairy. Condiments include miso, dashi (bonito- or pork-flavored broth), black sugar, *awamori* (an Okinawan brandylike liquor made from rice), soy sauce, and many assorted herbs, peppers, and spices. Let's take a closer look at some of these Okinawan power foods and see how they've helped elders like Ushi-san maintain a healthy weight and live such a long, healthy life.

Vegetables

One walk through an Okinawan market, and the sheer variety of healthy, delectable, and ingeniously prepared vegetables staggers the mind. It's definitely a case of the more the merrier, but when you're dealing with Okinawan dishes, it's hard to get in trouble. Even when they add high-CD ingredients like special peanut tofu or small side dishes of pork, the base of low-CD veggies keep their meals from getting too high on the CD pyramid. In their everyday cooking, Okinawans use plenty of deep yellow and antioxidant-rich dark green leafy veggies and high-fiber, cholesterol-lowering root vegetables. When we first arrived in Okinawa, we were amazed at how many vegetables were new to us. There was, for example, *karashina* (Japanese mustard greens), *kandaba* (sweet potato leaves), *shima ninjin* (a type of yellow carrot), *goya* (bitter melon), *hechima* (Chinese okra), *gobo* (edible burdock), and a bewildering variety of mushrooms and seaweed. We've since tried most of Okinawa's prized veggies, and while we can't think of a single one we don't like, a few top our list of favorites in terms of weight control, health, versatility, and taste.

IMO—SWEET POTATO (*Ipomoea batatas;* Satsuma-imo, Ryukyu-imo)

Nmu kamatooin?
Are you getting enough *imo?*

Let's start with Ushi-san's favorite. Sweet potatoes are the large tuberous root of a vine native to the tropics of Central America. They hail from the morning glory family—not, as one might suspect, from the nightshade family, which gives us white potatoes, tomatoes, and eggplants. First "discovered" by Columbus, sweet potatoes preceded white potatoes in Europe by at least a hundred years. In fact, at that time (the sixteenth century) the word *potato* referred to the sweet potato, not the white potato as it does today. The sweet potato has been an Okinawan staple for centuries. It's so highly regarded that in a small Okinawan town called Kadena a statue is dedicated to Sokan Noguni, the man credited with bringing the first sweet potato seedlings back from China some four hundred years ago. The hardy sweet potato was a godsend to the island kingdom, so often frequented by typhoons during harvest season, and a literal lifesaver to many Okinawans in the old days. According to an old Japanese report by the Department of Agriculture, in the late nineteenth century, the sweet potato was by far the largest single contributor to the daily diet of the Ryukyu Kingdom (Okinawa prefecture).[2] Perhaps that's why *"Nmu kamatooin"*—literally, "Are you getting enough *imo*?"—came to be a greeting synonymous with "How are you?"

Okinawans aren't alone in their reverence for the sweet potato. It's a staple food in many countries and has been cultivated in America's southern states for generations. (The mega-crowds at the annual Sweet Potato Festival in Vardaman, Mississippi, every fall attest to the sweet potato's popularity in the Deep South.) The two most common varieties in the United States are the pale sweet potato and a darker-skinned variety Americans mistakenly call *yam*. (The true yam is the tuber of a tropical vine from the plant family Dioscorea, which is native to Africa. They're drier, starchier, longer, and more cylindrical; have rougher skin; take about twice as long to mature; and are much lower in beta-carotene than sweet potatoes.)

Weight and health benefits. Prepared as a main dish or as a dessert, the sweet potato is a nutritional powerhouse as well as an economical food. One medium-size baked sweet potato (114 grams) provides 21,908 IU of vitamin A—about four times your mimimum daily needs—yet contains only 102 calories. That's real value in weight-watching terms. This nutritious vegetable also provides almost half of your daily vitamin C needs. It's low in sodium and a good source of fiber, calcium, potassium, iron, vitamins E and B_6, riboflavin, thiamin, pantothenic acid, and folic acid. The question isn't what the sweet potato has; it's what doesn't it have! A complex carbohydrate food source lower in GI than regular white potatoes, sweet potatoes also provide carotenoids (e.g., beta-carotene, lycopene), which may be a factor in reducing the risk of certain cancers and are good sources of saponins and flavonoids, healthy compounds also found in tea.[3]

How to use it. Sweet potatoes, like white potatoes, are always eaten cooked, but their sweetness makes them much more versatile. They can be baked, boiled, broiled, microwaved, canned, frozen, and used in baked desserts, breads, puddings, custards, casseroles, and stews. They go well with cinnamon, honey, lime, ginger, coconut, and nutmeg. To cut calories, serve sweet potato with little or no margarine or butter, and use nonfat milk or soymilk or unsweetened orange juice when preparing mashed sweet potatoes. To reduce calories in your favorite sweet potato recipe, experiment by reducing the sugar or fat by using the next lower measure on the measuring cup. For example, when a recipe calls for 1 cup of sugar or fat, reduce the amount to ¾ cup; for ¾ cup, reduce it to ⅔ cup, etc. When buying sweet potatoes, select firm, umblemished ones. Handle them carefully to prevent bruising. Store in a dry bin kept at 55–60°F. if possible. Don't refrigerate, as temperatures below 55°F. chill this tropical vegetable and give it a hard core and an unpleasant taste when cooked. Another tip: Bake a large pan of sweet potatoes to save time and energy. Freeze for later use, or store the baked potatoes in the fridge for up to ten days.

Where to find it. Okinawan *imo* (also called *beni imo,* or purple sweet potato) is generally available in major cities with large Asian populations. (In Hawaii, where 50,000 people of Okinawan descent live, it's carried in all supermarkets.) Orange-colored "yams," readily available in most markets, are actually a variety of sweet potato grown in the American South. We've tried "yams" in all our *imo* recipes, and the dishes are equally delicious—and nutritious.

GOYA—BITTER MELON
(*Momordica charantia;* African cucumber, balsam pear, *nigauri, fu gua*)

Goya is a strange-looking gourd, shaped something like a cucumber, with a rough, pockmarked skin. Its Latin name, *Momordica,* means "bite," which is quite apt, as it gives you a good bite of bitterness. Even so, *goya* is ubiquitous in Okinawan cuisine. It's used in salads (raw), stir-fry dishes, sandwiches, tempura; as juice and tea; and even in goya burgers and goya rings at fast-food restaurants. Some newcomers to Okinawan food are put off by goya's bitter bite, but after a while the taste seems to grow on you—at least it did with us—and you are hooked. And when goya is stir-fried with tofu, eggs, and canola oil, which is frequently the case, the other ingredients offset the tartness. *Goya,* like caviar, may be an acquired taste, but the more you eat it, the more you seem to want it.

Weight and health benefits. Goya is low in caloric density and high in fiber—one of our favorite combinations. It's also high in vitamin C, which it retains even when cooked at high temperatures—very rare in vegetables and fruit. Aside from culinary uses, goya has been used as a medicinal herb in China, Africa, and India, among other places. Like many other bitter-tasting traditional herbs, it is thought to be helpful for gastrointestinal problems. Therapeutically, it may be useful for diabetes, as it's been shown to lower the concentration of glucose in the blood.[4] Recent animal research from the University of Hong Kong has backed up these claims and added a further benefit by showing that bitter melon can reduce adiposity (fat levels), lower serum insulin, and normalize glucose tolerance, helping counteract the negative effects of a high-calorie diet.[5] It is not recommended for pregnant women or individuals with hypoglycemia (low blood sugar).

How to use it. Goya is a widely eaten food in Asia. Both the leaves and the fruit are used in the West to make teas and beer and to season soups. Blanching or soaking goya in water before cooking takes out some of the bite, as does pairing it with strong-flavored ingredients like black beans. One popular Chinese recipe features goya stuffed with pork, garlic, and mashed black beans and steamed to perfection. (Always remove and discard seeds before cooking.) Goya can also be pickled, cooked for salads, or just eaten raw. Try stir-frying it with tofu, tuna, eggs, pepper, sprouts, or other vegetables in a dash of canola oil; or try our Shiri-Shiri Carrot and Bitter Melon recipe on page 302.

Where to find it. Try Asian food stores or Chinese markets, where it's referred to as *chin-li-chih, goo-fa,* or *ku gua,* if not bitter melon. If you can't find goya, feel free to substitute any vegetable from the gourd family (of which goya is a member), such as zucchini, wax gourd, pumpkin, and squash.

KONNYAKU

(*Amorphophallus konjac;* devil's tongue, glucomannan, konjac mannan)
Konnyaku is a traditional Japanese jelly-like substance made from the starch of a tuber known as devil's tongue. No one is quite sure whether it came to Japan via China, Indochina, or Southeast Asia, but everyone agrees that it's been around for centuries. There are references to konnyaku in the *Wamyouruijou,* a Japanese dictionary printed in A.D. 930. Although konnyaku has no noticeable flavor of its own, it readily absorbs the flavors of other ingredients in simmered dishes when cooked long enough. The flour derived from this Japanese root is the key ingredient in konnyaku jelly, giving this much-loved food its signature texture

and nutritional value. Because of its high fiber content, Okinawans feel kon-nyaku "cleans your stomach." Konnyaku comes packaged two ways: as a small, dense, dark brown to hazy gray gelatinous cake, and as thick or thin noodles.

Weight and health benefits. Aside from being high in fiber, konnyaku is extremely low in caloric density (0.05) and contains practically no fat, making it an ideal food for weight control. It has, in fact, been studied as a weight loss agent, because it absorbs many times its weight in water, forming a bulky gel that helps create feelings of satiety. Konnyaku is 97 percent water and 3 percent glucommanan, a fiber similar to bran and pectin, making it an effective treat-ment for constipation[6] and high cholesterol,[7] and a beneficial adjunct treatment for type II diabetes[8] (due to its beneficial effects on blood sugar). It's also a rich source of calcium that is absorbed almost as easily as that in milk.

How to use it. In cooking, try konnyaku powder as a replacement for cornstarch and other starches. Konnyaku noodles work well in sukiyaki and *mizutaki* (chicken and vegetables in a pot), and chopped konnyaku cake is a natural in rice dishes. Konnyaku cakes, a delicious combination of konnayaku, white miso, vinegar, and sugar, are tasty snacks as well. Fruit-flavored konnyaku jelly, similar to our breakfast jelly, is popular in Japan as a fiber supplement.

As a fiber supplement and for treatment of high cholesterol and diabetes, take ¼ to ½ tablespoon powder with meals. Eat the packaged raw cubes (one to six per day) anytime, or substitute the noodles in any appropriate dish.

For weight loss, take 500 mg powder supplement 2 to 3 times per day, half an hour before meals. Konnyaku and glucomannan are generally regarded as safe because they've been used so long in Japan. As with most dietary fiber, excessive consumption of konnyaku may produce diarrhea, loose stools, bloating, and intestinal gas. Those on cholesterol-lowering or diabetes agents should take a lower dose because of additive effects. Never give the packaged cubes to infants or small children, as they may choke on them. And you should always drink at least six to eight glasses of water a day when taking it, as intestinal obstruction has been reported in patients who ingest excessive amounts of plant fiber with-out adequate liquid. Be sure to try our Sautéed Shiitake and Konnyaku on page 304. It's easy to prepare, takes about fifteen minutes, and is a fabulous intro-duction to the wonders of this versatile tuber.

Where to find it. Konnyaku can be found in the refrigerated section of most Asian food stores and in the international section of some supermarkets. Kon-nyaku powder is also available at many health food stores.

SHIITAKE MUSHROOM *(Lentinus edodes)*

The shiitake is a large, dark brown, umbrella-shaped mushroom. Long valued for its culinary and medicinal properties by Native Americans, it's been widely used for centuries by Asian cultures as well. Shiitake mushrooms are a major diet staple in some parts of China and were once considered an important source of protein in Japan and other parts of the Pacific Rim. They're especially beloved in Okinawa, where they're often dried, beautifully wrapped, and given as gifts on festive occasions. The rest of the world is catching on too—the shiitake, as well as other Japanese mushrooms (enoki and *maitake*), is currently experiencing a worldwide popularity boom.

Weight and health benefits. Dried shiitake mushrooms are an ideal ingredient for any low-fat, low-calorie, healthy dish. Shiitakes have practically no calories but are loaded with fiber, antioxidants, and vitamins A, B, B_{12}, C, niacin, and especially D (840 IU per 100 g). And shiitake contains all eight essential amino acids in comparable proportions to soybeans, meat, milk, and eggs. This amazing mushroom also has been shown to lower blood cholesterol levels and high blood pressure in laboratory animals and shows promise as a hypoglycemic (lowers blood sugar) with antiviral, antifungal, and antitumor effects.[9–11]

How to use it. The shiitake mushroom has a smoky, outdoor flavor that's a terrific complement to Asian seasonings such as soy sauce, miso, and oyster sauce. It's also a great addition to pasta dishes. In most Japanese homes, reconstituted shiitake mushrooms are added to wakame (seaweed) to create a variety of sea vegetable salads as well as entrées. Before adding dried shiitake to a recipe, soak it in a bowl of water at least fifteen minutes—and don't forget to save the soaking water! It adds welcome flavor to any recipe. Adding a few pinches of reconstituted shiitake to rice before cooking is a great way to add pizzazz. Larger, extra-thick fresh shiitake has a meaty texture and is well suited to stews and sandwiches and is perfect for slicing into salads and soups. You can also buy shiitake bouillon, which makes a tasty shiitake-flavored broth; 3 ounces (or 10 grams or 2 tablespoons) of the bouillon makes 1 quart broth. Add some of your favorite vegetables and a few cubes of tofu and you've got a healthy vegetarian soup.

Where to find it. Shiitake mushrooms are available in most grocery stores and all Asian food markets.

GOBO—BURDOCK (*Arctium lappa; ngau pong, harlock, eddick*)

Gobo (or burdock, as it's known in Europe and the United States) is a slender root vegetable with a rusty brown skin and grayish-white flesh. It's high in minerals (especially iron), and with its sweet, earthy flavor and crisp texture is considered a choice Okinawan vegetable. It's also a popular folk medicine in many parts of the world (considered a "blood purifier"). It's a member of the Compositae, or chrysanthemum, family, whose more familiar members include lettuce, artichoke, sunflower, chamomile, and marigold. Another species of wild burdock *(Arctium minus)* is a common American weed with burrs for seeds.

Weight and health benefits. Burdock root is low-CD and high in two kinds of fiber: inulin (up to 45 percent), and a spongy fiber called *mucilage,* a thick, glutinous substance, related to the natural gums used in medicine as emollients. This may explain burdock's purported soothing effects on the gastrointestinal tract. The high fiber content might also explain its popularity as a weight reduction remedy in Korea, where fresh burdock is cut into thin strips and marinated in vinegar before eating. Although there's no specific evidence for the efficacy of the burdock and vinegar diet, the beneficial effects of fiber on weight loss— especially in conjunction with a low-calorie diet—are well documented. Burdock has also traditionally been used as a blood purifier, liver tonic, and pain reliever. In animal studies it has been shown to reduce liver damage as well as to possess other anti-inflammatory properties,[12] and is being studied for its potential use in treating diabetes.

How to use it. Burdock's leaves and stems are edible when young. Prepare the leaves as you would spinach and the stems as you would asparagus. The best part of the plant, however, is the long, slender root. When very young, the roots are crisp and flavorful when peeled and eaten raw. They can also be peeled, chopped into matchstick pieces, and mixed with low-fat mayonnaise or a tofu-based mayo ("tofunnaise") as a salad. The mature root should be peeled, scalded, and cooked like carrots and parsnips. The flavor of burdock can vary with age and condition of the soil, but it is generally similar to Jerusalem artichokes and parsnips. Try our Fragrant Soy Go Vegetable Soup on page 241 as a nice intro- duction to burdock.

Where to find it. Burdock can be found in your local Asian market, health food stores, and some supermarkets. If you can't find it, substitute parsnip.

DAIKON—JAPANESE RADISH
(*Raphanus sativus;* Oriental or Chinese radish, *lobok*)

Daikon, from the Japanese words *dai* ("large") and *kon* ("root"), is a large Oriental radish with a sweet, tangy flavor that's milder than the small red radishes most of us know. It can be either creamy white or black on the outside and has crisp, juicy, white flesh inside. Daikon is a member of the Crucifereae, or mustard, family, which also includes broccoli, cabbage, turnips, watercress, kale, and cauliflower. Although most daikon weigh between one and five pounds, one variety, the *sakurajima,* has been known to grow to near one hundred pounds! An ancient crop in Japan, daikon was also used in Egypt as far back as 3,000 years ago.

Weight and health benefits. Daikon is free of fat and cholesterol, has an extremely low CD count (0.2), and is a good source of vitamin C and calcium (1 cup sliced raw daikon contains 22 mg vitamin C and 27 mg calcium). Daikon roots contain the enzyme diastase, a digestive aid, and may help prevent stomach and intestinal ulcers.[13] The leaves are also high in nutrition and contain vitamin A and calcium. It's an ideal food for weight control.

How to use it. In Japan, daikon is usually cooked or pickled as a side dish, but it can be used fresh in salads, crudités, and relishes. It is also terrific simmered in soups, added to stir-fries, sauces, and casserole dishes, used as garnish, and in cakes. The green tops can be braised, steamed, boiled, or used in soups. Daikon radish sprouts *(kaiware)* have a pleasant peppery-hot flavor and make a fine addition to sandwiches, salads, and stir-fries. Although daikon dry out and become limp quickly, they'll last up to a week when wrapped in plastic and kept in the vegetable crisper in the fridge.

Where to find it. Daikon can be found in your Asian market and in most large grocery stores. It is also known as Japanese radish, Chinese radish, and Satsuma radish.

Sea Vegetables

Seaweeds—or sea veggies, as we think of them—have been a dietary staple in Okinawa, Japan, China, and other parts of Asia for millennia. Okinawans are huge seaweed fans, and over a dozen varieties, including kombu, *aasa, mozuku, suunaa, hijiki,* wakame, *shinomata,* nori, and *gaana,* make up an indispensable part of Okinawan cookery. Although in the West we don't usually think of seaweed as a food source, chances are that you've probably consumed some sort of seaweed in the past couple of days without knowing it, as many foods contain seaweed polysaccharides (agars) that are used as thickening agents. Of course, you're getting minuscule amounts compared to the tons of seaweed consumed yearly in Okinawa. Seaweeds, like many of the Okinawan super-foods, have medicinal properties. They've been used to treat arthritis, colds, flu, and even cancer (although these claims have yet to be substantiated in clinical trials). There are thousands of species of seaweed worldwide. The varieties used most in Okinawan cuisine are *kombu, mozuku, wakame, hijiki* and *aasa.*

Weight and health benefits. Seaweed is a CD featherweight and wonderfully nutrient-dense. It's packed with protein, iodine, vitamin A, folate, magnesium, iron, calcium, phytoestrogens, and even vitamin B_{12}, which cannot be found in land plants. Iodine is essential to the function of the thyroid gland, which uses it to make hormones that regulate metabolism, thus it plays a substantial role in weight maintenance. Seaweed also is loaded with soluble fiber, which absorbs water and adds bulk, thus aiding regularity and favorably affecting cholesterol and blood sugar levels. Some animal experiments in Japan have supported traditional anti-cancer claims, although intensive clinical trials have yet to be carried out.[14] In areas of the world where soils are deficient in iodine, goiter (enlarged thyroid) is endemic, which is why iodine is added to table salt. Although seaweed supplements, such as kelp tablets, spirulina, and chlorella, are commonly sold as energy or immune boosters, there's no supporting evidence for these claims yet. Too much seaweed, in fact, can produce iron overload and thyroid toxicity—although it would be very difficult to eat enough seaweed to experience those effects. Those on sodium-restricted diets, though, should use caution. A half-cup of raw wakame contains approximately 900 mg sodium. The Unified Guidelines stress that daily sodium intake should not exceed 6 grams.

Where to find it. Seaweeds can be found in their dried form in many health food stores, Asian markets, and the international sections at large supermarkets. They're harder to find fresh. Your best bets are natural food stores and Asian markets.

KOMBU

This brown seaweed (or kelp) is especially popular in Okinawa. Along with *katsuobushi* (shaved dried bonito), *kombu* is one of the two basic ingredients in dashi (soup broth). Okinawans have been eating kombu since the eighteenth century, when ships used to make a pit stop in the islands en route to China from Japan's northernmost island prefecture, Hokkaido, where kombu grows in the cold waters. These days, Okinawans are among the top kombu consumers in all of Japan. Kombu is also a ritual food offered to the ancestors when visits are made to ancestral tombs.

We're as hooked on kombu as the Okinawans. We use it whenever we can in meat or fish dishes or as a vegetable with rice. The best kombu is dark, thick, and slightly sweet in flavor. It's also quite nice when dried and used in powder form in soup broth (dashi), sauces, and rice, along with spices.

How to use it. Kombu comes packaged in long, dried strips and is prepared by cutting the strips into smaller 2- to 3-inch strips and simmering them for about ten minutes. It's covered with a natural white powder that is the source of much of its flavor, so before cooking it should be lightly wiped off but not washed. After boiling, remove the kelp and use both the broth and rehydrated kombu in soups, salads, and other dishes.

Okinawans love kombu simmered with vegetables and tofu, served in miso soup; and as *kombumaki* or *osechi,* which is soaked in water, then wrapped around fish and vegetables seasoned with soy sauce, sake, and sugar. This dish is an integral part of the annual New Year feast. Kombu can also be pickled and used as a condiment. When stored unopened in a dry place, kombu will keep a very long time. Even after opening, it's good for six months or more when properly stored.

MOZUKU

This is another brown seaweed that's enjoyed throughout Japan. It's extensively farmed in Okinawa by simply implanting the hypha, or seedlings, on a net and then spreading the net over a coral reef on the seabed. Mother Nature and the Okinawan sun do the rest. The *mozuku* is harvested with a water pump from February through May and then sold in zipped plastic bags. It's mainly eaten with vinegar, in noodle dishes, with rice, or as jelly. The locals refer to it as "angel hair."

How to use it. Mozuku can be used in many dishes but is best eaten raw— straight from the package and flavored with a little vinegar. It makes a nice little side dish and can also be added to noodles and seasoned rice or made into jelly. If you're ever in Okinawa, try the mozuku jelly, dried mozuku noodles, or mozuku soup from the Mozuku Noodle Shop on Ou Island in Tamagusuku Village—it's worth the trip for that treat alone!

WAKAME

This is kelp that is blackish in color and leafy and mild in flavor: it turns green after soaking. It looks and tastes a lot like spinach lasagna. In Okinawa, it's traditionally added to miso soup along with tofu, but it's good in salads, with other vegetables (hot or cold), and in stir-fries or rice dishes as well. It also goes exceptionally well with soba noodles; wakame soba is popular throughout Japan.

How to use it. Wakame is best in raw form. Soak approximately 1 tablespoon dried wakame per person in water for about 1 minute. The seaweed will expand about ten times in size. Cut out the central vein after soaking. Drain and cut into small pieces and use it in your salad, as a topping for noodle dishes, or added to miso soup. Dried wakame should be kept in an airtight container in a cool, dry, and dark place. If cooked, wakame should be kept in the refrigerator. For an outstanding salad, try the recipe for Wakame Asparagusu salad on page 218.

HIJIKI

This is black in color and has a bittersweet taste that some liken to anise. It comes in short match-size strips. Okinawans like *hijiki* simmered with vegetables, whole soybeans, and *okara,* and as an ingredient in tofu burgers.

How to use it. Hijiki is best in dishes that require simmering or other types of slow cooking. In Okinawa, people simmer hijiki with soybeans, carrots, and other vegetables. Before using, they soak the soybeans and hijiki overnight, although two hours is usually enough. Try simmering hijiki with a bit of water, carrots, and *konnyaku;* season with soy sauce, sugar, and sake. Also, try our Hijiki Brown Rice recipe on page 327.

AASA

Aasa is yellow-green and grows on rocks along the tide line on most Okinawan beaches. Gathering the seaweed and storing it for later use in soups and tempura dishes is a common weekend activity in Okinawa. In Tamagusuku Village, on tiny Ou Island, there's even a festival to celebrate the start of the aasa seaweed season. Many people come from faraway Naha and central Okinawa to pick the seaweed at low tide.

How to use it. Aasa works best as an ingredient for soups or salads or in tempura dishes. *Aasajiru* is a favorite Okinawan dish that employs aasa seaweed combined with tofu in a soup base. Aasa keeps well if properly refrigerated.

Fruit

Okinawans generally don't eat a lot of fruit, although their diet does include bananas, oranges, pineapples, watermelon, dragon fruit, apples, and papaya. Even the fruits they do eat are often prepared as we would vegetables. Papaya, for example, is often picked when green and hard, then sliced and cooked with "other vegetables." Naturally, we don't mean to discredit fruit—in fact, we highly recommend it. Let's take a quick look at three of Okinawa's favorite fruits.

SHIKWASA (*Citrus depressa hayata; hirami* lemon)

Shikwasa, also called *hirami* lemon, is grown mostly in the north of Okinawa, and it is a difficult fruit to peg. It's somewhere between an orange, tangerine, and lemon. Like an orange, it's light green and tastes sour when immature, but it sweetens and becomes yellow-orange as it matures. There are a number of varieties. The most popular is almost a gold color when mature, and is in fact called *kugani,* which means "gold" in the Okinawan dialect. It has been gaining in popularity throughout Japan since researchers showed it might have anti-cancer effects. Citrus fruits, with their high amounts of vitamins A and C and flavonoids, have long been recognized for their health benefits—most notably for the prevention of scurvy. During the age of exploration, Portuguese, Spanish, Arab, and Dutch sailors planted citrus trees along their trade routes to avoid this nutritional deficiency disease.

Weight and health benefits. Research from Japan indicates that shikwasa can reduce both high blood sugar levels and high blood pressure; it also shows promise as an anti-cancer agent. Researchers credit the flavonoid nobiletin as the active agent.[15] Other research has supported anti-cancer effects for the flavonoid tangeretin as well as nobiletin in the test tube as well as in animal experiments.[16] Unfortunately, much of the flavonoids in citrus fruits are found in the inner peel of the fruit, the bitter part many people discard. Try to use as much of the whole fruit as possible.

How to use it. Shikwasa yield a unique juice that is simultaneously sweet and tangy. Add a hint of honey to the juice if it's too tart for your taste. It's also terrific added to sauces and dressings and squeezed over foods as you would a lemon.

Where to find it. You might find shikwasa in Asian markets, but if you can't, substitute limes, lemons, or tangerines.

PINEAPPLE (*Ananas comosus*)

Native to Central and South America (the word *pineapple* is derived from *piña* which is Spanish for "pine cone"), pineapples also thrive in southeast Asia, India, Hawaii, and throughout Okinawa—especially in the north. Pineapples have long been considered symbols of hospitality and used as an ornamental fruit; their scent alone can evoke images of tropical palm-fringed beaches.

Weight and health benefits. This amazingly sweet and chewy fruit is fat-free and low in calories (only 76 calories for 1 cup of fresh diced pineapple, or 60 calories for two slices.) Pineapple contains vitamin C, folate, iron, and vitamin B_6, and is a fair source of dietary fiber. It also contains an enzyme called *bromelain,* which some largely unsupported claims say help in protein and fat digestion; it has been used effectively as an anti-inflammatory agent to help heal minor injuries.[17]

How to use it. Pineapple is terrific as an anytime snack or dessert, and it goes well with pork, poultry, and seafood dishes—especially as pineapple salsa. It can be added to stir-fries, fruit salads, green salads, and smoothies, and even baked in breads. Selecting the right pineapple is key—they're best when ripe, but not overripe. Check for a nice, fragrant smell; avoid pineapples with sour or fermenting odors. Scales should have slightly brown tips, and if you can pull a leaf out of the top easily, the fruit is ripe. For peak sweetness, store at room temperature for a day or so before serving. Cut pineapple will do fine in the fridge for up to a week; it also freezes well.

Where to find it. Fresh pineapple is almost always available at supermarkets. Canned pineapple is a viable alternative; look for brands packed in water rather than heavyweight syrup.

WATERMELON

A favorite summertime game in Okinawa is called *suika wari.* Blindfolded, stick-wielding participants take turns finding a target watermelon as others shout out directions. Each player gets one shot at bashing the poor melon with his stick. If one player misses, it's on to the next contender. Of course, everybody is a winner because, once bashed, the watermelon is divided up and eaten by all. Okinawans aren't the only ones who know how to have fun with watermelons. There are dozens of watermelon festivals in the United States every summer. One of the most, uh, notable is the Watermelon Thump, in Luling, Texas, which hosts the world championship watermelon-seed-spitting contest every year. According to the *Guinness Book of World Records,* the seed-spitting distance set at the Thump currently stands at 68 feet, 9¼ inches—obviously a record accomplished by a terrific blowhard.

Weight and health benefits. Watermelon is fat-free and low in calories (less than 50 calories per cup, about 91 calories for a good-size slice). It's also an excellent source of vitamin C and vitamin A, and it contains vitamin B_6 and potassium as well. Perhaps most importantly, watermelon has more free-radical-fighting lycopene than any other fresh fruit or vegetable—fewer free radicals, of course, means less cellular damage and slower aging. All in all, watermelon is an ideal featherweight fruit, and it is considered by many to be a perfect diet food.

How to use it. Watermelon enthusiasts seem to find no limit to how this versatile fruit can be prepared and consumed. Some even suggest deep-frying it, currying it, and using the seeds for tea. We prefer it fresh as a nice slice, in fruit salads, or as part of other desserts. We also love it with Perrier and mint—try our Watermelon Fizz recipe on page 335.

How to select it. Look for a firm, symmetrical melon with no bruises, cuts, or dents. It should have a creamy yellow spot on its underside where it sat on the ground as it was ripened by the sun, and it should be heavy for its size. At 92 percent water, watermelon is one of the most water-rich foods around, and water is heavy.

Legumes

The high legume content in the Okinawan elders' diet is mostly in the form of soy products (made from soybeans), and it is undoubtedly another significant factor in their robust health. Soy is packed with plant compounds called phytoestrogens that are powerful antioxidants known for their heart-healthy and cancer-busting effects. Phytoestrogens (such as isoflavones from soy and lignans from flax) also have a positive effect on cholesterol concentration and blood clots, and they even make the blood vessels less stiff.[18] The tofu in Okinawa is lower in water content than Japanese tofu and higher in healthy fat and protein. This not only increases the flavor of the tofu but also increases its isoflavone content, which is very likely one of the reasons for the amazing low rates of cardiovascular disease and breast and prostate cancer in Okinawa.

OKINAWAN *DAIDZU* (soybeans)

In the old days, the elders relied on this simple bean as their main source of protein, and millions of people in China still do. The Okinawans love their soy as well. The elders have probably consumed more soy in the form of miso soup and tofu than people anywhere else in the world. Our studies show that they eat an average of 3 ounces of soy products a day, mostly tofu and miso (soy paste), but also in a few intriguing creations of their own, including a peanut "tofu," and a cheeselike sweet tofu that was considered so special in the days of the Ryukyu Kingdom that it was reserved for the royal family.

Weight and health benefits. Healthier hearts, lower risk for cancer, stronger bones—those are just a few of the potential benefits of soy. Soy protein has been shown to decrease levels of LDL cholesterol and triglycerides;[18] increase bone mass;[19] and even reduce the incidence of hot flashes.[20] In fact, the known health benefits of these healing beans are expanding with each passing day. A recent prospective (best evidence) Australian study[21] showed phytoestrogens like those in soy to be protective against breast cancer, further supporting the beneficial impact of dietary flavonoids on breast, prostate, and colon cancers.[22] In Japan, where soy consumption is high, women have minimal menopausal problems and less than a fifth of the rate of breast cancer of Westerners. Soy is a winner in terms of weight control too. It's a low-calorie food, and in Japan, some soy products have been patented specifically to promote weight loss. Here are a few of the ways soy is on your side in the battle of the bulge:

- It's high in fiber, which helps you to feel more satisfied and less hungry before your next meal.

- It rates extremely low on the Glycemic Index, which means it helps regulate blood sugar and insulin fluctuations.

- It contains more protein than milk does, but without the saturated fat or cholesterol.

- It may stimulate metabolism and inhibit fat absorption.[23]

- It may help control weight during menopause. (Researchers at Iowa State University report that "isoflavone-rich soy may attenuate the increase in fat deposition and prevent loss in lean tissue during menopause.")[24]

Where to find it. Soy products are as close as your nearest supermarket. You'll find traditional Asian soy foods like tofu and miso as well as westernized soy foods such as soy burgers, soy cheese, and soy hot dogs. You can also buy soy protein powder, which is probably the easiest and best way to get your soy protein and isoflavones if tofu and miso soup don't suit your taste. Just mix it into your orange juice. Okinawa tofu is still difficult to find in North America—although we're betting as more people are exposed to it, it'll become more readily available. Meanwhile, firm or extra-firm tofu is an excellent substitute. It is extremely high in cancer-fighting flavonoids and the closest in texture to its Okinawan cousin. You can find it in most supermarkets.

MISO SOUP

Miso is a soybean paste that has been a mainstay of Japanese cooking for hundreds of years. It has myriad uses, but the quintessential miso dish is traditional Japanese miso soup. This most popular soup in Japan is included in most typical Japanese meals—usually served in delicate small lacquer bowls with lids. Miso is made by mixing cooked soybeans, salt, grains (usually barley or rice), and a starter (fermenting agent) called *koji*. The process and ingredients vary somewhat among the types of miso.

Miso is classified according to color (white, red, brown, yellow); flavor (sweet or salty); and ingredients (the type of grain used). All miso is salty to some degree and can be smooth or chunky. Darker miso, which is usually red or brown, tends to be the saltiest. White miso has a somewhat sweeter flavor; yellow miso is usually made from rice and soybeans and falls in between. Some Western companies produce a pasteurized miso that contains preservatives, and a few manufacturers have come up with new types of miso that include non-traditional ingredients—dandelion-leek miso, for example. We prefer the traditional miso that is unpasteurized and aged over many months because it has a better flavor. It's also widely available.

Weight and health benefits. Because miso is a soy product, miso soup has all the health and weight control benefits associated with soy as well as the advantage of being a soup—which as you know, means low CD and high satiety.

How to use it. Miso can be enjoyed at any time of day—including breakfast. Traditional miso soup recipes start with a fish-based broth called dashi, but you can make simple homemade miso soup simply by simmering chunks of tofu and vegetables in broth or water. Then, just before serving, add ½ teaspoon of miso for each cup of water used. (Dissolve the miso in a little bit of warm water before adding.) Miso can also be used instead of salt in veggie or bean stews and soups. Although it's high in sodium, miso can actually help decrease sodium intake because it's more flavorful than salt, and thus less is used to season any particular dish. Or you can simply stick to low-sodium varieties, which are readily available.

The flavor of miso soup varies depending on the type of miso, broth, and ingredients, so it's best to experiment to find your favorites. We suggest the following ingredients for miso soup (use as many or as few as you like): tofu, daikon radish, wakame seaweed, clams, pumpkin, Chinese cabbage, spinach, potato, onion, green onion, green peas, cabbage, natto, enoki mushrooms, eggplant, thin (*somen*) noodles—but any other ingredient that appeals to your taste is fair game. Miso should be kept in the refrigerator, where it lasts for six months. The film of white mold that sometimes forms along the top is harmless and can be either scraped off or even stirred right into the miso if preferred.

Where to find it. Miso is always sold in natural foods stores and in Asian markets, and is becoming increasingly available in large supermarkets too. Look in the refrigerated section of stores.

BEAN SPROUTS (*Phaseolus aureus;* moyashi; *nga choy*)

The Chinese have been growing sprouts from the green-skinned mung bean for over 3,000 years. The crisp, flavorful bean sprouts are a key ingredient in Okinawan stir-fried dishes and one of the most widely used vegetables in Asian cuisine. They're plump, crunchy, delicately sweet, and readily available (mung bean sprouts are commonly referred to as *bean sprouts* in the West).

Weight and health benefits. Bean sprouts are low in calories (only 26 calories per cup) but high in protein, vitamins A and C, and folic acid—a dieter's dream food.

How to use it. Sprouts are terrific in salads, stir-fries, and almost any mixed vegetable dish. To maintain their crisp texture, they should be stir-fried no longer than about 30 seconds—add just before you're finished cooking. They're best when bought fresh (avoid any that look limp or are brownish in color), but they can be stored in the fridge in a sealed plastic bag with a bit of water for a day or two. To keep longer, put them in a jar, cover with cold water, and close the lid tightly. If you change the water every other day, they should last a week or so. Frozen bean sprouts are fine for cooking but not in salads. Soybean sprouts, which are bigger and beanier in flavor, and sunflower sprouts also work well in stir-fries and other cooked dishes.

Where to find it. Bean sprouts are carried by most supermarkets and are a favorite at farmers' markets. You can even sprout your own directly from the mung bean. It's easy: Wash, drain, and soak mung beans for about eight hours, drain again, put in a large jar, cover with cool water, and cover the jar with breathable fabric like cheesecloth. Change the water every day—and in a few days the sprouts will be plump and ready to eat.

ADZUKI BEANS (*Vigna angularis;* adzuki, *adanka*)

Adzuki beans have been grown in the Far East for millennia and used as a folk remedy for kidney problems for just about as long. They have a nutty, sweet flavor, and are extremely popular across Asia, where they're used to make red sweet bean paste. Although small in size (about 5 mm in diameter), adzuki beans are one of Japan's largest crops, with annual consumption of over 120,000 metric tons. You can recognize the dried adzuki bean by its dark reddish-brown color, pointed-oval shape, and the distinctive white ridge running along the side.

Weight and health benefits. High in protein and low in fat, beans provide a healthy alternative to animal protein. One cup of cooked beans contains only 224 calories. Like most beans, adzukis are rich in soluble fiber, which helps lower cholesterol, and are a good source of potassium, magnesium, iron, zinc, copper, manganese, and vitamin B_3. Their low sodium and high potassium levels help reduce blood pressure. Adzuki beans also contain protease inhibitors, which are thought to be anti-cancer agents.

How to use it. All dried beans require soaking before cooking, but adzuki beans need only a relatively short soak—about an hour. Adzuki beans also cook relatively quickly—also about an hour. Use about 4 cups water to 1 cup beans. In Okinawa they're often cooked with rice, which gives the rice a nice reddish-pink tinge. The dried beans should be kept refrigerated in a tightly sealed jar and, like mung beans or soybeans, also make tasty sprouts with a nutty flavor. Some people experience flatulence when they start to eat beans, so if you are not already a regular bean consumer, introduce them into your diet gradually. If you use canned beans, be sure to rinse them well before using, as most varieties are canned in a salt solution. The most popular use for adzuki beans in Japan is as *anko* (sweet beans), which is used for desserts and bread and cake fillings. Be sure to try our Mushi Manju dessert recipe (page 340) that makes wonderful use of adzuki beans.

Where to find it. Adzuki beans can be purchased at all health food stores and Asian markets.

Whole Grains

In southern Okinawa, it's said that there's an *utaki* (sacred grove) where the gods responsible for bringing the five sacred grains from across the seas dwell. You can often see shamans praying there, as it is believed to be a place of particularly high *shiji* (spiritual energy). The five sacred grains brought by the gods were *kome* (rice), *awa* (foxtail millet), *mugi* (barley, wheat), *hie* (quinoa-like millet), and *kibi* (broomcorn millet), and they've played an important part in Okinawan dietary and ritual life for centuries.

RICE (*Oryza sativa*)

Rice *(kome)* is a staple food of over half the world's population. It's so central to life in much of Asia that the word *rice* is almost synonymous with *food.* That's quite a contrast to the old days, when rice was so rare and valuable that it was used as an exchangeable form of currency and tax payments, and was available to common folk only for ceremonial occasions. Polished white rice was relatively unknown, but as time passed and incomes rose, it became a symbol of higher status, and brown rice became associated with the poor and uncultured.

> A meal without rice is really not a meal.
> *Japanese proverb*

In modern Okinawa, white rice has almost completely replaced the sweet potato as the staple food, and brown rice has only recently resurfaced as a healthy alternative. Although some of the elders eat a traditional mixture of white rice, brown rice, millet, barley, and other whole grains, others complain that they ate too much of that "brown chewy rice" when they were young and poor and are quite fond of the white kind. We, of course, recommend you go for the brown chewy stuff, as it has so much more nutrition and fiber than white rice—and we find it much more delicious. A little white rice with sushi is fine, but if you eat rice regularly, go brown.

BROWN RICE

There are literally thousands of varieties of rice grown throughout the world but in the United States rice is referred to by length of grain. Long-grain is typically *Indica* rice while short-grain is typically *Japonica*. Long-grain *Indica* rice is usually grown in hotter climates (mostly in India, Thailand, Vietnam, and southern China). When the rice is cooked, it's fluffy and doesn't stick together. Short-grain *Japonica* rice is usually grown in temperate climates (especially in Japan); its grains are round, less likely to crack or break, and when cooked, it is sticky and moist. Either type can be processed into white rice, and include nonglutinous and glutinous varieties. Nonglutinous rice is the kind usually used in rice dishes in the West—just cook it in water and serve plain and fluffy. Sticky glutinous rice is commonly used to make rice cakes, sushi, desserts, and snacks.

Weight and health benefits. Because rice has no cholesterol and little fat and provides only about 160 calories per cooked cup, it's a viable low-CD food choice (brown rice CD 1.1) for healthy weight. Its nutritional value depends primarily on the type of processing it's gone through. Brown rice provides complex carbohydrates, B vitamins and vitamin E, calcium, iron, phosphorus, and significant levels of fiber. (A cup of brown rice adds nearly 3.5 grams of fiber, while a cup of white rice has less than 1 gram.) Semipolished rice, which still has the whole germ, contains high amounts of the grain's original nutrients and fiber. Polished rice, the type most of us generally eat, has had the husk and bran completely removed and contains fewer vitamins, minerals, oils, and fiber than either semipolished or brown rice. Brown, obviously, is the nutritional winner. A big advantage of rice as a grain in general is that fewer people are allergic to it than they are to wheat and other grains.

How to use it. Rice dishes can be spicy or tangy, savory or sweet. Traditionally eaten with legumes, such as tofu and other types of beans, rice soaks up gravies and sauces and cools and refreshes the palate when served with spicy food. Rice can be boiled, baked, roasted, fried, and pressure-cooked. We like using an automatic rice cooker because it's extremely easy and ensures consistent results. Rice is best cooked immediately before serving, but cooked rice can be kept in the refrigerator for up to about five days and can quickly become the base for a rice salad, fried rice, a rice/vegetable dish, or with additions, a savory meal. Waste not; want not. If cooked rice starts to dry out (which it can on about the third day), you can either scrape off and discard the top crusty layer or add a few tablespoons of moisture before reheating. Because rice so readily absorbs water, it triples in bulk when cooked (1 cup of rice produces 3 cups of cooked rice.) The amount of water required for cooking varies with the type of rice used. Long-grain rice, for instance, generally needs less water than short-grain rice.

Where to find it. Well-stocked supermarkets and natural foods stores offer over a dozen varieties of rice, from short-grain brown to aromatics such as basmati and jasmine.

MILLET

(*Setaria italica*, or foxtail, *awa, aa; Pancium miliaceum*, or broomcorn, *kibi; Echinocloa crus-galli*, or barnyard millet, *hie*)

Millet, a grain popular in birdseed mix in America, is actually a cereal staple for almost a third of the world's population. It is very common in Africa and Asia. Millet looks like a tiny yellow ball—about a millimeter in diameter—and comes in many varieties, two of which, *awa* (foxtail millet, or *Setaria italica*) and *kibi* (broomcorn millet, or *Panicum miliaceum*), have been part of the Okinawan diet for over a thousand years (according to archeological finds). Millet's popularity in Okinawa is most likely partially due to the fact that it's a hardy grain that adapts relatively easily to the environmental problems that have traditionally plagued Okinawa, such as infertile soils, droughts, and typhoons. It was widely eaten throughout the Japanese archipelago up until the 1970s; now few younger people know of it other than from history books.

Weight and health benefits. Millet is rich in protein and other nutrients. Of all the grains, it has the highest amounts of iron, thiamin, and riboflavin. Millet—and, in fact, all whole grains—contains high amounts of fiber and phytochemicals such as lignans, phenolic acids, and phytosterols, which help lower cholesterol, improve sensitivity to insulin, and help prevent colon cancer. Millet is also gluten-free, which makes it a valuable substitute for people with wheat allergies.

How to use it. Millet has a mild flavor that lends itself well as a background to seasonings. It's prepared like rice by boiling in water and is used to make hot cereal and dishes like pilaf. Ground millet is used as flour to make puddings, breads, and cakes.

Where to find it. All health food stores and Asian markets carry millet, as do some supermarkets

QUINOA (*Chenopodium quinoa*)

Although most grains are from the grass family, a few broadleaf plants such as quinoa and amaranth are also considered grains (or pseudo-cereals) because their seeds are used for cereal and for making flour. Closely resembling millet in shape, quinoa originated in the highlands of Peru to become the staple crop of the Incas and is still very popular in South America. Quinoa (pronounced keen-wah) cooks quickly and has a mild nutty flavor and a delightful, slightly crunchy texture. Quinoa comes in colors ranging from pale yellow to red to black.

Weight and health benefits. Because it contains a lot of the amino acids methionine and lysine, it provides more of a complete protein than many other cereal grains. Gluten-free, it makes a good substitute for people with gluten allergies. It's also high in fiber, vitamin E, and calcium. In fact, one cup of quinoa has more calcium than a quart of milk.

How to use it. Quinoa is a good substitute for rice. Wash and rinse well before using to remove its bitter natural coating. Quinoa can be eaten as a hot breakfast cereal, eaten in salads, used in soups (like barley), or in stews to thicken, in casseroles, or also in desserts.

Where to find it. Quinoa is available at all health food stores and some supermarkets.

AMARANTH (*Amaranthus spp.*)

Another "pseudo-cereal" used in much the same way as quinoa. The Aztec and Mayan civilizations enjoyed this pleasant-tasting peppery "grain" as a dietary staple and it remains popular in South and Central America as well as among health food consumers in North America. In China and India the leaves of this plant are used as a spinachlike vegetable (it's actually called Chinese spinach).

Weight and health benefits. With a higher protein content than wheat, rice, or corn (around 16 percent) and gluten-free, it makes for a good substitute for those who may be allergic to wheat or corn. Like millet and quinoa, amaranth is also high in calcium, iron, and potassium.

How to use it. The seeds can be flaked like oatmeal or popped like corn. Baking it in bread adds a nutty flavor and a delicious aroma. Makes a good substitute for quinoa, millet, or rice.

Where to find it. Amaranth is available in any health food store and in some larger supermarkets or international-food markets.

BARLEY (*Hordeum vulgare; omugi*)

While this hardy grain has a long history of worldwide use, it has gradually come to be regarded as a "poor man's grain." Even in Okinawa there are folktales associating barley with the poor and uncultured, and, for the most part, it's used as animal fodder, or to make beer and whiskey. (One notable exception to this trend is barley's continuing role in soups like Scotch broth.) Whole-grain barley is referred to as *hulled barley* or *barley groats,* and because only the thick outer hull is removed, it's the most nutritious form of the grain. Scotch barley has had the outer hull removed and has been further refined by stripping the nutritious bran layer, but since the inner pearl of the kernel and endosperm remain intact, it's still nutritious. Pearl barley is the most common form—and unfortunately, the most refined as well. It's had the outer hull, bran layer, and endosperm removed and has been steamed and polished, leaving only the "pearl." Still, despite all the processing, it still miraculously retains some viable nutrients.

Weight and health benefits. As barley is among the lowest in fat of all the grains, it makes a great diet food. The beta-glucans and the antioxidants in barley contribute to reducing cholesterol, and the soluble fiber can help regulate blood glucose levels in type II diabetics. When combined with water and lemon, pearl barley is used to make barley water, an old-fashioned remedy for general malaise.

How to use it. Barley is most often used in soups and stews, where it serves as both a puffy grain and a thickener, but it also makes a nice side dish or salad. Rolled barley is a nutritious cereal like rolled oats, but with less than half the fat of rolled oats. Barley flour or barley meal is ground from pearl barley and must be combined with a gluten-containing flour, such as wheat, in order to make bread that rises.

Where to find it. All markets carry fast-cooking polished pearl barley. Hulled barley and barley groats are generally found in health food stores. These types are healthier and chewier and take longer to cook.

WHEAT (*Triticum aestivium; komugi*)

Wheat, the world's largest cereal crop, has grown wild since paleolithic times and has been cultivated by human beings for at least 6,000 years. As a world food staple, it's second only to rice in popularity. Unlike other cereals, wheat contains a relatively high amount of gluten, the protein that allows bread to rise. Wheat bread (known as *pan* throughout Japan) was first introduced to Okinawa by the Portuguese in the fifteenth century, although it took the American postwar presence for it to be more than an item of curiosity there.

Wheat 101. There are three major types of wheat: high-protein, gluten-rich hard wheat, which is used for making bread; soft wheat, with less protein and gluten, which is better suited to biscuits, cakes, and other baked goods; and durum wheat, which is generally ground into semolina, and used to make pasta.

All kinds of wheat start with the unprocessed wheat kernel, or wheat berry, which consists of three major parts: the bran, germ, and endosperm. Wheat bran, the rough outer covering, has little nutritional value but plenty of fiber. During milling, the bran is removed from the kernel. It's sold separately and used to add flavor and fiber to baked goods. Wheat germ, the embryo of the berry, is a concentrated source of vitamins, minerals, and protein. It has a nutty flavor and is very rich in oil, which causes it to turn rancid quickly. Removing the germ and bran led to longer-lasting but less nutritious white flour. Wheat germ is sold in both toasted and natural forms, and it is used to add nutrition to a variety of foods. Wheat germ oil, an extraction of the germ, is a strongly flavored and expensive health food supplement high in vitamin E. The wheat endosperm, which makes up the majority of the kernel, is full of starch, protein, niacin, and iron and is the primary source of many wheat flours. In addition to flour, wheat is available as whole-wheat berries, cracked wheat (the berry broken into coarse, medium, and fine fragments), and bulgur wheat, which is whole wheat that's been soaked and baked to speed the cooking time. It's especially popular in the Middle East, where it's used to make tabouli and pilafs.

Weight and health benefits. Among the cereal grains, whole wheat (hard) is among the highest in protein, calcium, thiamin, and niacin. However, refining whole wheat into white bread removes about 25 percent of the protein, over half the calcium, over 70 percent of the thiamin and niacin, and over 80 percent of the fiber and other important vitamins, minerals, and micronutrients. For health and taste, go brown!

How to use it. Most wheat is ground into flour, but whole or cracked grains are used in pilafs and salads, and wheat flakes are made into hot cereals or granolas. We like to sprinkle wheat bran in cereal for extra fiber and to top yogurt with a bit of crunchy toasted wheat germ. Another great idea: Soak a cup of bulgur in cool lemon water for a few hours, then drain and add cut-up red peppers, green beans, zucchini, tomatoes, and other veggies for wonderful fresh low-CD, summer salad. Also try our Nuts 'n' Seeds Bread recipe on page 212 to experience using whole-wheat flour in baking.

Where to find it. These days, whole-wheat products are available just about everywhere. Wheat berries, cracked wheat, and bulgur can be found in health food stores and many supermarkets.

BUCKWHEAT (*Fagopyrum esculentum;* soba)

Buckwheat has been enjoyed for hundreds of years throughout Asia in the form of soba noodles made from buckwheat flour. Although usually thought of as a grain, buckwheat is actually an herb of the buckwheat family, Polygonaceae. It's been cultivated in China for more than 1,000 years and was brought to Europe during the Middle Ages. Small groats (crushed grains) roasted in oil are called kasha in Russia and are an East European staple.

Weight and health benefits. Buckwheat is high in protein, contains all eight essential amino acids, and is rich in B vitamins (especially niacin), calcium, iron, phosphorus, and potassium. For people with gluten intolerance or wheat allergies, buckwheat is a good substitute, as it is gluten-free.

How to use it. Buckwheat has a pleasing, delicately nutty taste. It can be used for a variety of baked products, including pancakes, muffins, bagels, cookies, and breads. It's also a popular addition to breakfast cereals and poultry stuffing in North America; Europeans use buckwheat groats (crushed grains) in porridges, soups, and breakfast cereals. Buckwheat breads are dark brown, light, and airy; buckwheat pancakes have a wonderful taste and a slightly rougher texture than conventional pancakes. Be sure to try our Buckwheat Flax Pancakes on page 216.

Where to find it. Buckwheat can be found at any health food store and many supermarkets.

Fish

Although the 160 or so islands of the Ryukyu archipelago that make up the Okinawa prefecture fall well within the temperate zone, the warm waters of the Kuroshio current produce a humid, subtropical marine climate all year round. The cobalt blue seas and surrounding coral reefs are home to over 2,000 species of fish, so it's not surprising that marine life has always supplemented the Okinawa diet. A walk through the colorful fish market is testimony to the variety of seafood consumed in these islands. You'll see bubbling tanks filled with mollusks, crabs, and lobsters; piles of squid and octopus; and row upon row of incredibly colorful and exotic green, blue, and red fish. Stalls are decorated with hanging ropes of coiled dried black eel and the puffed-up skins of poisonous spiny blowfish. In some ways, it's as much theater as market!

The Okinawans enjoy all kinds of fish, ranging from lighter white fish like sea bream and fusilier to fattier, more omega-3-rich fish, such as mackerel, tuna, and salmon—no doubt a factor in their low rate of heart disease. Fish can be divided into three basic categories according to their fat content: lean, moderate-fat, and high-fat. Lean fish, such as cod, flounder, haddock, halibut, pollock, perch, red snapper, and trout, have mild light-colored meat and contain less than 2.5 percent fat (the fat is concentrated in the fish's liver rather than being distributed through the body). Moderate-fat fish usually have less than 6 percent fat; this category includes barracuda, swordfish, and bonito tuna. High-fat fish have about a 12 percent fat content, although some Okinawan heavies like eel *(irabu)* can be as high as 30 percent fat. Compare this 12 percent fat to the 17 percent fat in extra-lean beef, and you can see that the fat in fish is usually much lower—and healthier—than in most supermarket meat. Popular high-fat fish are Atlantic herring, mackerel, salmon, sturgeon, and yellowtail. The wider distribution of fat in moderate-fat and high-fat fish gives their flesh a darker color, firmer texture, and more distinctive flavor—and, of course, a higher dose of heart-healthy omega-3 fatty acids.

OKINAWA'S FAVORITE FISH

In Okinawa, the coastal villages of Minatogawa, Itoman, and Motobu stand as famous centers of the fishing industry. It was in the latter of these three villages that we met Nakamura-san, a tanned, extremely fit eighty-seven-year-old fisherman who offered to show us the traditional Okinawan method of dive-fishing with nets. We put on our dive suits, helped Nakamura-san pack up the equipment, and headed out to the edge of the reef in his small wooden boat. Then we all dove in. Once under water, we watched as Nakamura-san placed nets between crevasses in the reef, effectively forming a net circle with only a small opening at one end. We were only at about twenty feet but still found it hard to keep up with the old fisherman. Adding to our embarrassment at being unable to keep up with a man pushing ninety was that although we had on our diving gear, our fearless leader swam without flippers, mask, snorkel, or air tank. His only equipment were his handmade goggles and wetsuit. We could only watch with amazement as he held his breath and dove to the bottom to set the nets. After just a few trips to the surface for breath, the nets were in place. Then Nakamura-san picked up a long bamboo pole topped with colorful flags and dove back down to the bottom to drive the fish into the corral of nets. In no time at all the nets were full of the blue, green, red, orange, and yellow fish that make the warm tropical seas their home. After gathering up the nets and the catch, we rowed back to shore, and that night at Nakamura-san's house we dined on the freshest, most delicious sashimi we'd ever tasted.

GURUKUN

(*Pterocasio diagramma;* banana fish; *takasago;* fusilier)

This small, colorful tropical fish is so familiar to Okinawans that it's been given the special distinction of prefectural fish of Okinawa. It's one of the most popular fish for making the *kamaboko* (fish cake) that is served alongside stir-fried vegetables. *Gurukun* are about eight to ten inches long, are either blue or red, and have two banana-like yellow streaks running the length of their bodies and black-tipped tails. And these fish get around. *Gurukun* have been spotted in warm waters from southern Japan to Australia and often show up in Indonesia, New Caledonia, and India. In Okinawa, *gurukun* prefer the coral reefs and are easily caught throughout the year by the traditional Okinawan net-fishing technique.

Weight and health benefits. A very light fish, low in fat and calories but rich in protein, calcium, and vitamin A, with moderate levels of omega-3 fatty acids.

How to use it. As sashimi, or steamed, baked, broiled, or fried. If fried, the fish should be patted with paper towels to remove as much of the oil as possible. Also, try it as prepared fish paste with stir-fried vegetable dishes.

Where to find it. Fish paste from light white fish can be found in the frozen food section of most large grocery stores or in the fish market. Gurukun may be difficult to find in the states, but substitutes for gurukun include sea bream and other white fish. Try our Poached White Fish with Honey-Lime Sauce and our Ryukyu Fish Curry on pages 258 and 260.

KATSUO (*Sarda spp.;* bonito; skipjack tuna)

It's difficult to imagine Okinawan or Japanese food without *katsuo.* It's used to make broth for miso soup and stews and sauce for tempura or noodle dips, and it is sprinkled on stir-fried dishes, just to name a few of its multitudinous uses. *Katsuo-bushi* (bonito flakes) is, in fact, used every day throughout Japan. Although dried bonito fills the main market in downtown Naha City, you'd most likely walk right by it. It looks much more like a block of wood or a large piece of charcoal than a fish. It all makes sense when you consider that the fish is boiled whole; then, with head, tail, bones, and skin removed, it is dried in the sun and smoked over and over again. Curing bonito can take half a year! Using a plane, shavings are collected into clear plastic bags and sold as a broth ingredient or to be sprinkled on food as a seasoning. Up to a few years ago, every household in Okinawa had a plane for shaving dried bonito; today most people just head to the market or grocery store and buy the shavings ready-made, or even substitute powdered or liquid seasonings.

Weight and health benefits. Tuna is known for its high levels of heart-healthy omega-3 fatty acids. Bonito is a low-calorie tuna that contains less fat than other tunas but similar levels of niacin and iron. It also contains taurine, which promotes decomposition of cholesterol.[25]

How to use it. Bonito is terrific as sashimi and eaten with soy sauce, vinegar, grated ginger, and slices of garlic. Bonito flakes (*katsuo-bushi*) are one of the key ingredients in Japanese cuisine for soup broths or seasoning. Try our tuna dishes as well, such as Teriyaki Yellowtail on page 266 and Hawaiian Lemon–Ahi Poke on page 260. Canned albacore tuna is great for salads or sandwiches.

Where to find it. *Katsuo* can be found at your local Asian market, fish market, or in the international food section of larger supermarkets. For cooked dishes, substitute other kinds of tuna that you can find more easily in your area, such as yellowtail.

SEA BREAM (*Gymnocranius euanus;* Japanese sea bream, *tai, shiruiyu*)
Sea bream is a name given to any of several similar species of freshwater and saltwater fish, such as Japanese sea bream *(tai),* the French *daurade,* or the American porgy. Sea bream (called *taman* in Okinawa) is meaty, not unlike red snapper, and lends itself well to Okinawan cuisine. Although it's popular for weddings, festivals, and other special occasions in mainland Japan, it's more commonly eaten in Okinawa, especially in local soup dishes.

Weight and health benefits. Sea bream are similar to other white fish: low in fat and calories but rich in protein, calcium, and vitamin A, with moderate levels of omega-3 oils.

How to use it. In general, sea bream can be steamed, grilled, baked, and fried, and it makes a great fish soup. Cooking in foil is also easy and helps retain flavors. People who find heads and bones unappealing should get filleted bream, but the skin should always be kept on to keep the flesh as moist as possible. Be sure to try our recipe for Sea Bream Carpaccio with Turmeric Sauce on page 256.

Where to find it. Sea bream is fairly common, so you should be able to find it at your local fish market. If not, substitute red snapper, trout, or cod.

EATING FISH DURING PREGNANCY

According to a USDA Consumer Advisory (USDA, March 2001), fish should be limited or avoided if you are pregnant or could become pregnant, are breast-feeding, or have small children. Some fish contain high levels of a form of mercury called methylmercury that may harm an unborn child's developing brain if eaten regularly. These findings are controversial, since recent research suggests this mercury is not as harmful as usual mercury. Still, almost all fish contain trace amounts of methylmercury, through small quantities are not harmful to humans and it is eliminated from your body over time. But long-lived, larger fish accumulate the highest levels of methylmercury and pose a greater potential risk to you and your unborn child.

Importantly, fish is still a great food that is high in protein and heart-healthy oils—and so long as you choose the right variety, you are safe. If you are pregnant, you can safely eat 12 ounces per week of cooked fish. A regular serving of fish is around 3 to 6 ounces.

Eat anytime (up to 12 oz./week)	Eat once a week	Eat once every two weeks	Do not eat
Clams	Canned tuna	Yellowfin tuna or bigeye tuna (light pink meat)	Pacific blue marlin
Crabs	Cod		Shark
Farm-raised fish	Grouper		Swordfish
Mullet	Halibut		
Octopus	Mahimahi		
Opelu	Orange roughy		
Salmon	Pollock		
Scallops	Skipjack tuna (red meat)		
Shrimp			
Small fish (fits in a frying pan whole)	Striped marlin, or *nairagi*		
Squid			

From: Consumer Advisory, USDA, March 2001; Harris et al., *Science* 2003; 301:1203.

Meat and Dairy

MEAT

People familiar with Japanese cuisine are surprised the first time they walk into any restaurant in Okinawa specializing in local cuisine. Pork seems to dominate the meat part of the menu—pork soba, tenderloin medallions coated in roasted sesame, boiled pig's feet, entrail soup, shredded pig ears in vinegar slaw, and pork mixed with various vegetable dishes are just a few of the more notable dishes to be found. The local expression "Pigs can be eaten from nail to tail—everything but the voice" is pretty accurate. In the past, when fat intake was extremely low, Okinawans even saved the lard from the pork to use in their cooking. When cheap (and healthy) cooking oil made from vegetable oil became available in the 1950s, it quickly became the cooking oil of choice, and when pork is cooked today, the fat is mostly thrown away.

Pork, has, in fact, been an important part of Okinawan cuisine for centuries. Some credit Chinese influences, but the fact that there are indigenous wild boars on the islands suggests the preference for pork may predate even the Chinese. Furthermore, Okinawans, more shamanistic than Buddhist, have none of the historical Japanese religious-based prejudices against eating meat.

The westernization of the Okinawan diet has meant an increase both in meat choices and in intake, which has resulted in interesting fusion-style cuisine. At *yakiniku* grill restaurants, for instance, thin slices of filet mignon are marinated in miso sauce and *kalbi* steak is grilled at your table alongside seafood and vegetables. Other fusion dishes have been influenced by the American military bases. One notable example is "taco rice," a hybrid American-Mexican-Okinawan dish that is essentially a dish of rice topped with seasoned hamburger meat, lettuce, tomatoes, taco sauce, and various condiments. And the ubiquitous canned pork luncheon meat, a quick and easy substitute for traditional pork, has been readily adapted to stir-fried vegetable dishes.

But despite increased meat consumption compared to the traditional Okinawan diet, the elders still consume only about a quarter of the meat we do in America. Because meat was eaten mostly on religious occasions before World War II, the Okinawan elders have consumed very little meat over the course of their lives and still get the bulk of their protein from vegetable sources.[26] Increased meat consumption is much more widespread among the younger generations, and this CD heavyweight is now contributing to the epidemic of obesity among Okinawan youth. Boiled meats are also popular among the elders, which results in lower overall saturated fat and cholesterol intake, lower caloric density, and less exposure to possible carcinogens formed by grilling or frying meat. If you eat meat, take a lesson from the elders: Eat it sparingly, boil it, and toss the fat away!

DAIRY AND EGGS

Along with more meat in the Okinawan diet came a big increase in milk consumption—but, as in the case of meat, this increase is more pronounced in the younger generations. In fact, the only dairy product that most elders in Okinawa regularly consume is a yogurt drink, but they do enjoy their eggs. Eggs were an important source of protein in the past, and they are still popular in Okinawa and throughout Japan. In fact, Japan now has one of the highest per-capita rates of egg consumption in the world. The elders, of course, ate free-range eggs, high in omega-3 fatty acids and vitamin B_{12}, which were all that was available when they were growing up. Eggs, though, were not part of their daily fare but rather eaten on occasion, as they were believed to improve strength and stamina.

Spices and Herbs

Cutting fat, salt, or sugar from a recipe may be healthy, but it doesn't make food tasty. All three provide lots of flavor, and when they're left out, food can be terribly boring and bland. Enter herbs and spices. These are terrifically effective in giving foods more depth and complexity of taste. Herbs and spices not only boost the flavor and richness of any dish but also provide great health benefits. Some are rich in powerful phytonutrients that can protect against a wide range of cancers, cardiovascular disease, and other chronic illnesses.

Using herbs in cooking is a safe and tasty way to incorporate them into your diet—as opposed to taking them in supplement pill form. Fresh herbs are best. A rule of thumb for using fresh herbs is to double the amount when a recipe calls for the herb in dried form. The many herbs, spices, and flavorings in the Okinawans' cooking arsenal not only contribute extraordinary flavor to various foods but offer weight and health benefits as well. Chili peppers, for example, a common ingredient in Okinawan cuisine, have been found to reduce appetite[27] and increase the metabolism of dietary fats.[28] Most of the herbs and spices we include here also contain antioxidants and phytonutrients that help combat the ravages of time and give your system an extra boost of healing power. Some of them even help the body to use insulin more efficiently. Although most of the health claims for these herbs and spices are drawn from traditional Okinawan folk medical practice and are untested at this point, other claims have been borne out in clinical trials. Add these herbs and spices to vegetables rather than butter, margarine, cheese, or sour cream, and watch the caloric density of your meal drop!

UCCHIN—TURMERIC (Curcuma longa; ukon, jiang huang, Indian saffron)
Turmeric, or *ucchin,* is an herb that every Okinawan is intimately familiar with. Many drink it as a tea, others take it in tablet form, but most simply use it in their cooking. Its wonderful orange-yellow color gives saffron rice and yellow curries their distinctive taste and yellow hue. Originally from India, turmeric belongs to the ginger family.

Weight and health benefits. Turmeric is frequently used in Ayurvedic medicine and traditional Okinawan medicine as a metabolism booster, and when combined with bitter herbs such as barberry, it is said to eliminate "excess fat." It's also used as an antimicrobial, liver protectant, and stimulant for poor digestion. Scientists have studied turmeric for antioxidant properties,[29] for use as an anti-cancer agent,[30] with respect to heartburn and stomach ulcers,[31] and as a treatment for arthritis,[32] high cholesterol,[33] and HIV.[34] Turmeric's medicinal potential is mainly due to its major active component, curcumin, thought to stimulate the body's ability to release the hormone cortisol, which regulates metabolism, maintains blood pressure, and decreases inflammation. (People considering using turmeric in amounts greater than commonly found in food should consult their health-care provider.)

How to use it. It's great as a spice for curries, soups, fish, and most Indian dishes. You can also add turmeric to tea—it works well with oolong. We use it to perk up our chicken and vegetable soups and tuna and bean salads, and to add zip and color to salad dressings.

Where to find it. Turmeric can readily be found in Asian and international markets as well as in regular supermarkets.

HIHATSU (Piper hancei; Okinawan pepper; *hippazu)*
The little red fruit from this vine-like plant can be dried and ground for use as pepper. It is a prime ingredient in the hot, spicy dishes that came to Okinawa from southern China. The leaves of the plant are also used in tempura dishes, and the herb can often be found in the apothecary of traditional herbal medicines.

Weight and health benefits. Traditional medicine frequently uses peppers and hot spices such as *hihatsu* as well as cayenne, black pepper, ginger, garlic, and turmeric to increase metabolism. In Okinawan herbal medicine, *hihatsu* has been used to treat stomach problems and gout among other ailments. There has been some limited research support for red chili pepper's ability to raise metabolic rates and possibly accelerate the rate of body fat loss,[35] but these claims need further study. Pepper has also been shown to have antioxidant and antimicrobial properties,[36] and numerous clinical trials attest to its efficacy as a topically applied analgesic (in cream form).[37]

How to use it. Hihatsu powder adds a uniquely stimulating taste and a fresh scent to most foods, including rice, pasta, soups, and vegetables. Sprinkle the powder on noodles and soups, salads, rice, and vegetables, or simply use when cooking as you would pepper.

Where to find it. Hihatsu is most always available in large Asian food stores. Fresh ground black pepper or ground chili peppers makes a good substitute.

KOREGUSU (*Capsicum annuum; togarashi;* chili pepper in *awamori* liquor)

Koregusu is a unique-tasting liquid seasoning made by dipping chili peppers in *awamori* (Okinawan sake). It's especially popular for Okinawa soba (noodle) dishes or soups, and you'll find a tiny bottle of it in every Okinawa soba shop. The taste of this hot pepper is a signature of Okinawa cuisine and is a big contributor to its reputation as "Japanese food with salsa."

Weight and health benefits. The chili peppers in koregusu contain capsasinoids (an antioxidant), high levels of carotenoids, and vitamins A and C. Internally, capsasinoids act as a circulatory stimulant and are used to stimulate digestion. Topical capsaicin preparations are used for the relief of pain associated with shingles and arthritic and rheumatoid conditions.[37] Claims for peppers as metabolism boosters have received some limited support from the research literature.[35]

How to use it. Add a dash of this seasoning whenever you need to spice up a meal or recipe. It goes well with seafood, in barbecue sauce, or in dressings.

Where to find it. Koregusu is available at some Asian food stores. Red-hot chili peppers are a close relative and make a good substitute.

SHICHIMI—SEVEN-SPICE POWDER

Shichimi is a mixture of chili peppers, hemp seeds, dried orange peel, nori seaweed flakes, white sesame seeds, perilla leaf, and *sansho* leaf.

Weight and health benefits. Because one of chili's phytonutrients, capsaicin, is believed to be a "fat burner" in Japan, some young Japanese use this powder to season everything they eat. Some limited research has supported capsicums' ability to increase metabolic rates,[35] reduce appetite,[27] and increase metabolism of dietary fats,[28] but this requires further study. The hemp seeds provide omega-3 fatty acids; the seaweed is very high in calcium; and the mixture offers a host of other phytonutrients from carotenoids to flavonoids.

How to use it. Sprinkle shichimi on any food that needs a bit of flavor. Try it with soup, grilled fish, noodles, and simmered vegetables. It even makes a nice addition to plain rice and potatoes.

Where to find it. Shichimi is readily available at grocery stores with international food sections and at all Asian food stores.

OBAKO (*Plantago asiatica;* plantain, ribwort)

The leaves of *obako,* or plantain, as it is commonly known in the West, have been one of Okinawa's traditional, popular green leafy vegetables. They are used in myriad dishes—especially soups and tempura. Obako should not be confused with the bananalike plants of the same plantain family (Plantaginaceae) that also grow throughout Okinawa.

Weight and health benefits. As a traditional herbal medicine, the leaves of obako have been used to treat stomach troubles, kidney ailments, inflammation of the bladder and urinary tract, and coughs. The seeds have a mild laxative effect, similar to the seeds of another plantain, psyllium *(Plantago ovata).* Indeed, Metamucil and similar products use psyllium husks to treat constipation. Studies have found that psyllium is a useful addition to weight-loss regimens because the bulk it creates helps contribute to feelings of satiety.[38] It also lowers LDL cholesterol,[39] improves blood sugar levels in some people with diabetes,[40] and may be helpful for ulcerative colitis.[41]

How to use it. Obako, and similar species of young plantain leaves such as ribwort *(Plantago lanceolata),* makes a pungent and healthy addition to salads and dips. The leaves taste best before the plant has flowered and can also be used as a vegetable in stir-fries, as cooked greens similar to spinach, in soups, and as an herbal tea. For intestinal health and regularity, try the psyllium husks that come from the dried seeds of plantains such as ribwort, known commonly as *psyllium powder.* Mix 1 teaspoonful of psyllium powder with juice or water and have it before meals once or more a day.

Where to find it. Ribwort is an old-world plantain that grows wild on lawns, fields, and roadsides throughout Europe and North and Central Asia; in recent centuries it has spread throughout most of the United States and southern Canada. It's especially common in the east-central states, where it is known as a perennial weed with large, broad, green, ribbed leaves and pale greenish-yellow and brown flowers on long spikes. Dried ribwort leaves and teas can be found in health food stores. Psyllium products like Metamucil can be found in any supermarket.

SHIRUMINNA (*Stellaria media; midori hakobe,* chickweed)

Shiruminna, or chickweed, as it is commonly known throughout the West, is a traditional ingredient for soups and stews in Okinawa. The leaves, stems, and flowers have been used medicinally throughout Europe and in Okinawa as well. A native of temperate regions everywhere, chickweed likes damp, shady gardens, lawns, and open fields. It is, in fact, a common backyard herb and one of the most prolific "weeds" in the world.

Weight and health benefits. Chickweed holds a reputation as a folk remedy for obesity and as a topical treatment for skin conditions throughout old Europe. In Okinawan folk medicine, it has been used to increase milk production in young mothers, to decrease appendicitis inflammation, as a treatment of kidney problems, and as a remedy for scurvy. Research has confirmed high amounts of vitamin C and flavonoids in chickweed,[42] which helps explain its effectiveness in treating skin irritations and scurvy. It has also been found to have diuretic properties and to contain both anti-inflammatory saponins and spongy, fiberlike mucilage (like psyllium), which might explain its reputation as a diet aid.

How to use it. Chickweed is a wonderful, crispy green that we often add to fresh salads. It is also a fine addition to soups, stews, pasta dishes, and breads.

Where to find it. Chickweed grows abundantly across North America and can often be found in moist, shaded areas in yards, cultivated land, and woodlands throughout the year. It has straggling, trailing stems up to twelve inches tall, with green paired leaves and numerous tiny white flowers, each with five deeply lobed petals. The fruit is small and reddish-brown. You can also buy chickweed in health food stores as a dried herb, in tea bags, or as an ointment or extract.

ICHOBA—FENNEL (*Foeniculum vulgare; uikyo,* sweet fennel, *hui xiang*)

Fennel, a tall, hardy, aromatic perennial of the parsley family, has been traditionally used in Okinawa both as a vegetable and an herbal medicine. It's also been a popular herb in Europe since ancient times. The Romans called this native Mediterranean plant *foeniculum,* which means "fragrant hay." Often confused with dill, the stalk looks something like celery. "Fennel seeds," which are served after dinner in Indian restaurants, much as mints are in the West, are actually the dried fruit of the common fennel. Anise, dill, cumin, and caraway all belong to the same plant family, Apiaceae, and have similar shapes and scents.

Weight and health benefits. Fennel "seeds" have a traditional reputation as an aid to weight loss and longevity. In the Greek legend of Prometheus, fennel granted its user immortality. A nice thought—but no supporting evidence for that one. Medicinal claims, though, do have some heft. In Okinawa, locals have found *ichoba* useful for curing upset stomach, heartburn, and gas and for treating urinary stones. That makes sense, as fennel has been shown to contain terpenoids in its volatile oils, which inhibit spasms in smooth muscles such as the intestinal tract.[43] That's most likely why this sweet-smelling herb was formerly classified as an official drug in the United States and listed for use in cases of indigestion.[44] Fennel is also thought to possess diuretic,[45] pain-reducing,[46] fever-reducing,[47] and antimicrobial actions, and it may act as an estrogenic agent.[48]

How to use it. Fennel is popular in meat and seafood dishes, pickles, and vinegar dishes, and it goes well with the earthy aroma of bread.

Where to find it. Fennel seeds are available in any grocery store.

TEA *(Camellia sinensis)*

Far better to be without food for three days than tea for one.
—*Ancient Chinese proverb*

People have been drinking tea since its "discovery" more than 5,000 years ago—when, legend has it, some tea leaves blew into the pot of water that was being boiled for the Chinese emperor. Ever since then, delicious tea has been an integral part of Chinese culture and has spread to every part of the world. Buddhist priests traveling between Japan and China introduced this drink to Japan, and the famous Japanese tea ceremony was perfected with the help of Ch'a Ching (*The Tea Book,* written by the Chinese scholar Lu Yu).

The Ryukyu Kingdom, with its close ties to China, was an early benefactor of the wonders of tea, which has been used for centuries as both a tasty beverage and as part of the herbal apothecary of the Okinawans. Now science is showing that tea may even help prevent cancer, heart disease, and stroke and help slow the aging process itself. But before we get into the health benefits of this amazing drink, we should note that not all teas are created equal. In fact, some "teas" are not teas at all. "Herbal teas," for instance, are made from herbs, not tea leaves, so they don't really qualify.

Essentially, there are only three types of tea—black, green, and oolong—and they come from the leaves of the tropical evergreen tea plant called *Camellia sinensis.* Black tea is made from tea leaves that have been fermented, heated, and dried to produce the characteristic English tea flavor and a red-brown to black color. Green tea, which has a slightly bitter taste and is a greenish-yellow color, is produced from leaves that are steamed and dried but not fermented. Oolong tea is produced from leaves that are partially fermented, a process that creates teas with a flavor, color, and aroma that falls between black tea and green tea. Other distinguishing characteristics depend on where the tea is grown, the processing method, and whether other botanicals or flavorings are added. The size of the leaf is also an important distinguishing characteristic of tea; younger, more tender leaves are generally considered best. There are over 2,000 varieties of specialty teas flavored with spice or flower additions, such as jasmine or chrysanthemum blossoms and orange or lemon peel. The favorite tea of the Okinawan elders is *sanpin* tea, a combination of green tea and jasmine flowers, which gives the tea a beautiful aroma and flavor. It can be found in North American supermarkets as jasmine tea.

Weight and health benefits. Given that tea has virtually no calories or fat, hundreds of tantalizing flavors, and dozens of health benefits, its worldwide popularity is easy to understand. A simple cup of tea, in fact, may be one of the best defenses against illness, aging, and disease. Research has linked tea consumption with a reduction in heart attacks,[49] better bone health,[50] cancer prevention,[51] better cholesterol control,[52] and relief of arthritis and other inflammatory conditions.[53] Many of these health benefits are due to the high levels of antioxidants and flavonoids found in tea. Both black and green teas contain potent levels of these compounds, although green tea has more of a certain kind of flavonoid called *catechins,* which are potent antioxidants. One of these catechins, called *epigallocatechin gallate* (EGCG), may help weight loss by increasing energy expenditure. According to a recent paper appearing in the *American Journal of Clinical Nutrition,* healthy young men who took two green tea capsules (containing 50 mg caffeine and 90 mg EGCG) three times a day had significantly more energy and fat oxidation than those who took caffeine alone or a placebo.[54] If these preliminary observations hold, help with weight control will be just one more benefit of this already incredibly healthful plant.

How to use it. Pick your tea according to your own taste and steep bags or leaves in a pot for a tasty brew. Tea can also be used in cooking. *Matcha,* or ground green tea leaf powder, is a favorite ingredient in Japanese desserts. Try our Green Tea Panna Cotta and Sweet Potato Mousse with Green Tea Sauce on pages 339 and 345.

Where to find it. Both black teas (in leaf and tea-bag form) and instant teas are readily available in all supermarkets. Other teas can be found in great variety in health food stores, Asian markets, and stores specializing in tea and coffee.

A CAUTIONARY NOTE REGARDING NATURAL HERBAL "DIET" AIDS

Most people tend to take herbs less seriously than prescriptions drugs. This is a serious mistake. Herbal medicine is not risk-free, and the pharmacological properties of herbs can interact with doctor-prescribed medications. So you must be careful. To give you an example of the importance of taking herbs seriously, here's the scoop on the most popular herb for weight loss.

Ma huang, or *ephedra,* as it is commonly known, is a shrublike plant found in desert regions of northern China and Mongolia. The Chinese have used the dried green stems of the plant medicinally for more than 5,000 years, primarily for lung and bronchial constriction, edema, coughs, and shortness of breath. The active constituent, ephedrine, was isolated in the late nineteenth century and became popular with doctors in the United States in the 1920s for treating asthma and bronchial congestion. Ephedrine and its over-the-counter synthetic counterparts, variously labeled as Metabolife, Metab-O-LITE and Metabomax, did a booming business as diet pills. In 1998, Metabolife alone racked up sales of more than $600 million!

Although ephedra can suppress the appetite and raise your metabolism, which may help lead to short-term weight loss, it can also cause side effects, including raised blood pressure, insomnia, seizures, heart attacks, strokes, and, possibly, death. A recent paper appearing in the *New England Journal of Medicine* reviewed 140 reports of cardiovascular and central nervous system adverse reactions and concluded that two-thirds of adverse health reports were definitely, probably, or possibly related to the herbal formulas.[55] In all the cases cited, the people took ephedra together with either caffeine or drugs with cardiovascular side effects, such as theophylline and phenylpropanolamine.

The FDA has limited control over the use of these types of products, since they're classified as "herbal diet supplements" rather than "drugs." So it's up to you to be a savvy consumer. As a rule, we believe that rational herbal medicine has fewer side effects than conventional medicine, as herbs are generally more diluted, but you have to be careful when an herb is removed from its cultural context. Such is the case with ma huang, where despite 5,000 years of use in Chinese medicine, the herb was synthesized, dosed up, and combined with other stimulants like caffeine to create products much more powerful and potentially dangerous than the original herb.

Bottom line: We don't recommend the use of ephedra-type diet pills or similar weight-loss products. Their short-term safety is questionable, and long-term effects have not been explored enough for our liking. In fact, in May 2003, Illinois became the first state in the United States to ban the sale of ephedra products, and other states are following suit. It's always a good idea to consult your physician before taking any herbal supplements, just as you would before taking any other medicine. As for herbs you have picked yourself, if in doubt of what they are, you can usually send them to your nearest herbarium or botanical gardens for identification. Often they will identify it free of charge, but you will need to follow specific instructions for proper handling. Better safe than sorry. And always talk to your doctor before embarking on any diet regimen. As we've pointed out, the moderate use of herbs in cooking, teas, or infusion is the safest way to incorporate them into your diet. When it comes to herbal weight-loss plans—or, in fact, any health-promoting product—remember, if it sounds too good to be true, it probably is. *Nuchi gusui!*

Chapter 6

FINDING BALANCE: YOUR PERSONALIZED WEIGHT CONTROL PLAN

It's Never Too Late: Tama Nakajima's Story

When Tama Nakajima, a wiry Okinawan grandmother, turned sixty-six years old, she decided that a change was in order. She had worked hard all her life as a farmer and raised seven children and a brood of grandchildren, but she wanted to eat better and become more active. Tama had been athletic in her youth and had always stayed lean, but middle age and the new ways were catching up with her. While she had happily filled up on homemade miso soup (her favorite food), veggies, and other low-CD lightweights in the old days, now processed, sugar-laden foods were a big part of the picture. She decided to leave them behind and return to her roots. Fortunately, Tama didn't see her age as a barrier to change, but rather as a challenge. She went back to her childhood diet and began to walk—then run, then jump. Soon there was no stopping her. She began entering races, tournaments, and even long-jump meets. "My younger friends taught me how to jump, telling me 'Grandma, you jump from here, like this,'" she says with a laugh—and a mini-demonstration. Now Tama not only holds the national record in the seventy-five-year-old class for the 100-meter dash and the 800-meter distance run, but the world record in her class for the long jump. And at eighty-four years old, with twenty grandchildren and seven great-grandchildren, she feels younger and more fit than she ever did at sixty-six. "I thought I'd be weaker as I aged, but actually I improved," she muses. "It doesn't make sense, but it makes me very happy."

To us, of course, it makes a lot of sense. Recent research from our colleagues at Harvard Medical School has shown that flavonoids can induce the same longevity-inducing enzyme changes seen in animals on calorically restricted regimens,[1] and with Okinawa sweet potatoes and tofu dominating her traditional diet, Tama's getting plenty of flavonoids. But there's another ingredient in her winning formula that shouldn't be over looked: her indefatigable spirit. "We all need to have fondness and courage for what we do," she says. "Although you may be good at something, if you don't like it or have no courage, it is no good. Everything depends on your heart." Amen.

Before we move along to our menu plans and tempting recipes, we want to briefly address some of the other fundamentals of weight maintenance. While eating the right food is, of course, the core of any healthy weight-loss plan, a positive mental attitude and regular physical activity play important roles as well. They are, in fact, crucial not only to losing your unwanted pounds but also to keeping them off long-term.[2] Combine these two elements with your smart eating choices and you'll have a winning total health program and be well on your way to achieving the balance of mind, body, and spirit the Okinawan elders feel is essential to life—and that is integrated with everything they do.

Balancing Mind and Spirit

GETTING INTO THE RIGHT MIND-SET

To one degree or another, we all have a negative inner voice that gives us faulty advice about what to think and how to act. To truly get control of our eating and exercise habits, that voice needs to be harnessed and reprogrammed to give positive advice—not just about diet and exercise but also about life and, ultimately, about ourselves. Self-love is an essential step toward that goal. When you love yourself, you want to do good things for yourself. You'll want to lose excess weight because it is a good, healthy thing to do for yourself, not in order to become someone you can love. Obviously there's a lot to the psychology behind all this—but that's another book. Here, we just want to give you food for thought and some helpful tips to keep in mind to start you on this new journey.

• **Praise yourself; don't criticize.** Self-criticism breaks the inner spirit. Praise builds it up. Tell yourself how well you are doing as you start to apply the principles of our diet. Refuse to criticize yourself, and try to accept yourself exactly as you are. We all change throughout our lives, but when you criticize yourself, changes tend to be negative; when you approve of yourself, changes are positive. If you feel a bout of self-flagellation coming on, immediately switch gears and think of something you did well.

- **Be gentle, kind, and patient with yourself.** Positive change takes time as old habits are broken and new ones develop. Treat yourself as you would a beloved friend who needs support.

- **Change your negatives into positives.** Many unhealthy eating habits were developed to fulfill a need. Now you are finding new, positive ways to fulfill those needs. So lovingly release the old negative patterns. Creating positive self-talk is important to your long-term success. Try this exercise: Sit in a comfortable quiet place and listen to your internal dialogue. Does your self-talk calm or stress you? If a word triggers a negative association, try to reroute it by immediately thinking of something positive. Repeat out loud, "I am a good person." Repetitive positive reinforcement helps replace the negative thoughts.

- **Find new outside support.** Reach out to friends and allow them to help you. Join a weight-loss support group or an athletic club, and engage in group activities.

- **Love your mirror image.** This is an amazingly powerful exercise. Look into the mirror and into your own eyes. Openly express the growing sense of love you feel for yourself. Forgive yourself for bad habits and past mistakes. At least once a day, look in the mirror and say to yourself, "I love you; I really love you!" (You can even talk to your parents this way and forgive them, too.)

- **Take care of your body.** Learn about nutrition; this book is a great start. Become fully informed and conscious of the kinds of fuel your body needs for optimum energy and vitality. Learn more about exercise and zero in on the kinds you enjoy. Cherish and revere the temple you live in.

- **Start now.** Don't wait until you lose the weight, or get the new job, or find the new relationship. Begin *now*—do the best you can.

DEFINE YOUR MOTIVATION

It really helps to accurately define and state your motivations for losing weight. See if you can write down at least five reasons you're starting this diet. Do you just want to look and feel better about yourself? Do you have or want to prevent a specific health condition such as heart disease, high blood pressure, or diabetes? Are you a highly trained athlete trying to eliminate unnecessary fat and build muscle? Are you out to push your energy efficiency to its limits, to gain the maximal benefits of caloric restriction? Or do you simply want to drop ten pounds of fat? Different motivations and goals mean different levels of diligence, commitment, and end points, so you need to be realistic.

Carry your list of reasons for healthy weight with you for a day or so and think about it throughout the day. Then, when you're doing something that's part of your plan, like limiting your portion sizes or choosing fruit over an ice-cream sandwich, say to yourself, "I'm doing this *for my health and heart*," or whatever personal motivating factors you listed. When you find yourself slipping, it's particularly helpful to remember all of your important health and personal reasons for losing weight and to have coping strategies that work well for you.

DESCRIBE YOUR GOAL

It's equally important to have a specific goal in mind: the number of pounds you want to lose, for instance, or the dress size or suit size you'd like to be able to wear again. Again, write down specifically what you want to accomplish. You'll find it much easier to stay focused on your goal, and the means of achieving it, once you've clearly defined it. Your goal will become more real and more attainable.

Also, set a realistic timeline for yourself. Remember that it took a lifetime to accumulate most of the weight, and it will take a long-term plan to get it off and keep it off. Generally, weight lost rapidly tends to return rapidly. Losing one to three pounds a week is a sound, realistic goal.[2] A prudent approach is to aim for a loss of 5 to 10 percent of your total body weight and then to allow your body time to adjust to that weight for at least a few weeks before trying to lose more weight.

EAT ONLY WHEN HUNGRY

This is not as easy as it sounds. People eat for all sorts of emotional reasons: anger, loneliness, boredom, anxiety, family problems, nervousness, social pressures—you name it. Even though we've provided plenty of low-cal snacks that you can eat while sticking to your plan, it's still important to identify your personal triggers so you can establish strategies for coping with them. A few ideas:

Common Pitfalls and Coping Strategies

Eating Pitfall	Coping Strategy
Anger	Talk to the person or address the problem, take a walk, call a friend.
Anxiety	Do deep breathing, yoga, meditation.
Boredom	Exercise, see a movie.
Fatigue	Take a nap.
Loneliness	Call or e-mail a friend.

VISUALIZE SUCCESS . . . BUT EXPECT SETBACKS

You *will* fail or slip occasionally; everyone does. But once you realize this fact and are prepared for it, you can move on, stronger, more focused, and more determined than before. Expecting occasional slips also helps you focus on the long term and helps you keep things in perspective. One effective strategy for getting back on track after a relapse is to put an old picture of yourself at your starting weight near the refrigerator or on your computer screen. That will definitely help fix your goal firmly in your mind. Visualize, several times a day, exactly what it will be like when you accomplish your weight-loss goal. What will you feel like? Will you be more outgoing? More energetic? Will you carry yourself with more confidence and pride? This exercise does wonders for maintaining motivation or reinvigorating the plan. Impressing your new image on your subconscious helps you mobilize the willpower and energy to follow through with your plan.

Keeping a food and exercise record is also highly motivating, and if the pounds aren't coming off as anticipated, it helps you figure out why and how to make adjustments to the plan. (Try using our energy balance record on page 172.) Our list of tips should also prove a big help.

Tips to Keep You Going

Obstacle	Tips
Exercise	Determine to make exercise your priority.
	Schedule your exercise session in your daily planner.
	Get up earlier and exercise first thing in the morning.
	Do 10-minute mini-sessions several times a day—e.g., at lunchtime and coffee breaks.
	If you are not really watching TV, use the time to exercise, or exercise while watching TV.
	Place a book rack on an exercise machine and use your reading time for exercise.
	Incorporate calorie-burning activity into your life—climb stairs, get off at a farther bus stop, park a greater distance from work, buy a pedometer and walk 10,000 steps a day. It's easier than you think!
Fattening Snacks	Nibble throughout the day on low-CD snacks.
	Try to eat fruit, chew gum, or suck on a mint before or while grocery shopping.
	Always be conscious of what you are about to eat—a lot of snacking is done unconsciously, "because it was "in front of me."

Obstacle	Tips
Finding Time to Shop and Prepare Meals	Be organized—divide shopping list into categories so that you don't have to come back to the same row in the store.
	Stock your cupboards, fridge, and freezer with our pantry foods (page 186) to pull together nutritious, healthy meals in a hurry.
	Use commuting time to think about what to cook, what to buy, and the most efficient cooking procedure—this saves up to 30 percent of kitchen prep time.
	Place the menu on a refrigerator door so that your children can start helping you when they are home.
	When you have time, check out the availability of healthy prepared foods in your grocery store (e.g., sushi, veggie pizza, low-fat and low-sodium prepared soup, etc.)
	Know that healthy meals are not necessarily complicated meals—e.g., sauté fish with spices or herbs, steam some veggies, and serve healthy canned soup—it's a meal!
	Check out our quick recipes in chapter 8; also visit recipe websites to find quick recipe ideas.
	Cook a week's worth of each meal and freeze portions for your busier days.
Hunger	Ensure you are getting enough protein throughout the day (e.g., add low-CD protein between meals, such as small yogurts, soy wieners, and low-cal protein bars).
	Have a bowl of low-CD fruit handy.
	Drink a cup of tea.
	Avoid high-GI snacks (chocolate bars, white bread, jelly beans).

CELEBRATE YOUR SUCCESS

As you chart your progress at the end of the day or week (or whenever you need a little boost), celebrate your success. Give yourself a mental pat on the back; do a happy little dance; spend some quiet time in the den with a good book or movie; or get a fabulous massage. Treating yourself feeds into your brain's reward system and keeps the mental and spiritual energy flowing to keep you moving toward your goal. Also, share your success stories with friends, coworkers, and family members. As they share in your joy, it will stoke your enthusiasm and propel you along.

BELIEVE IN YOURSELF

Some people may say you're denying yourself too much or that you're getting *too* thin. Sometimes a spouse may even get jealous because you're turning more heads now. Don't allow your goal to be undermined by this type of feedback. Remember that it's where *you* want to be that counts, not where others want you to be.

SEE THE BIG PICTURE

Your success at weight control is the result of meeting many small, achievable goals. A few mistakes along the way can't undo all the positive changes you are making—changes that will benefit not only you but your family too. Not only will you feel better about yourself, and be healthier, but you'll be a better role model for other family members. It's all about quality of life—yours and theirs.

MEDITATE

Meditation is a centering experience. It does wonders to relax the mind and relieve the stress that can lead to overeating, missing workouts, and imbalance. The easiest way to begin is to sit quietly for five to ten minutes at a time, breathe deeply, and try to empty your mind of thoughts. As new thoughts come, picture them floating through your mind and out, and refocus on the emptiness. It takes practice, but is definitely worth the time spent. (*The Okinawa Program* can help you explore this further.)[3]

READ INSPIRATIONAL STORIES

Find stories about people who have been successful in weight loss or other areas of life who can inspire you. Having a role model can make all the difference.

Balancing your Body and Energy

Achieving weight control is all about the energy balance we discussed in chapter 2. In order to lose weight, your energy output (physical activity) has to surpass your energy input (the calories you eat). In other words, you have to burn more calories than you consume—and that boils down to this simple mathematical equation: To lose one pound a week, you have to consume 3,500 fewer calories per week than you expend. This amounts to creating a caloric deficit of 500 calories a day. The best way to do that is to decrease caloric intake and increase energy expenditure through exercise.

Most of us will begin to lose weight if we keep our caloric intake below 1,500 calories/day and do aerobic (cardio, or "fat-burning") exercise for at least thirty minutes, three to four times a week. You already know how to reduce your caloric intake by following the CD rules from chapter 3, so let's talk a bit about the other side of the energy equation.

Determine Your Energy Balance

Step 1: Baseline Output

How much are you burning? Determine your baseline calorie burn.

Get your number from the Baseline Calorie Burn table (opposite) that corresponds to your gender and occupation. Multiply by your current weight.

Example: You are a woman working as a computer programmer (desk work) and your weight is 140 pounds.

$$12 \times 140 = 1,680 \leftarrow \text{This is how many calories you burn}$$
in a typical day without exercise.

Step 2: How Many Calories Do You Burn from Exercise?

Using our Great Aerobic (Cardio) Calorie Burners table on page 174, figure out approximately how many calories you burn from exercise.

Example: You weigh 140 pounds and walk briskly (approximately 3 mph) to and from your work, one hour in total (thirty minutes each way).

$$260 \leftarrow \text{Calories you burn by one hour of brisk walking}$$

Determine Your Input

Step 3: How Much Should You Eat?

To lose one to two pounds per week, you need a daily calorie input approximately 500 to 1,000 calories less than your calorie output.

Example: You are burning 1,940 calories per day
(work = 1,680 calories; 1 hour brisk walk = 260 calories).

$$1,940 - 500 = 1,440 \leftarrow \text{this is your Calorie Input Level}$$

Choose the 1,400-calorie plan and you will lose approximately 1 pound of fat per week, because you have a 540-calorie-per-day deficit.

UNDERSTAND YOUR BASELINE CALORIE LEVEL

When starting on any weight-loss program, it helps to know approximately how many calories you burn in a typical day without additional exercise. We call this your Baseline Calorie Burn, and a number of factors influence your individual burn number. To keep this simple and practical, we've distilled it down to three major factors: gender, current body weight, and occupation.

The table below makes it easy to determine your routine daily calorie expenditure (your baseline calorie burn). The number in the last column represents the amount of calories you burn per pound of body weight during your typical daily routine. Select your appropriate gender and occupation, then multiply the calorie level by your weight. So, for example, if you're a woman who spends most of the day doing computer or other desk work and you weigh 140 pounds, you'd multiply 12 × 140, which would give you 1,680 calories; that's how many calories you burn during your usual daily routine. If you want to maintain your current weight, you cannot eat more than 1,680 calories—unless you increase your activity level. If you eat a little less than that and increase your activity a bit, you will lose weight. (As you can see from the table, men have it easier; sedentary men burn about the same number of calories per pound of body weight as a woman with a moderately strenuous job!)

Baseline Calorie Burn[4]

Gender	Baseline Activity	Calorie Level/Pound
Female	Sedentary work (desk work)	12
Female	Moderately active work (teacher, shopkeeper, nurse, etc.)	14
Female	Very active work (outdoor work, exercise instructor, contractor, etc.)	16
Male	Sedentary work (desk work)	14
Male	Moderately active work (teacher, shopkeeper, nurse, etc.)	17
Male	Very active work (outdoor work, exercise instructor, contractor, etc.)	20

While you could use this formula to simply reduce your calories without exercising, we very strongly recommend you do both—cut the calories *and* exercise—because the combination allows you to lose more fat, maintain more muscle, and shape your body against the inevitable sag of gravity. Our Great Aerobic (Cardio) Calorie Burners table (on page 174) will give you a good idea of just how many calories you'll burn at your current weight with different kinds of exercise. In thirty minutes, for instance, the table shows that our 140-pound

Great Aerobic (Cardio) Calorie Burners

Activity	Calories Burned in 30 Minutes, by Body Weight							
	100 lbs.	*120 lbs.*	*140 lbs.*	*160 lbs.*	*180 lbs.*	*200 lbs.*	*220 lbs.*	*240 l*
Aerobics, light	115	147	173	195	220	246	271	294
Aerobics, hard	169	203	237	256	290	327	365	400
Bicycling, moderate	180	216	252	288	324	360	396	432
Golf (no cart)	124	149	173	198	223	248	272	297
Karate	225	270	315	360	405	450	495	540
Kickboxing	245	293	342	390	440	490	539	582
Rope jumping	228	274	319	365	410	456	502	547
Rowing machine	161	190	223	255	289	326	364	400
Running (12-minute mile)	180	216	252	288	324	360	396	432
Running (10-minute mile)	225	270	315	360	405	450	495	540
Running (8-minute mile)	285	342	395	450	503	559	614	668
Squash	239	279	326	382	419	465	512	570
Stationary cycling (medium)	158	189	221	252	284	315	347	378
Stationary cycling (hard)	236	264	331	378	425	473	520	567
Swimming (slow)	180	213	247	283	318	354	387	417
Swimming (fast)	218	263	305	349	393	446	480	528
Tai chi	90	108	126	144	162	180	198	216
Tennis (singles)	180	216	252	288	324	360	396	432
Tennis (doubles)	135	162	189	216	243	270	297	324
Walking (2 mph)	61	74	89	101	114	127	140	153
Walking (3 mph)	91	108	130	143	160	180	196	213
Walking (4 mph)	118	140	161	186	210	235	257	278
Water aerobics	101	122	142	162	182	203	223	243
Weight training (circuit)	180	216	252	288	324	360	396	432
Weights (free weights)	125	150	175	201	225	250	276	300
Yoga	86	105	121	139	156	174	192	209

woman will burn 173 calories doing light aerobics, 252 calories biking or jogging, 130 calories for walking, and 121 calories doing yoga.

As we've discussed, to lose one to two pounds a week, your daily calorie input needs to be approximately 500 to 1,000 calories less than your calorie output. Let's say you're our 140-pound office worker. We've established that your baseline calorie level is 1,680 calories—that's how much you burn just sitting there working at your desk. But you've wisely decided to walk half an hour to and from work, so add another 260 calories to the amount of calories burned: 1,680 + 260 = 1,940 calories burned. Now subtract 500 calories, which is the amount of calories needed to lose a pound per week (500 cal × 7 days = 3,500 calories = 1 pound of fat). You get 1,440 calories. Result: Eat about 1,440 calories a day, and you should lose about a pound of fat a week—which is easy to do when you eat the Okinawa way.

Remember that these are estimates only. Obviously, in practice it would be difficult to run a deficit of *exactly* 500 calories per day for weeks on end. We all tend to underestimate what we eat to a degree; we all miss our workouts on occasion; and we all have slightly different metabolisms. And when winter hits, there go our brisk walks. So don't drive yourself crazy counting every single calorie. Just set the idea of energy balance firmly in your mind and aim for a calorie deficit of between 500 and 1,000 calories a day through a combination of less input and more output. It will involve some trial and error, but for most women starting at a calorie level of 1,000 to 1,200 calories per day, exercising for a calorie burn of at least 150 calories daily (say, half an hour of brisk walking) will result in healthy weight loss. For most men, 1,400 to 1,600 calories a day is a good place to start. Adjust the numbers up or down depending on how it's going —the rate you're losing or not losing weight. You will also have to readjust your calorie input every few weeks as your weight loss progresses. As you lose weight you will become more energy efficient and lose fewer calories. Every ten pounds of weight loss is a good time to recalculate your food intake.

Keeping Track–Useful Tools

One great way to keep track of all this—especially in the beginning as you're forming new habits—is to keep a daily journal noting what you ate, your activities, your feelings and goals, and your energy balance. On pages 180–81 we show an example of what this journal might look like. You can make your own chart or photocopy ours. You'll find it an effective tool. (Calorie amounts and CD ratings for specific foods are found in the Caloric Density Index on page 59.)

Another way of keeping tabs is by using a personal CD pyramid like the one on page 180. It's ideal when combined with your journal record. It's set up like our regular CD pyramid, with low-CD featherweight foods at the bottom, lightweights and middleweights in the center, and the heavyweights at the top. Just check the pyramid boxes as you go or at the end of the day to remind yourself how many servings from each tier you've had. It's a terrific way to get accustomed to thinking in terms of caloric-density categories. You can check the CD Serving Guide below to see approximately how many servings from each category you should eat according to your calorie input level (which you just tallied). You'll know you're heading in the right direction when you see most of your checks in the featherweight and lightweight categories. (Because featherweights have so few calories, you can pretty much eat them to your heart's content. And when you eat a lot of them, you'll tend to eat less of the other foods.)

The easiest tracking method of all is to simply photocopy the Caloric Density Pyramid (page 58) and stick it to your fridge as a reminder to eat three-fourths of your foods from the featherweight and lightweight categories and one-quarter from the other categories. No muss, no fuss, and the pounds will still melt away.

CD Serving Guide

	Calorie Input Level						
Category	1000	1200	1400	1600	1800	2000	2200
Featherweights	4 or more	5 or more	5 or more	6 or more	6 or more	7 or more	7 or more
Lightweights	4	4	5	5	7	7	8
Middleweights	2	3	3	4	4	5	5
Heavyweights	1/2	1/2	1	1	1	1	1½

*Note: There will be some water loss and lean body mass (muscle) loss in any weight-loss plan. To minimize this, we recommend you plan for no more than three pounds per week fat loss and plan an intake of at least 1,000 calories per day for women and 1,400 calories per day for men.

Your Fitness Program

A good health program helps you maintain hydration and lose stored fat while maintaining as much lean body mass (muscle) as possible. It has to include a balanced eating pattern—which, of course, we've discussed—and a well-rounded program of physical activity that includes some strength training. Physical activity boosts metabolic rate and burns calories; strength training plays an important role in building and preserving muscle as you burn fat; and weight-bearing activities such as walking help to maintain and improve bone density.

WHAT YOU NEED TO KNOW ABOUT BODY FAT

Lean body mass. Lean body mass is commonly used to describe the muscles in your arms, legs, back, neck, and abdomen. But the term also includes your heart muscle and the tissues of your other internal organs as well as water and bone. This is the part of your body you want to preserve or expand. The amount of lean body mass you have is the most important factor in determining your metabolism (the rate at which you burn calories). The higher the amount of lean body mass in your body, the higher your metabolic rate and the more calories you'll burn when you are sitting or lying down. So a nice, high metabolic rate makes it easier to lose weight and maintain weight loss.[5]

Long-term calorie burn (muscle strengthening and toning). A regular program of resistance training, or strength training, helps you preserve lean muscle, tone your muscles, and ultimately lose less muscle as you are dropping fat pounds. Strength training exercises include either working out with weights (free weights or machines) or doing exercises that involve using your own body weight against itself, such as push-ups, lunges, sit-ups, and dips. Muscle-building exercises like these are important because muscles burn more calories than fat. Even after you're finished with your workout, your muscles will still be burning calories! Resistance training also strengthens your bones (thereby preventing osteoporosis) and helps sculpt your body. Try to do it two or three times a week for twenty to sixty minutes (include a five- to ten-minute warm-up and cool-down period.) Recent research has shown that as little as one set of eight to ten repetitions per major body part results in significant gains in strength and muscle tone.[6] A little bit goes a long way. Although we adults gain both lean body mass and storage fat when we put on weight, the amount of fat gained usually far exceeds the amount of lean body mass gained. The exception: when we're involved in a training program specifically aimed at increasing muscle mass. Think of resistance training as a necessary part of resisting age-related muscle loss and the sag of gravity.

Immediate body fat burn (cardio). When you combine resistance training with at least thirty minutes of aerobic (cardio) exercise three to four times per week, you're set. Pick a cardio exercise you like. It could be brisk walking, jogging, riding a stationary bike, swimming, tennis, or even dancing. You can vary your cardio workouts for variety—a walk on Monday, tennis on Wednesday, and dancing Friday night. The trick is to choose activities you can do easily most days of the week, that you'll look forward to, and that will get your heart pumping—that means exercising with enough intensity to sweat. See the Target Heart Rate table on page 182 to gauge your exercise intensity.

Weight Loss Winners

A recent project recruited 784 individuals (629 women, 155 men) for the National Weight Control Registry (NWCR), the largest database of individuals who have successfully achieved prolonged weight loss. Criteria for NWCR membership are that participants be eighteen years or older and that they have maintained weight loss of at least 30 pounds for one year or longer. Participants averaged 66 pounds of weight loss, and 14 percent lost more than 100 pounds. Members maintained the required minimum 30-pound weight loss for a 5.5-year average.

About half of the NWCR members used either a formal program or professional assistance to lose weight; the rest succeeded on their own. Regarding weight-loss methods, 89 percent modified food intake and maintained relatively high levels of physical activity (2,800 kcal weekly on average) to achieve target weight loss. Only 10 percent relied solely on diet, and 1 percent used exercise exclusively. The diet strategy of nearly 90 percent of participants restricted intake of certain types and/or amounts of foods—44 percent counted calories, 33 percent limited fat intake. Forty-four percent ate the same foods they normally ate but in reduced amounts (see table). Note the lack of use of low-carb diets.

The Key Points

- 80 percent of the subjects are women; average age is 45 years
- 90 percent of the subjects had been unsuccessful in past weight-loss attempts
- 50 percent were overweight as children and most had overweight parents
- Average weight loss was 66 pounds
- Subjects have maintained that loss for more than 5.5 years on average
- 90 percent modified both diet and exercise
- Three common strategies were employed:
  1. Diet moderate in fat, protein, and carbohydrates (equivalent to Unified Dietary Guidelines)
  2. Regular physical activity
  3. Frequent self-monitoring

Comparative Lifestyle of NWCR Members and Okinawa Elders

Group	Calories/day	Carbs	Protein	Fat	Main Exercise
Okinawan elders	1358/day	57%	17%	25%	Walking
NWCR	1381/day	56%	19%	24%	Walking

Specific Dietary Principles

- Low-calorie (CR) diet with energy balance
- Macronutrient balance (no restriction of any single macronutrient)
- Fewer than 1 percent ate a low-carb diet
- Those who ate a low-carb diet (fewer than 24 percent calories as carbs) were less physically active and maintained the loss for a shorter time
- Most averaged five meals a day (grazed rather than gorged)
- Most ate at restaurants fewer than three times a week; most ate at fast-food outlets less than once a week

Activity Strategies

- 91 percent used exercise to assist them with weight loss and maintenance
- For exercise, women burned 2,545 calories a week and men 3,293 calories a week (equivalent to walking 20 to 30 miles a week)
- Most increased both regular activity (e.g., climbed more stairs) and regularly structured exercise
- 77 percent used walking as main exercise
- 20 percent engaged in weight training

Monitoring Strategies

- Most monitored their diets (calories) regularly, especially if they noticed weight gain
- Three quarters weighed themselves daily or weekly

Failure (Weight Regain) Triggers

- Increased fat intake
- Decreased physical activity, by average 800 calories per week
- Reduced self-monitoring

1. What I Ate   **Date:**_____

	FOOD	FOOD GROUP	AMOUNT	CD PYRAMID SERVING	CALORIES
BREAKFAST					
SNACK					
LUNCH					
SNACK					
DINNER & LOW-CAL DESSERT					
TOTAL					

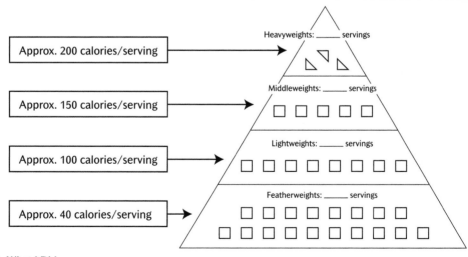

Approx. 200 calories/serving → Heavyweights: _____ servings

Approx. 150 calories/serving → Middleweights: _____ servings

Approx. 100 calories/serving → Lightweights: _____ servings

Approx. 40 calories/serving → Featherweights: _____ servings

2. What I Did

Today's Exercise: _____ Minutes: _____ Calories Burned: _____

3. What I Thought

Thoughts and Goals: _____

Today's Energy Balance: Input _____ - Output (_____ + _____) = _____

Baseline Burn   Exercise Burn   GOAL = -500 to 1,000

1. What I Ate   Example: 140-pound female computer programmer.   **Date:** June 16

	FOOD	FOOD GROUP	AMOUNT	CD PYRAMID SERVING	CALORIES
BREAKFAST	Ryukyu Scrambled Eggs II (page 286)	Feather	1 serving	2	81
	Whole Grain Toast	Middle	2 toast	2	160
	Jasmine Tea		1 cup	0	0
SNACK	Oatmeal Cookie, Fat-Free	Heavy	1 ounce	0.5	92
	Green Tea		1 cup	0	0
LUNCH	Pita Bread with Hummus	Middle	1 pita/ 2 tbsp. hummus	2	192
	Vegetable Soup, Fat-Free	Feather	1 cup	2	80
	Pear	Feather	1	2	98
	Jasmine Tea		1 cup	0	0
SNACK	Yogurt, fat-free	Feather	6 ounces	2	95
	Green Tea		1 cup	0	0
DINNER & LOW-CAL DESSERT	Miso Salmon with Vegetables (page 265)	Feather	1 serving	4	188
	Garden Greens with Balsamic Vinaigrette (page 218)	Feather	1 serving	1	26
	Side Pasta with Tomato Sauce	Light	½ cup	1	100
	October Pumpkin Soufflé (page 343)	Light	1 serving	1.5	144
	Jasmine Tea		1 cup	0	0
TOTAL					1,256

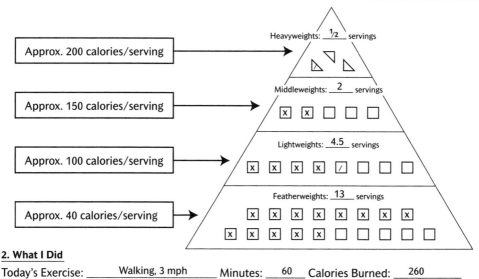

2. What I Did

Today's Exercise: _____Walking, 3 mph_____ Minutes: ___60___ Calories Burned: ___260___

3. What I Thought

Thoughts and Goals: ___Felt recharged after my walk; waist looks slimmer! Yea!___

Today's Energy Balance: Input _____1,256_____ - Output (__1,680__ + __260__) = ___- 684___

Baseline Burn*   Exercise Burn   GOAL = -500 to 1,000

*Baseline burn: 140-pound woman x 12 calories = 1,680 calories (see page 172 for details).

Target heart rate. To make the most of your workouts, you need to know how hard to work. Contrary to popular belief, more is not always better. Check your pulse during a workout to find the point at which you maximize calorie burn and get your heart pumping.

Target Heart Rate

Age	% Allowable Maximum				
	60%	70%	75%	80%	85%
Under 20	21	25	26	28	30
20	20	23	25	27	28
25	20	23	24	26	28
30	19	22	24	25	27
35	19	22	23	25	26
40	18	21	23	24	26
45	18	21	22	23	25
50	17	20	21	23	24
55	17	19	21	22	23
60	16	19	20	21	22
65	16	18	19	21	22
70	15	18	19	20	21
75	15	17	18	19	21

1. Choose either your carotid or radial artery to check your pulse (carotid artery is just to either side of the center of your neck; radial artery is your wrist). Apply light pressure with your fingers, but don't use your thumb.

2. Count the beats you feel in 10 seconds.

3. Refer to the table to see if you're within your proper training range.

LOSE FAT, NOT WEIGHT

When you lose weight, you lose water, other lean body mass (mostly muscle), and storage fat. To replace lost water, it's important to maintain proper hydration. From a health and metabolic standpoint, it's better to preserve as much lean body mass as possible as you reduce your body fat. Experts have determined that during the early weeks of weight loss, at least 75 percent of the weight you lose should be fat and not more than 25 percent should come from lean body mass. As you continue to lose weight, especially if you do regular weight-bearing exercises, about 90 percent of the weight lost should be fat and only 10 percent should come from lean body mass. Low-carb dieters tend to lose only about 35 percent of their weight as fat (see table below). One recent study showed that those who performed aerobic exercise *and* weight training while dieting lost 97 percent of their "weight" as body fat.[5]

Type of Weight Loss on Moderate vs. Low-Carbohydrate Diets

Diet	Type of Weight Loss (%)		
	Water	Fat	Protein
Moderate carbohydrate (45% carbs)	37.1%	59.0%	3.9%
Low carbohydrate (5% carb—e.g., Atkins' Diet)	61.1%	34.8%	4.1%

Note: The problem with low-carbohydrate diets is that most of the weight loss is essential water. Low-carb diets also cause more protein loss, whereas on the more healthy moderate carbohydrate diets you lose mainly fat. These results are based on a study of human volunteers who followed the diets for approximately six weeks. See Yang, M., and Van Itallie. *J. Clin Invest* 1976; 58:722–30.

To chart your progress, we recommend you track your body fat percentage as well as your weight, as it tells you how much fat you're losing in relation to water or muscle and gives you a more precise method for goal-setting.[7] Although you can approximate your body fat with body mass index (BMI; see Figure 1.2, page 6), an even easier way is with a BIA (bioelectrical impedance analysis) scale, which makes tallying body fat as easy as pushing a button.[8] BIA scales are available online and in sports and department stores. BIA works by sending a very low-level electrical signal through your body when you stand on the foot sensors. The signal travels quickly through lean tissue (muscle), which has a high percentage of water and thus conducts electricity well, and more slowly through fat, which has a lower percentage of water. A validated equation calculates your body fat, based on sex, height, weight, and a fat standard. The standard may vary somewhat depending on your ethnicity and whether or not you are highly athletic. Because the electrical signal varies with your hydration status, whether you have just exercised (perspiration conducts better), if you are wearing clothing, and the time of day, try to keep the conditions the same when you measure yourself and look at weekly trends rather than daily differences.

We all need some essential body fat for healthy functioning. In men, essential fat (as opposed to storage fat) is approximately 2–4 percent of body weight; in women, it's about 10–12 percent.[8] So that's a good base to remember. A good, prudent body fat number to aim for is between 10 and 20 percent for men and 15 and 25 percent for women (see figure 6.1). If you stay within those numbers, you should be in excellent shape. As we get older, we tend to have more fat—although as you've seen with the Okinawans, it's not inevitable. Trained

Figure 6.1

HEALTHY BODY FAT RANGES FOR ADULTS

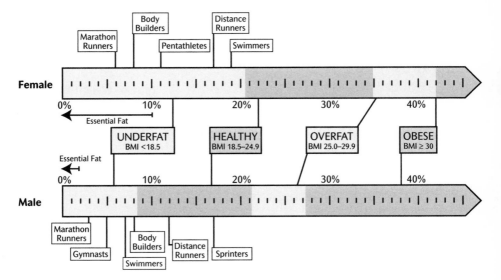

Note: There is much that is still unknown about body fat levels, health, and longevity, particularly at the lower ranges. As seen in this figure, a BMI of less than 18.5 is considered underfat by most expert bodies, including the WHO, yet many athletes, who are quite healthy, are below these ranges. Studies on caloric restriction (CR) also show that CR animals achieve exceptionally low body fat levels, which may be one of the reasons for their exceptional longevity. Based on Clinical Guidelines on the Identification, Evaluation, and Treatment of Overweight and Obesity in Adults, NIH, 1998. Gallagher et al. *Am J Clin Nutr* 2000; 72: 694–701.

competitive athletes, of course, have a lot less. Most experts start to get nervous when body fat falls below what is commonly considered "essential storage levels," and menstrual irregularities occur more often when levels dip below about 15 percent, although this is highly individual. For most of us, we dare say, the danger is in too much fat rather than in too little.

CHART YOUR PROGRESS

It may take you several weeks or months to reach your goal, and there may be roadblocks along the way. To stay motivated, keep a record of your progress in a notebook, calendar, or your personalized energy balance chart. When you start to feel discouraged because you're *still* not where you want to be, or because you've slipped up, look over your notes and take pride in the progress you have made. Rome wasn't built in a day. And don't forget to make notes about the smart choices you made at the grocery store, or how you ate only one Oreo instead of a whole bag, or how you went to two aerobics classes *and* took a hike in the forest. Ignore the obstacles and give yourself credit for each little successful step. All those little steps ultimately add up to a successful journey.

Chapter 7

THREE DIET MENU PLANS: THE OKINAWAN/EASTERN, EAST-WEST FUSION, AND WESTERN TRACKS

Starting something new—especially a new diet or a new way of eating—can be overwhelming. To make it as easy as possible for you, we've created three low-CD eating plans, complete with vegetarian alternatives. Each provides meal suggestions for two weeks, and all the recipes are in the chapter immediately following the plans. We think of these menu plans like training wheels on a bike. They ease you into a new skill and help you adjust to a new way of balancing your meals. They make new food concepts easy. After a few weeks of following the plans, you'll have enough experience to take off the training wheels and continue confidently on your culinary journey.

Which of the three plans you decide to follow is entirely up to you—and your taste buds and spirit of adventure. Each track is tilted toward a particular eating style. The Okinawan/Eastern track reflects a more traditional Okinawan diet sprinkled with Japanese and other Asian styles and is best suited for the more adventuresome palate. If you're used to Asian cooking or want to be daring and try something entirely new, this one is great fun. The East-West Fusion track, as the name suggests, is a blend of Eastern and Western cooking styles. It's similar to the fusion style that's so popular in Hawaii and California and is most like the Okinawan elders' current diet. If you're used to eating Western food but enjoy eating out in Japanese, Thai, Chinese, or other Asian restaurants occasionally, you'll love this one. The Western track is most like U.S. fare; it features more lean meat dishes (without overdoing it) and more familiar ingredients. It's designed for those of you who want to follow the basic principles of healthy low-CD eating but are still a little tenuous about leaving all your old habits behind. The Western track allows you to dip your toes in while remaining safely on shore.

Needless to say, you can switch between tracks whenever the mood hits you. If you start with the Western track and really start to enjoy the new tastes (which we know you will), you can try a meal or two from the Fusion track—or even get brave and swing over to the Okinawan track. And if you ever want to substitute for a particular recipe, you can also use the recipe index in Appendix B (page 367) to select another option with a similar caloric value.

Whichever track you choose, if you stay within the plans, you'll get slimmer— and healthier. Each plan is geared toward a weight loss of two or three pounds a week if you simply follow the plan and don't calculate calories (although there will be individual variations). Each plan is set at a base of about 1,000 calories a day; this can be ramped up according to your activity levels and unique needs. (Each meal provides about 300 calories; snacks are about 100 calories. Where specific dishes are given, we intend one serving, which you can determine from the recipe yield.) You can add any foods or snacks to bring you up to your desired level. If you plan on eating about 1,400 calories a day, for instance, simply add 400 calories to the base plan.

Before you get on track, of course, you'll have to go shopping for the proper ingredients. A pantry list follows with all the specific ingredients called for in the recipes. That truly can be part of the adventure—especially if you've never been to a good natural foods store or an Asian market. Then we've provided a list of easy snack ideas, which includes their caloric density and other nutritional information. You can use this list whenever the menu plans call for a low-calorie snack. A whole new world is about to open to you—in the stores, in your kitchen, and at your table.

The Okinawa Diet Pantry

Essential Staples	Where to Find
Grains, beans, and nuts	
Brown rice, medium grain	Regular grocers or health food stores
Soba buckwheat noodles, dry	Health food stores and Asian food stores
Whole-wheat spaghetti	Regular grocers and health food stores
Buckwheat flour	Regular grocers and health food stores
Whole-wheat flour	Regular grocers
All-purpose, unbleached flour	Regular grocers

Flax seeds	Health food stores
Walnuts and almonds (raw, unsalted)	Regular grocers and health food stores
Peanuts, raw, unsalted	Regular grocers and health food stores
White sesame seeds	International food section of regular grocers and Asian food stores

Dried vegetables

Wakame seaweed, dried flakes	International food section of regular grocers and Asian food stores
Kombu seaweed, or kelp, dried strips	Health food stores and Asian food stores
Nori seaweed, or laver, dried sheets (unseasoned, unoiled)	Health food stores and Asian food stores
Shiitake mushrooms, dried	Health food stores and Asian food stores

Flavorings, condiments, and oils

Rice vinegar	International food section of regular grocers and Asian food stores
Apple cider or white wine vinegar	Regular grocers
Balsamic vinegar	Regular grocers
Soy sauce, low-sodium	International food section of regular grocers, health food stores and Asian food stores
Miso, white	International food section of regular grocers and Asian food stores
Sake rice wine (no color, clear)	International food section of regular grocers and Asian food stores
Mirin sweet rice wine (light yellow, clear)	International food section of regular grocers and Asian food stores
White and red wine (do not buy "cooking wine" due to its high sodium content)	Regular grocers and liquor stores
Soy or canola mayonnaise, low-fat	Some large grocers or health food stores
Dijon mustard	Regular grocers
Turbinado or brown sugar	Regular grocers or health food stores
Kudzu powder or arrowroot powder	International food section of regular grocers and Asian food stores
Agar-agar powder or flakes	Health food stores and Asian food stores
Bonito flakes, dried, or bonito powder (choose non-MSG if bonito powder)	International food section of regular grocers and Asian food stores

Vegetable bouillon, low-sodium, or vegetable broth, low-sodium	Regular grocers and health food stores
Chicken broth, low-fat, low-sodium	Regular grocers or health food stores
Sea salt	Regular grocers or health food stores
Turmeric, ground	Regular grocers
Ground cinnamon	Regular grocers
Cayenne pepper	Regular grocers
Cumin seeds, dried	Regular grocers
Red chili flakes	Regular grocers
Chili powder	Regular grocers
Vanilla beans	Regular grocers
Canola oil, nonstick spray	Regular grocers
Canola oil	Regular grocers
Olive oil, spray	Regular grocers
Olive oil	Regular grocers

Teas

Green tea powder or matcha	International food section of regular grocers or Japanese food stores
Green tea (loose or tea bag)	International food section of regular grocers and Asian food stores
Jasmine tea (loose or tea bag)	International food section of regular grocers and Asian food stores
Black tea (decaf if you prefer)	Regular grocers

Prepared, ready-to-eat healthy foods

Vegetarian burgers	Regular grocers and health food stores
Fat-free or low-fat vegetable soups and bean soups	Regular grocers and health food stores
Cereals with more than 3 grams of fiber per serving, preferably multigrain	Regular grocers and health food stores
Vegetarian bean burritos	Regular grocers and health food stores

Perishables

Eggs, free-range, omega-3	Regular grocers and health food stores
Tofu, water-packed, firm-lite, or silken	Regular grocers, health food stores, and Asian food stores
Konnyaku yam cake	Some large grocers and Asian food stores
Daikon white radish	Some large grocers and Asian food stores

Edamame green soybeans, frozen (with or without pods)	Frozen-food section of regular grocers, health food stores, and Asian food stores
Shiitake mushrooms	Regular grocers, health food stores, and Asian food stores
Bananas	Regular grocers
Bitter melon	Asian food stores
Garlic	Regular grocers
Ginger	Regular grocers
Green onions (scallions)	Regular grocers
Lemon, lime	Regular grocers
Mung or soybean sprouts	Regular grocers
Spinach	Regular grocers
Strawberries	Regular grocers
Tomato	Regular grocers

Easy Low-Cal Snack Suggestions

Protein

Soy Cheese, 1 slice (28 g)	Caloric Density 2.5; Calories 69; Protein 3; Carbohydrate 7; Fat 4
Cottage Cheese, 2% fat, 1/4 cup	Caloric Density 0.9; Calories 51; Protein 8; Carbohydrate 2; Fat 1
Cream Cheese, fat-free, 2 tablespoons	Caloric Density 1.0; Calories 29; Protein 4; Carbohydrate 2; Fat 0
Feta Cheese, 1 ounce	Caloric Density 2.6; Calories 74; Protein 4; Carbohydrate 1; Fat 6
Yogurt, plain, nonfat, 1 6-ounce container	Caloric Density 0.6; Calories 95; Protein 10; Carbohydrate 13; Fat 0
Soy yogurt	Caloric Density 0.7; Calories 112; Protein 4; Carbohydrate 18; Fat 3
Soymilk, plain, 3/4 cup	Caloric Density 0.5; Calories 105; Protein 5; Carbohydrate 14; Fat 3
Soymilk, vanilla, light, 3/4 cup	Caloric Density 0.5; Calories 90; Protein 2; Carbohydrate 16; Fat 2
Milk, low-fat, 3/4 cup	Caloric Density 0.4; Calories 77; Protein 6; Carbohydrate 9; Fat 2
Milk, skim, 3/4 cup	Caloric Density 0.4; Calories 64; Protein 6; Carbohydrate 9; Fat 0
Cream Cheese and Tofu Dip, 1 serving; 2 tablespoons silken tofu and 1 tablespoon fat-free cream cheese	Caloric Density 0.5; Calories 24; Protein 4; Carbohydrate 1; Fat 1
Diced Tofu for soups, 1/3 cup small cubes	Caloric Density 0.5; Calories 40; Protein 6; Carbohydrate 0; Fat 1
Soy Sausage, 1 sausage (60 g)	Caloric Density 1.2; Calories 71; Protein 14; Carbohydrate 3; Fat 1

Tuna, canned in water,
2 tablespoons   Caloric Density 0.7; Calories 15; Protein 5; Carbohydrate 0; Fat 0

Turkey Ham, 1 slice (1 oz)   Caloric Density 1.3; Calories 36; Protein 5; Carbohydrate 1; Fat 1

Fruits

Apple, 1 medium   Caloric Density 0.6; Calories 81; Protein 0; Carbohydrate 21; Fat 1

Applesauce, unsweetened,
½ cup   Caloric Density 0.8; Calories 97; Protein 0; Carbohydrate 25; Fat 0

Apricots, 4 apricots   Caloric Density 0.5; Calories 67; Protein 1; Carbohydrate 16; Fat 1

Banana, ½ banana   Caloric Density 0.9; Calories 54; Protein 1; Carbohydrate 14; Fat 0

Fig, Fresh, 2 figs   Caloric Density 0.7; Calories 74; Protein 1; Carbohydrate 19; Fat 0

Frozen Fruit or Juice Bar, 1 bar Caloric Density 0.8; Calories 75; Protein 1; Carbohydrate 19; Fat 0

Fruit Cocktail, canned in juice,
½ cup   Caloric Density 0.5; Calories 55; Protein 1; Carbohydrate 14; Fat 0

Fruit Salad, 1 cup, ¼ cup canta-
loupe, honeydew, orange, grape   Caloric Density 0.4; Calories 66; Protein 1; Carbohydrate 17; Fat 0

Grapefruit, ½ grapefruit   Caloric Density 0.3; Calories 37; Protein 1; Carbohydrate 9; Fat 0

Mango, ½ mango   Caloric Density 0.7; Calories 67; Protein 1; Carbohydrate 18; Fat 0

Melon Balls, frozen, 1 cup   Caloric Density 0.3; Calories 57; Protein 2; Carbohydrate 14; Fat 0

Orange, 1 orange   Caloric Density 0.5; Calories 62; Protein 1; Carbohydrate 15; Fat 0

Papaya, ½ papaya   Caloric Density 0.4; Calories 59; Protein 1; Carbohydrate 15; Fat 0

Peaches, canned in juice, ½ cup   Caloric Density 0.4; Calories 55; Protein 1; Carbohydrate 14; Fat 0

Pear, 1 pear   Caloric Density 0.6; Calories 98; Protein 1; Carbohydrate 25; Fat 1

Pineapple Chunks, canned in
juice, ½ cup   Caloric Density 0.6; Calories 70; Protein 0; Carbohydrate 17; Fat 0

Plum, 2 plums   Caloric Density 0.6; Calories 73; Protein 1; Carbohydrate 17; Fat 1

Strawberries, 1 cup   Caloric Density 0.3; Calories 50; Protein 1; Carbohydrate 12; Fat 1

Tangerine, 1 tangerine   Caloric Density 0.4; Calories 37; Protein 1; Carbohydrate 9; Fat 0

Vegetables

Asparagus, 1 cup boiled
or steamed   Caloric Density 0.2; Calories 43; Protein 5; Carbohydrate 8; Fat 1

Baby Carrots, 8 carrots   Caloric Density 0.4; Calories 30; Protein 1; Carbohydrate 7; Fat 0

Baby Sweet Corn, whole,
canned, 3 ounces baby corn
with 1 teaspoon brown mustard   Caloric Density 0.6; Calories 50; Protein 3; Carbohydrate 8; Fat 1

Baked Sweet Potato, ⅓ cup   Caloric Density 1.0; Calories 69; Protein 1; Carbohydrate 16; Fat 0

Bean Sprouts, ¾ cup steamed
with 1 tablespoon Thai
peanut sauce   Caloric Density 0.6; Calories 54; Protein 4; Carbohydrate 8; Fat 1

Bell Peppers, ½ cup raw,
chopped   Caloric Density 0.3; Calories 20; Protein 1; Carbohydrate 5; Fat 0

Broccoli, ½ cup raw   Caloric Density 0.3; Calories 12; Protein 1; Carbohydrate 2; Fat 0

Brussels Sprouts, ½ cup
boiled or steamed   Caloric Density 0.4; Calories 30; Protein 2; Carbohydrate 7; Fat 0

Cabbage, ¾ cup shredded   Caloric Density 0.3; Calories 17; Protein 1; Carbohydrate 4; Fat 0

Cauliflower, ½ cup raw   Caloric Density 0.3; Calories 13; Protein 1; Carbohydrate 3; Fat 0

Celery, 3 small stalks   Caloric Density 0.2; Calories 14; Protein 1; Carbohydrate 3; Fat 0

Cucumber, ½ cucumber   Caloric Density 0.1; Calories 17; Protein 1; Carbohydrate 4; Fat 0

Hawaii Mountain Yam or
Taro, ¾ cup, steamed   Caloric Density 0.8; Calories 89; Protein 2; Carbohydrate 22; Fat 0

Lentil and Carrot Soup,
canned, fat-free, 1 cup   Caloric Density 0.4; Calories 100; Protein 10; Carbohydrate 25; Fat 0

Sugar Snap Peas, 1 cup boiled
or steamed with 1 teaspoon
soy mayonnaise   Caloric Density 0.5; Calories 79; Protein 5; Carbohydrate 12; Fat 2

Radish, 1 cup   Caloric Density 0.2; Calories 23; Protein 1; Carbohydrate 4; Fat 1

Tomato Juice, no salt, 1 cup   Caloric Density 0.2; Calories 41; Protein 2; Carbohydrate 10; Fat 0

Vegetable Soup, fat-free, 1 cup   Caloric Density 0.3; Calories 80; Protein 6; Carbohydrate 17; Fat 0

Yellow Sweet Corn, boiled,
½ cup   Caloric Density 1.1; Calories 89; Protein 3; Carbohydrate 21; Fat 1

Grains

Bagel, Whole-Wheat, with
Cream Cheese, ½ bagel with
1 tablespoon fat-free
cream cheese   Caloric Density 1.7; Calories 100; Protein 5; Carbohydrate 20; Fat 1

Bread, Whole-Wheat, Garlic,
1 slice (28 g) bread, 2 sprays
olive oil, rubbed with garlic   Caloric Density 2.8; Calories 80; Protein 2; Carbohydrate 14; Fat 2

Cream of Wheat Cereal, ¾ cup
cooked with water   Caloric Density 0.4; Calories 82; Protein 2; Carbohydrate 17; Fat 0

English Muffin, Whole-Wheat,
with Egg, ½ muffin with
1 cooked egg white   Caloric Density 1.3; Calories 84; Protein 6; Carbohydrate 13; Fat 1

English Muffin, Whole-Wheat,
with Jam, ½ muffin with
1 teaspoon fruit preserves   Caloric Density 2.2; Calories 86; Protein 3; Carbohydrate 18; Fat 1

Pasta, Whole-Wheat, with
Tomato Sauce, ½ cup cooked
pasta, 1½ tablespoons sauce   Caloric Density 1.1; Calories 100; Protein 4; Carbohydrate 20; Fat 1

Pita Bread, Whole-Wheat, with
Hummus, ½ pita bread,
1 tablespoon hummus, ¼ cup
alfalfa sprouts, 1 slice tomato   Caloric Density 1.3; Calories 96; Protein 5; Carbohydrate 18; Fat 2

Pumpernickel Toast, 1 slice
with 1 teaspoon apricot jam   Caloric Density 2.5; Calories 96; Protein 3; Carbohydrate 20; Fat 1

Brown Rice Cakes, plain,
low-sodium, 2 rice cakes
(9 g each)   Caloric Density 3.8; Calories 70; Protein 2; Carbohydrate 15; Fat 1

Tortilla, Whole-Wheat, fat-free,
with vegetables, 1 fat-free
tortilla (37 g), 2 teaspoons soy
mayonnaise, 1 cup shredded
romaine lettuce, ¼ cup
diced tomato   Caloric Density 0.7; Calories 100; Protein 3; Carbohydrate 16; Fat 3

Salty

Feta Cheese with Lettuce,
1 ounce cheese with 1½ cups
romaine lettuce   Caloric Density 0.8; Calories 89; Protein 5; Carbohydrate 3; Fat 6

Hummus, 1 tablespoon   Caloric Density 1.7; Calories 24; Protein 1; Carbohydrate 3; Fat 1

Lentil and Carrot Soup,
canned, fat-free, 1 cup   Caloric Density 0.4; Calories 100; Protein 10; Carbohydrate 25; Fat 0

Turkey, Roasted, with
Cranberry Sauce, 2 small pieces
(1¼ oz) with 1 tablespoon
cranberry sauce   Caloric Density 1.6; Calories 97; Protein 13; Carbohydrate 7; Fat 2

Turkey Ham with Endive,
2 slices (1 oz each) turkey
ham with 1 cup endive   Caloric Density 0.6; Calories 88; Protein 12; Carbohydrate 4; Fat 3

Vegetarian Chili, canned,
½ cup   Caloric Density 0.7; Calories 85; Protein 7; Carbohydrate 15; Fat 1

Whole-Wheat Herb Crackers,
fat-free, 8 crackers (6 g each)   Caloric Density 1.8; Calories 80; Protein 3; Carbohydrate 18; Fat 0

Sweets

Chocolate Soy Ice Cream, ⅓ cup	Caloric Density 1.5; Calories 87; Protein 1; Carbohydrate 15; Fat 3
Fig Bar, Whole-Wheat, fat-free, 1 bar (19 g)	Caloric Density 3.2; Calories 60; Protein 1; Carbohydrate 13; Fat 0
Gelatin, low-cal, sugar-free, 1 cup with ¼ cup strawberries	Caloric Density 0.1; Calories 32; Protein 2; Carbohydrate 3; Fat 0
Italian Ice or Gelato, with Fruit, ½ cup	Caloric Density 0.5; Calories 61; Protein 0; Carbohydrate 16; Fat 0
Oatmeal Cookie, fat-free, 1 ounce	Caloric Density 3.3; Calories 92; Protein 2; Carbohydrate 22; Fat 0

Creamy

Cream of Broccoli or Mushroom Soup, fat-free, ½ can condensed, prepared with 1 cup water	Caloric Density 0.2; Calories 80; Protein 2; Carbohydrate 12; Fat 3
Frozen Yogurt with Fruit, fat-free, ½ cup	Caloric Density 1.0; Calories 100; Protein 3; Carbohydrate 23; Fat 0
Peach Ice Cream, nonfat, ½ cup	Caloric Density 1.5; Calories 100; Protein 3; Carbohydrate 22; Fat 0
Yogurt, plain, nonfat, 1 6-ounce container	Caloric Density 0.6; Calories 95; Protein 10; Carbohydrate 13; Fat 0

Drinks

Café Latte, 1 shot espresso with 6 ounces 2% milk	Caloric Density 0.4; Calories 92; Protein 6; Carbohydrate 9; Fat 4
Café Mocha, 2 teaspoons thin chocolate syrup, 1 shot espresso, and 6 ounces skim milk	Caloric Density 0.4; Calories 93; Protein 7; Carbohydrate 17; Fat 0
Cocoa-Flavored Soymilk, ¾ cup	Caloric Density 0.5; Calories 90; Protein 2; Carbohydrate 17; Fat 1
Herbal Tea, sweetened, 1 cup	Caloric Density 0.3; Calories 70; Protein 0; Carbohydrate 17; Fat 0
Herbal Tea, unsweetened, 1 cup	Caloric Density <0.1; Calories 2; Protein 0; Carbohydrate 1; Fat 0
Hot Chocolate, fat-free mix prepared with 1 cup water	Caloric Density 0.2; Calories 50; Protein 4; Carbohydrate 9; Fat 0
Rice Drink, Vanilla, ¾ cup	Caloric Density 0.5; Calories 98; Protein 1; Carbohydrate 21; Fat 2
Tea Drink, Peach Flavor, 1 cup	Caloric Density 0.4; Calories 100; Protein 0; Carbohydrate 26; Fat 0
Tea, Green, sweetened, 1 cup	Caloric Density 0.3; Calories 70; Protein 0; Carbohydrate 18; Fat 0
Tea, Jasmine, Green or Black, unsweetened, 1 cup	Caloric Density <0.1; Calories 3; Protein 0; Carbohydrate 1; Fat 0
Tomato Juice, no salt, 1 cup	Caloric Density 0.2; Calories 41; Protein 2; Carbohydrate 10; Fat 0

The Okinawan/Eastern Track

For those who are already fans of Asian cuisine or who are more culinarily adventurous, here is where you will discover a delightful choice of Okinawan, Japanese, and other Asian dishes that are consistent with the healthy low–caloric density diet of traditional Okinawa. So dive in, enjoy, and watch the pounds melt away. Recipes for all dishes in boldface are provided in the next chapter. For low-cal snacks, choose any of the options on pages 189–193.

Nutrition Facts of the Week
Calories: 1033 • Protein: 62g • Carbohydrate: 170g • Fat: 16g

Monday

Breakfast	Lunch	Dinner
1/2 cup cooked brown rice **Basic Miso Soup (wakame potato)** jasmine tea	**Hijiki Brown Rice** **Shiri-Shiri Carrot and Bitter Melon** jasmine tea	**Spicy Tofu and Summer Vegetables (veg.)** *or* **Nsunaba Sukiyaki (beef)** **Cucumber and Wakame Vinaigrette** 1/2 cup cooked brown rice 1/2 papaya 2 tablespoons low-fat ice cream or soy ice cream jasmine or decaf tea
Mid-A.M. Snack 1 low-cal snack green tea	**Mid-P.M. Snack** 1 low-cal snack your favorite tea	

Tuesday

Breakfast	Lunch	Dinner
Soy Spinach Congee jasmine tea	**Goya Sushi Roll** jasmine tea	**Ginkgo-Tofu Supreme (veg.)** *or* **Hawaiian Lemon-Ahi Poke (fish)** **Nankwa Nbushi** 1/2 cup cooked brown rice **Fuchiba Nantu** jasmine or decaf tea
Mid-A.M. Snack 1 low-cal snack green tea	**Mid-P.M. Snack** 1 low-cal snack your favorite tea	

Wednesday

Breakfast	Lunch	Dinner
3 oz. silken tofu with low-sodium soy sauce **(veg.)** *or* **Grilled Fish with Grated Radish (fish)** 1/2 cup cooked brown rice 1 pear jasmine tea	**Fragrant Soy-Go Vegetable Soup** 1/2 cup cooked brown rice jasmine tea	**Teriyaki Tofu Fingers (veg.)** *or* **Walnut-Dressed Chicken (chicken)** **Cumin-Chili Cauliflower** 1/2 cup cooked brown rice 1/8 cantaloupe wedge 1/2 cup soy yogurt or low-fat plain yogurt jasmine or decaf tea
Mid-A.M. Snack 1 low-cal snack green tea	**Mid-P.M. Snack** 1 low-cal snack your favorite tea	

Thursday

Breakfast	Lunch	Dinner
½ cup cooked brown rice **Basic Miso Soup** (mustard greens) jasmine tea	**Soba Salad** **Basic Miso Soup** (wakame tofu) jasmine tea	**Asparagus Tofu Stir-Fry (veg.)** *or* **Pork Daikon (pork)** **Creamy Split Pea and Sweet Potato Soup** ½ cup cooked brown rice **Mochi on a Leaf**
Mid-A.M. Snack	**Mid-P.M. Snack**	jasmine or decaf tea
1 low-cal snack green tea	1 low-cal snack your favorite tea	

Friday

Breakfast	Lunch	Dinner
½ cup cooked brown rice **Gumbo à la Okinawa** jasmine tea	4 pieces of your favorite store-bought sushi (no egg sushi) 1 pear jasmine tea	**Yuki's Indian Tofu Curry (veg.)** *or* **Teriyaki Yellowtail with Rice (fish)** **Asian Okra and Tomato** 1 peach
Mid-A.M. Snack	**Mid-P.M. Snack**	2 tablespoons low-fat vanilla ice cream or soy ice cream
1 low-cal snack green tea	1 low-cal snack your favorite tea	jasmine or decaf tea

Saturday

Breakfast	Lunch	Dinner
½ cup cooked brown rice **Basic Miso Soup** (wakame tofu) jasmine tea	**Baby Bok-Choy Stir-Fry** ½ cup cooked soba noodle, served with bok-choy jasmine tea	**Goya Delight (veg.)** *or* **Chilled Chicken Wontons (chicken)** **Wakame Asparagusu** ½ cup cooked brown rice **Tapioca Sweet Potato Dessert**
Mid-A.M. Snack	**Mid-P.M. Snack**	jasmine or decaf tea
1 low-cal snack green tea	1 low-cal snack your favorite tea	

Sunday

Breakfast	Lunch	Dinner
Ogimi Village Sweet Potato Leaf Risotto Cantaloupe jasmine tea	**Snacking Pita Pizza (veg.)** *or* **Salmon with Nuts and Rice (fish)** jasmine tea	**Buddhist Temple Tofu (veg.)** *or* **Traditional Tsumire Soup (fish)** **Roasted Vegetables with Miso-Sesame Sauce** ½ cup cooked brown rice **Sweet Amagashi Beans**
Mid-A.M. Snack	**Mid-P.M. Snack**	jasmine or decaf tea
1 low-cal snack green tea	1 low-cal snack your favorite tea	

Monday

Breakfast	Lunch	Dinner
½ cup cooked brown rice **Basic Miso Soup (mustard greens)** jasmine tea **Mid-A.M. Snack** 1 low-cal snack green tea	**Baked Sweet Potatoes** jasmine tea **Mid-p.m. Snack** 1 low-cal snack your favorite tea	**Sloppy Veggie Tofu (veg.)** *or* **Sloppy Tofu with Beef (beef)** **Sautéed Shiitake and Konnyaku** ½ cup cooked brown rice 1 cup cantaloupe cubes sprinkled with 1 teaspoon lime juice ⅓ cup soy yogurt or low-fat plain yogurt jasmine or decaf tea

Tuesday

Breakfast	Lunch	Dinner
Soy Spinach Congee jasmine tea **Mid-A.M. Snack** 1 low-cal snack green tea	1 vegetarian noodle dish at your local Japanese or Chinese restaurant, with ½ cup noodles and plenty of vegetables jasmine tea **Mid-P.M. Snack** 1 low-cal snack your favorite tea	**Asparagus Tofu Stir-Fry (veg.)** *or* **Chicken and Peanut Stir-Fry in Oyster Sauce (chicken)** **Cucumber and Wakame Vinaigrette** ½ cup cooked brown rice 1 cup unsweetened fruit salad jasmine or decaf tea

Wednesday

Breakfast	Lunch	Dinner
½ cup cooked brown rice 1 sheet nori laver seaweed, cut into eighths ½ cup steamed spinach with ½ teaspoon low-sodium soy sauce jasmine tea **Mid-A.M. Snack** 1 low-cal snack green tea	**Fresh Tofu Spring Roll (veg.)** *or* **Papaya and Shrimp Spring Roll (seafood)** jasmine tea **Mid-P.M. Snack** 1 low-cal snack your favorite tea	**Sweet Potato Miso Soup (veg.)** *or* **Sea Bass Fennel Soup (fish)** **Gumbo à la Okinawa** ½ cup cooked brown rice **Sweet Potato Mousse with Green Tea Sauce** jasmine or decaf tea

Thursday

Breakfast	Lunch	Dinner
½ cup cooked brown rice	Soba Salad	Genmai Tea Shiitake Potato
Yuki's Yonaguni Pickles	1 orange	**Medley (veg.)** *or* **Pork Daikon**
3 ounces silken tofu block	jasmine tea	**(pork)**
with minced green onion and		**Asian Okra and Tomato**
½ teaspoon low-sodium soy	**Mid-P.M. Snack**	½ cup cooked brown rice
sauce	1 low-cal snack	½ papaya
jasmine tea	your favorite tea	2 tablespoons low-fat vanilla
Mid-A.M. Snack		ice cream or soy ice cream
1 low-cal snack		jasmine or decaf tea
green tea		

Friday

Breakfast	Lunch	Dinner
½ cup cooked brown rice	4 pieces of your favorite	**Soy-Sake Shiitake Mushroom**
Basic Miso Soup (wakame	store-bought sushi (no egg	**Steak (veg.)** with ½ cup
potato)	sushi)	cooked brown rice *or*
jasmine tea	1 apple	**Nasi Goreng Ayam (chicken)**
Mid-A.M. Snack	jasmine tea	**Shiri-Shiri Carrot and Bitter**
1 low-cal snack	**Mid-P.M. Snack**	**Melon**
green tea	1 low-cal snack	1 banana, halved lengthwise
	your favorite tea	and sprinkled with
		½ teaspoon brown sugar
		jasmine or decaf tea

Saturday

Breakfast	Lunch	Dinner
Basic Miso Soup, cooked with	**Sweet Potato Miso Soup**	**Fragrant Soy Go Vegetable**
½ cup cooked brown rice,	**(veg.)** *or* **Chicken Tom**	**Soup (veg.)** *or* **Salmon Miso**
crumbled silken tofu, and	**Yummy Goong (seafood)**	**Soup (fish)**
spinach	½ cup cooked brown rice	**Goya Delight**
jasmine tea	jasmine tea	½ cup cooked brown rice
Mid-A.M. Snack	**Mid-P.M. Snack**	**Darjeeling Pudding**
1 low-cal snack	1 low-cal snack	jasmine or decaf tea
green tea	your favorite tea	

Sunday

Breakfast	Lunch	Dinner
3 ounces silken tofu with	**Sprouts Stir-Fry**	**Buddhist Temple Tofu (veg.)**
low-sodium soy sauce **(veg.)**	½ cup cooked brown rice	*or* **Beef in Oyster Sauce**
or **Grilled Fish with Grated**	Fresh grapes	**(beef)**
Radish (fish)	jasmine tea	**Wakame Asparagusu**
½ cup cooked brown rice	**Mid-P.M. Snack**	**Dandelion Spring Rice**
1 pear	1 low-cal snack	**Mochi on a Leaf**
jasmine tea	your favorite tea	jasmine or decaf tea
Mid-A.M. Snack		
1 low-cal snack		
green tea		

The East-West Fusion Track

This is for the semi-adventurous. It is where East meets West, where healthy versions of scrambled eggs are equally at home with tofu and miso soup, and hearty granola meets delicate jasmine tea. After two weeks on this track your taste buds will be satisfied but your waistline noticeably smaller. Recipes for the bold-faced dishes appear in the following chapter. Select low-cal snacks from the list on pages 189–193.

Nutrition Facts of the Week
Calories: 1021 • Protein: 63g • Carbohydrate: 161g • Fat: 20g

Monday

Breakfast	Lunch	Dinner
Ryukyu Scrambled Eggs II	4 pieces of your favorite store-bought sushi (no egg sushi)	**Honey Mustard Tofu (veg.)** *or* **Simple and Easy Tandoori Chicken (chicken)**
1 slice whole-grain toast		
jasmine tea	1 apple	**Dandelion Spring Rice**
	jasmine tea	**Tropical Mango Pudding**
Mid-A.M. Snack		jasmine or decaf tea
1 low-cal snack	**Mid-P.M. Snack**	
green tea	1 low-cal snack	
	your favorite tea	

Tuesday

Breakfast	Lunch	Dinner
½ cup cooked brown rice	**Tofu and Veggie Pita Sandwich**	**Sloppy Veggie Tofu (veg.)** *or* **Ryukyu Fish Curry (fish)**
Basic Miso Soup (mustard greens)	jasmine tea	**Fava Beans and Tomato Salad**
jasmine tea	**Mid-P.M. Snack**	½ cup cooked brown rice
Mid-A.M. Snack	1 low-cal snack	**Cucumber and Wakame Vinaigrette**
1 low-cal snack	your favorite tea	1 peach
green tea		2 tablespoons low-fat vanilla ice cream or soy ice cream
		jasmine or decaf tea

Wednesday

Breakfast	Lunch	Dinner
Hearty Granola *or* ½ cup granola	1 whole-grain roll	**Creamed Spinach and Broccoli on Soba (veg.)** *or* **Chicken Edamame Curry (chicken)**
Your favorite fruits	1 cup of your favorite vegetable dish at local grocery store (spinach, bean sprouts, potato salad, etc.)	
⅔ cup lite soymilk		**Daikon Shrimp Som Tam Salad** (substitute tomato for shrimp, if vegetarian)
jasmine tea	1 orange	
	jasmine tea	**Fruitful Frozen Yogurt**
Mid-A.M. Snack		jasmine or decaf tea
1 low-cal snack	**Mid-P.M. Snack**	
green tea	1 low-cal snack	
	your favorite tea	

Thursday

Breakfast	Lunch	Dinner
Soy Spinach Congee jasmine tea	**Vegetarians' Cheese Quesadilla** jasmine tea	**Turmeric-Marinated Tofu with Chard** (veg.) or **Bambou Short Ribs** (beef)
Mid-A.M. Snack 1 low-cal snack green tea	**Mid-P.M. Snack** 1 low-cal snack your favorite tea	**Stuffed Summer Tomato** 2 whole-grain rolls 1 cup strawberries 3 tablespoons soy yogurt or low-fat plain yogurt jasmine or decaf tea

Friday

Breakfast	Lunch	Dinner
Apricot-Yogurt Soy Smoothie ½ whole-grain bagel with 1 tablespoon fat-free cream cheese or soy cream cheese jasmine tea	1 6-inch turkey breast or vegetarian sandwich on wheat bread with plenty of veggies and light mayo but without cheese jasmine tea	**Fresh Garden Quiche** (veg.) or **Shrimp and Broccoli Penne** (seafood) **Sweet Potato Salad** 1 cup unsweetened fruit salad jasmine or decaf tea
Mid-A.M. Snack 1 low-cal snack green tea	**Mid-P.M. Snack** 1 low-cal snack your favorite tea	

Saturday

Breakfast	Lunch	Dinner
½ cup cooked brown rice **Basic Miso Soup** (wakame potato) jasmine tea	**Tomato Broth Soba Noodles** jasmine tea	**Nsunaba Sukiyaki Vegetarian** (veg.) or **Nsunaba Sukiyaki** (beef) ½ cup cooked brown rice
Mid-A.M. Snack 1 low-cal snack green tea	**Mid-P.M. Snack** 1 low-cal snack your favorite tea	**Tofu Key Lime Pie** jasmine or decaf tea

Sunday

Breakfast	Lunch	Dinner
Easy, Hearty Vegetarian Pancakes Your favorite fruits jasmine tea	**Edamame Basil Spaghetti** 1 apple jasmine tea	**Mediterranean Ratatouille** (veg.) or **Miso Salmon with Vegetables** (fish) **Garden Greens with Balsamic Vinaigrette** ½ cup cooked pasta with 2 tablespoons low-sodium tomato-based pasta sauce
Mid-A.M. Snack 1 low-cal snack green tea	**Mid-P.M. Snack** 1 low-cal snack your favorite tea	**October Pumpkin Soufflé** jasmine or decaf tea

Monday

Breakfast	Lunch	Dinner
Basic Miso Soup, cooked with ½ cup cooked brown rice, crumbled silken tofu, and spinach	**Fresh Tofu Spring Roll (veg.)** *or* **Papaya and Shrimp Spring Roll (seafood)**	**Creamy Garlic Portobello (veg.)** with ½ cup cooked brown rice *or* **Nasi Goreng Ayam (chicken)**
jasmine tea	jasmine tea	**Baby Bok-Choy Stir-Fry**
Mid-A.M. Snack	**Mid-P.M. Snack**	1 cup strawberries
1 low-cal snack	1 low-cal snack	3 tablespoons soy yogurt or low-fat plain yogurt
green tea	your favorite tea	jasmine or decaf tea

Tuesday

Breakfast	Lunch	Dinner
Green Tea Steamed Bread	1 vegetarian noodle dish at your local Japanese or Chinese restaurant, with ½ cup noodles and plenty of vegetables	**Ginkgo-Tofu Supreme (veg.)** *or* **Balsamic Pork with Mushrooms (pork)**
½ grapefruit		**Cucumber and Wakame Vinaigrette**
jasmine tea	jasmine tea	½ cup cooked brown rice
Mid-A.M. Snack	**Mid-P.M. Snack**	1 banana, halved lengthwise and sprinkled with ½ teaspoon brown sugar
1 low-cal snack	1 low-cal snack	
green tea	your favorite tea	jasmine or decaf tea

Wednesday

Breakfast	Lunch	Dinner
1 cup flax cereal	**Soba Salad**	**Shima Tofu and Vegetable Terrine (veg.)** *or* **Traditional Tsumire Soup (fish)**
½ cup skim or soy milk	1 orange	
Strawberries	jasmine tea	**Cumin-Chili Cauliflower**
jasmine tea	**Mid-P.M. Snack**	½ cup cooked brown rice
Mid-A.M. Snack	1 low-cal snack	**Darjeeling Pudding**
1 low-cal snack	your favorite tea	jasmine or decaf tea
green tea		

Thursday

Breakfast	Lunch	Dinner
½ cup cooked brown rice	1 6-inch turkey breast or vegetarian sandwich on wheat bread with plenty of veggies and light mayo but without cheese	**Teriyaki Tofu Fingers (veg.)** *or* **Spicy Garlic Shrimp (seafood)**
1 sheet nori laver seaweed, cut into eighths		**Goya Delight**
½ cup steamed spinach with ½ teaspoon low-sodium soy sauce		**Basic Miso Soup** with wakame seaweed
jasmine tea	jasmine tea	½ cup cooked brown rice
Mid-A.M. Snack	**Mid-P.M. Snack**	½ papaya
1 low-cal snack	1 low-cal snack	2 tablespoons low-fat vanilla ice cream or soy ice cream
green tea	your favorite tea	jasmine or decaf tea

Friday

Breakfast	Lunch	Dinner
1 cup hot porridge with brown sugar to taste	**Baked Sweet Potatoes**	**Yuki's Indian Tofu Curry (veg.)** *or* **Chicken Edamame Curry (chicken)**
1 apple	jasmine tea	**Garden Greens with Balsamic Vinaigrette**
¼ cup skim or soy milk	**Mid-P.M. Snack**	1 cup cantaloupe cubes sprinkled with 1 teaspoon lime juice
jasmine tea	1 low-cal snack	⅓ cup soy yogurt or low-fat plain yogurt
Mid-A.M. Snack	your favorite tea	jasmine or decaf tea
1 low-cal snack		
green tea		

Saturday

Breakfast	Lunch	Dinner
Soy Spinach Congee	**Tofu and Veggie Pita Sandwich (veg.)** *or* **Veggie Pork Pita (pork)**	**Honey Mustard Tofu (veg.)** *or* **Sea Bream Carpaccio with Turmeric Sauce (fish)**
jasmine tea	jasmine tea	**Roasted Vegetables with Miso Sesame Sauce**
Mid-A.M. Snack	**Mid-P.M. Snack**	½ cup cooked brown rice
1 low-cal snack	1 low-cal snack	**Tapioca Sweet Potato Dessert**
green tea	your favorite tea	jasmine or decaf tea

Sunday

Breakfast	Lunch	Dinner
Buckwheat Flax Pancakes	**Daikon Shrimp Som Tam Salad** (substitute tomato for shrimp, if vegetarian)	**Tofu Shish Kabobs (veg.)** *or* **Spicy Stewed Chicken (chicken)**
Blueberries	½ cup rice noodles, soaked in hot water until soft and seasoned with ¼ teaspoon fish or soy sauce, lime juice, and fresh cilantro	**Sweet Potato Salad**
½ tablespoon maple syrup	jasmine tea	½ cup brown rice or 2 whole-grain dinner rolls
jasmine tea		**Green Tea Panna Cotta**
Mid-A.M. Snack	**Mid-P.M. Snack**	jasmine or decaf tea
1 low-cal snack	1 low-cal snack	
green tea	your favorite tea	

Western Track

This track sticks to the principles of tasty, low–caloric density eating while offering you the occasional chance to slip in a little soy here and there, but always provides a delectable choice for both the vegetarian *and* the carnivore. Just the plan for the less adventurous diner who wishes to eat better and lose fat, but is not ready for yoga or tai chi. You'll find the recipes for all bold-faced dishes in the next chapter, and suggestions for low-cal snacks on pages 189–193. Bon appetit!

Nutrition Facts of the Week
Calories: 1080 • Protein: 66g • Carbohydrate: 173g • Fat: 21g

Monday

Breakfast	Lunch	Dinner
Banana-Vanilla French Toast	**Brilliant Vegetarian Chili**	**Roasted Tomato Pasta (veg.)**
1 orange	*or* 1 cup low-fat,	*or* **Okinawan Coq au Vin**
jasmine tea	low-sodium chili	**(chicken)**
	1 cup green salad	2 whole-grain dinner rolls
Mid-A.M. Snack	1 whole-grain roll	1 cup cantaloupe cubes
1 low-cal snack	jasmine tea	sprinkled with 1 teaspoon
tea or coffee		lime juice
	Mid-P.M. Snack	1/3 cup soy yogurt or low-fat
	1 low-cal snack	plain yogurt
	your favorite tea	jasmine or decaf tea

Tuesday

Breakfast	Lunch	Dinner
1 cup hot porridge with	**Tofu and Veggie Pita**	**Special Herb Potato Gratin**
brown sugar to taste	**Sandwich (veg.)** *or* **Veggie**	**(veg.)** *or* **Cheesy Scallop and**
1 apple	**Pork Pita (pork)**	**Potato (seafood)**
1/4 cup skim or soy milk	jasmine tea	**Slimming Tomato Cabbage**
jasmine tea		**Soup**
	Mid-P.M. Snack	2 whole-grain dinner rolls
Mid-A.M. Snack	1 low-cal snack	**Can't-Be-Easier Chocolate**
1 low-cal snack	your favorite tea	**Fruit Pudding**
tea or coffee		jasmine or decaf tea

Wednesday

Breakfast	Lunch	Dinner
Apricot-Yogurt Soy Smoothie	1 whole-grain roll	**Hearty Bean Stroganoff**
1/2 whole-grain bagel with	1 cup of your favorite	**(veg.)** *or* **Beef à la Crème**
1 tablespoon fat-free cream	vegetable dish at local	**(beef)**
cheese or soy cream cheese	grocery store (spinach, bean	1/2 cup cooked brown rice or
jasmine tea	sprouts, potato salad, etc.)	your favorite whole-grain
	1 orange	noodles
Mid-A.M. Snack	jasmine tea	1/2 papaya
1 low-cal snack		2 tablespoons low-fat vanilla
tea or coffee	**Mid-P.M. Snack**	ice cream or soy ice cream
	1 low-cal snack	jasmine or decaf tea
	your favorite tea	

Thursday

Breakfast

1 cup flax cereal
½ cup skim or soy milk
Strawberries
jasmine tea

Mid-A.M. Snack

1 low-cal snack
tea or coffee

Lunch

Bean and Rice Burritos
jasmine tea

Mid-P.M. Snack

1 low-cal snack
your favorite tea

Dinner

Creamy Garlic Portobello (veg.) *or* **Poached Chicken with Herb Dressing** (chicken)

Cumin-Chili Cauliflower

Hearty Vegetable Soup

2 whole-grain dinner rolls

Roasted Summer Peach

jasmine or decaf tea

Friday

Breakfast

2 strips soy bacon (veg.) *or* 1 egg, any style except fried (egg)
2 slices whole-grain toast
½ grapefruit
jasmine tea

Mid-A.M. Snack

1 low-cal snack
tea or coffee

Lunch

1 6-inch turkey breast or vegetarian sandwich on wheat bread with plenty of veggies and light mayo but without cheese
jasmine tea

Mid-P.M. Snack

1 low-cal snack
your favorite tea

Dinner

Tofu-Stuffed Mushrooms (veg.) *or* **Sea Bream Carpaccio with Turmeric Sauce** (fish)

½ cup cooked brown rice

Garden Greens with Balsamic Vinaigrette

1 cup unsweetened fruit salad

jasmine or decaf tea

Saturday

Breakfast

Buckwheat Flax Pancakes
Blueberries
½ tablespoon maple syrup
jasmine tea

Mid-A.M. Snack

1 low-cal snack
tea or coffee

Lunch

Vegetarians' Cheese Quesadilla
jasmine tea

Mid-P.M. Snack

1 low-cal snack
your favorite tea

Dinner

Painted Bean Casserole (veg.) *or* **Veggieful Beef Stew** (beef)

Herbed Zucchini

2 whole-grain dinner rolls

Cantaloupe and Grapefruit Sorbet

jasmine or decaf tea

Sunday

Breakfast

Sweet Potato Orange Muffins
1 pear
jasmine tea

Mid-A.M. Snack

1 low-cal snack
tea or coffee

Lunch

Garlic Mussels with White Wine Sauce (seafood) *or* **Teriyaki Tofu Fingers** (veg.)

Cumin-Flavored Fava Bean

1 whole-grain roll
jasmine tea

Mid-P.M. Snack

1 low-cal snack
your favorite tea

Dinner

Shima Tofu and Vegetable Terrine (veg.) (2 servings) *or* **Chicken Asparagus Cordon Bleu** (chicken)

Mediterranean Ratatouille

½ cup of your favorite whole-grain noodles or pasta

Tofu Key Lime Pie

jasmine or decaf tea

Monday

Breakfast	Lunch	Dinner
Banana-Vanilla French Toast 1 orange 1 cup jasmine tea	**Bean and Rice Burrito** jasmine tea	**Edamame Basil Spaghetti (veg.)** *or* **Chicken and Mushroom Linguine (chicken)** **Stuffed Summer Tomato** ½ papaya
Mid-A.M. Snack 1 low-cal snack tea or coffee	**Mid-P.M. Snack** 1 low-cal snack your favorite tea	2 tablespoons low-fat vanilla ice cream or soy ice cream jasmine or decaf tea

Tuesday

Breakfast	Lunch	Dinner
1 cup hot porridge with brown sugar to taste 1 apple ¼ cup skim or soy milk jasmine tea	1 whole-grain roll 1 cup of your favorite vegetable dish at local grocery store (spinach, bean sprouts, potato salad, etc.) 1 orange jasmine tea	**Spicy Tofu and Summer Vegetables (veg.)** *or* **Poached White Fish with Honey-Lime Sauce (fish)** **Garden Greens with Balsamic Vinaigrette** 2 whole-grain dinner rolls
Mid-A.M. Snack 1 low-cal snack tea or coffee	**Mid-P.M. Snack** 1 low-cal snack your favorite tea	1 cup unsweetened fruit salad jasmine or decaf tea

Wednesday

Breakfast	Lunch	Dinner
Apricot-Yogurt Soy Smoothie ½ whole-wheat bagel with 1 teaspoon fat-free cream cheese or soy cream cheese jasmine tea	**Vegetarians' Cheese Quesadilla** 1 cup jasmine tea	**Creamy Garlic Portobello (veg.)** *or* **Beef à la Crème (beef)** **Dandelion Spring Rice** 1 cup prepared vegetable soup
Mid-A.M. Snack 1 low-cal snack tea or coffee	**Mid-P.M. Snack** 1 low-cal snack your favorite tea	1 banana, halved lengthwise and sprinkled with ½ teaspoon brown sugar jasmine or decaf tea

Thursday

Breakfast	Lunch	Dinner
1 cup flax cereal ½ cup skim or soy milk Strawberries jasmine tea	1 6-inch turkey breast or vegetarian sandwich on wheat bread with plenty of veggies and light mayo but without cheese jasmine tea	**Brilliant Vegetarian Chili (veg.)** *or* **Baked Salmon Mousse (fish)** **Herbed Zucchini** 2 whole-grain dinner rolls
Mid-A.M. Snack 1 low-cal snack tea or coffee	**Mid-P.M. Snack** 1 low-cal snack your favorite tea	1 serving low-calorie applesauce jasmine or decaf tea

Friday

Breakfast	Lunch	Dinner
2 strips soy bacon (veg.) *or* 1 egg, any style except fried (egg)	Brilliant Vegetarian Chili *or* 1 cup low-fat, low-sodium chili	Mediterranean Ratatouille (veg.) *or* Cheesy Scallop and Potato (seafood)
2 slices whole-grain toast	1 cup green salad	Hearty Vegetable Soup
½ grapefruit	1 whole-grain roll	2 whole-grain dinner rolls
jasmine tea	jasmine tea	1 cup cantaloupe cubes sprinkled with 1 teaspoon lime juice
Mid-A.M. Snack	**Mid-P.M. Snack**	⅓ cup soy yogurt or low-fat plain yogurt
1 low-cal snack	1 low-cal snack	jasmine or decaf tea
tea or coffee	your favorite tea	

Saturday

Breakfast	Lunch	Dinner
Buckwheat Flax Pancakes	Zucchini and Mushroom Pancakes	Roasted Tomato Pasta (veg.) *or* Shrimp and Broccoli Penne (seafood)
Blueberries	1 apple	Creamy Split Pea and Sweet Potato Soup
½ tablespoon maple syrup	jasmine tea	Tropical Mango Pudding
jasmine tea		jasmine or decaf tea
Mid-A.M. Snack	**Mid-P.M. Snack**	
1 low-cal snack	1 low-cal snack	
tea or coffee	your favorite tea	

Sunday

Breakfast	Lunch	Dinner
Sweet Potato Orange Muffin	Special Herb Potato Gratin	Hearty Bean Stroganoff (veg.) with ½ cup cooked brown rice *or* Poached Chicken with Herb Dressing (chicken) with 2 whole-grain dinner rolls
1 pear	Fresh grapes	1½ cups Caesar salad with low-fat dressing, nonfat croutons, and low-fat Parmesan cheese
jasmine tea	jasmine tea	Cantaloupe and Grapefruit Sorbet
Mid-A.M. Snack	**Mid-P.M. Snack**	jasmine or decaf tea
1 low-cal snack	1 low-cal snack	
tea or coffee	your favorite tea	

Chapter 8

THE OKINAWA DIET RECIPES

Yaasaru Maasaru.
Food is delicious when one is hungry.

"If we nourish the spirit through proper food and drink, illness will cure itself." These words from the *Textbook of Herbal Medicine (Gozen Honzou)* were written in 1832, by Dr. Tokashiki Tsuka, physician to the King of the Ryukyus (present-day Okinawa). They embody the concept of *nuchi gusui*—the healing power of food. Today the *nuchi gusui* spirit still permeates the Okinawan psyche and has made its way into the Okinawan kitchen—and now into yours. In ancient China, the diet doctor received top ranking, and it's said that the first medical textbook was actually a cookbook. To us that makes total sense. We are firm believers in the healing power of good food. We hope our program and the recipes we present here will not only help you put healthy delicious food on your table, but also keep the doctor at bay, and serve as a powerful tool for lifelong weight control. The recipes exemplify the healing power of good food and splendidly reflect Okinawan culture and its unique historical position as the former crossroad of Asian cultures. As an independent kingdom, Okinawa traded with China, Korea, Japan, Siam, Java, and other ancient kingdoms of Southeast Asia, and Okinawan cooking, with its main *chample* style and multinational seasonings, incorporates the best of all these cultures. Familiar and unfamiliar feather-weight vegetables, anchored by lean protein from soy, fish, lean meats, and other foods, arrange and rearrange themselves in brilliant and novel combinations guaranteed to keep your appetite satisfied and your weight down.

A good number of these wonderful recipes come from the elders themselves and have been passed from generation to generation. Many others were provided by some of the world's top Okinawan and Asian fusion chefs, and still others come from our files and from the personal collections of Okinawan cooks around the world. They've been adapted and taste-tested and perfected to please your palate and to respond to your needs. But equally important, they were assembled with a plentiful serving of *yuimaru*—people helping each other—another powerful philosophical hallmark of Okinawan culture. Without that spirit, this endeavor would not have been possible.

The right foods and lifelong balance have helped the Okinawan elders stay lean and fit, and have played an essential role in their extraordinarily healthy longevity. Now it's your turn. Allow their spirit to inspire you as it has us. And always remember no matter where you are in life, it is never too late to start new eating habits—or exercise regimes, or spiritual practices. There is an Okinawan proverb, *Acha nu neen chi ami.* It means, "Tomorrow is a new day." Every day *is* the beginning of the rest of your life—eat healthy, and enjoy it to its fullest.

If Asian cooking is new to you, just dive in and take the challenge. Don't question the ingredients; don't question the methods. Just go for it—there's a good chance you'll love it so much that your eating and cooking habits will change for good. After preparing some of our recipes, be adventurous and try cooking up your own creations. You never know—you might come up with a culinary masterpiece. One thing is for sure, eating the Okinawa way will help you enjoy your food more and will make it much easier to stay slim and healthy for life. Be sure to let us know how your adventure goes. Bon appétit, and *nuchi gusui!*

Bread and Baked Foods

Bread is a relatively recent, and minor, addition to the Okinawa diet. It's now available in most all neighborhood groceries, and even the elders indulge themselves occasionally—usually just a small slice with cooked vegetables and a cup of tea a few times a week. Bakeries have also sprung up all over Okinawa, most of them specializing in muffin-size "stuffed bread," which is filled with curried vegetables, sweet potato, or bean paste—and is quite delicious.

Healthy Tips: Whenever you bake, use whole grains, heart-healthy omega-3 eggs, and monounsaturated fats like canola oil, and try to avoid butter, lard, and trans-fat-rich margarines. Feel free to jazz up recipes with seeds, spices, and other healthy ingredients such as soy cheese, fruits, and vegetables. Whenever a recipe calls for sugar, use lower-GI turbinado sugar, which is steam-cleaned raw sugar, instead of brown sugar, which is almost always white sugar with molasses.

Turmeric and Rosemary Grissini

Green Tea Steamed Bread

Vegetarians' Cheese Quesadilla

Nuts 'n' Seeds Bread

Banana-Vanilla French Toast

Sweet Potato Orange Muffins

Easy, Hearty Vegetarian Pancakes

Buckwheat Flax Pancakes

Turmeric and Rosemary Grissini

SERVES 4

Grissini are thin, crispy breadsticks that originated in Turin, Italy. Served as an antipasto or appetizer, the thin shape is designed to keep guests occupied without filling them up too much to enjoy the rest of the meal. *Grissini* can be pencil-thin or cigar-fat, and either plain or coated with olive oil, sprinkled with cheese, or infused with spices or herbs. Try them with the main dish instead of regular bread, or as part of a light lunch with crudités and fat-free dips. Also great for entertaining—turmeric, one of our favorite healthy spices, turns these breadsticks into colorful, edible art. Stick them in tall glasses as a festive treat.

1¼ cups warm water (100 to 115°F)	2 cups whole-wheat flour
1 package (¼ ounce) active dry yeast	½ teaspoon sea salt
1 tablespoon turbinado or brown sugar	1 tablespoon ground turmeric
2 tablespoons olive oil	2 tablespoons dried rosemary
1 cup all-purpose unbleached flour	Canola oil spray

Pour the warm water in a small mixing bowl and stir in the yeast and turbinado sugar. Dissolve and let stand for 4 to 5 minutes, or until foamy, to make sure the yeast is active.

Stir in the olive oil.

In a large mixing bowl, mix both flours and the salt, make a hole in the center, and pour in the dissolved yeast. Mix well. Transfer the dough to lightly floured working surface and knead until the dough is smooth and elastic, approximately 10 minutes. Cover with a dish towel and let rest for 40 minutes.

Preheat the oven to 400°F.

Add the turmeric to the dough and knead for 10 more minutes. Shape the dough into a 14 × 4-inch rectangle. Cover and let rest for 10 more minutes.

Sprinkle the rosemary on top of the dough and cut horizontally into twenty 4-inch strips, about ⅔ inch thick. Stretch and roll the dough into 8- to 10-inch sticks, rolling in the rosemary.

Coat baking sheets with canola spray. Place the sticks a few inches apart on the sheets and bake for 15 to 20 minutes or until golden and of your desired degree of crunchiness. Cool on racks. Serve as an appetizer, for lunch with salad, or for a light snack.

NUTRITION FACTS: 1 BREADSTICK; Caloric Density 2.2; Calories (Kcal) 80; Protein (g) 2; Carbohydrate (g) 14; Total Fat (g) 2; Saturated Fat (g) 0.3; Monounsaturated Fat (g) 1.1; Polyunsaturated Fat (g) 0.3; Dietary Fiber (g) 2.0; Flavonoid and Other Phyto (mg) 0.0; Cholesterol (mg) 0; Sodium (mg) 48; Vitamin A (IU) 11; Vitamin C (mg) 0; Calcium (mg) 12; Iron (mg) 1.1; PERCENTAGE (%) Protein 11.8; Carbohydrate 69.3; Fat 18.9

Green Tea Steamed Bread

SERVES 4

Eating tea, or drinking ground tea leaves without infusing, is one of the great cultural traditions of Japan. Although tea was introduced to Japan from China in the early sixth century, it wasn't until the twelfth century that a Japanese monk who had studied in China returned with the method of mixing hot water with green tea powder to create a drink. Until then, only the fruit of tea plants was used by monks and the upper class as medication for fever, swellings, and fatigue. Now, in modern Japan, using tea powder as a cooking ingredient is immensely popular, not least because of its healthy catechins, powerful antioxidants that protect against heart disease and cancer. Okinawans also combine tea powder with native tropical ingredients to produce culinary wonders like tea powder–pineapple cakes and tea powder–raw sugar candies. Steamed breads are also common in Okinawa and Japan. The steaming creates an unusually smooth texture, preserves the original color of the ingredients, and keeps the bread from going stale. This recipe puts a fresh twist on two wonderful old traditions.

½ cup all-purpose unbleached flour	1 free-range omega-3 egg or ¼ cup egg
¼ cup whole-wheat flour	substitute or egg white
1 teaspoon baking powder	⅓ cup water
¼ cup turbinado or brown sugar	1 teaspoon green tea powder
Pinch of sea salt	Canola oil spray

Prepare a steamer. If using a pan, use a flat 10-inch pan with a lid.

Place the two flours, the baking powder, the sugar, and the sea salt in a large mixing bowl and mix.

Mix the egg, the water, and the green tea powder in a small mixing bowl.

Combine the two mixtures and stir with a whisk until smooth.

Spray 4 nonstick mini tin cups (about 2½ inches deep, 2½ inches in diameter, preferably with a fluted edge) or ramekins with canola oil. Pour the batter to fill about half of each cup.

Steam for 10 minutes. Remove from the cups, cool on a rack, and serve.

NUTRITION FACTS: 1 SERVING, 1 BREAD; Caloric Density 2.1; Calories (Kcal) 141; Protein (g) 4; Carbohydrate (g) 28; Total Fat (g) 2; Saturated Fat (g) 0.4; Monounsaturated Fat (g) 0.5; Polyunsaturated Fat (g) 0.3; Dietary Fiber (g) 1.8; Flavonoid and Other Phyto (mg) 0.1; Cholesterol (mg) 28; Sodium (mg) 179; Vitamin A (IU) 279; Vitamin C (mg) 1; Calcium (mg) 111; Iron (mg) 1.7; PERCENTAGE (%) Protein 11.7; Carbohydrate 78.6; Fat 9.7

Vegetarians' Cheese Quesadilla

SERVES 4

Quesadilla, which means "cheesecake" in Spanish, is essentially a toasted or fried flour tortilla filled with any combination of shredded cheese, cooked meat, or refried beans and folded in half into a turnover shape. But there's a lot more nutrition (and a lot fewer calories) in this version than in the regular kind—and it's definitely healthier than any cheesecake we've ever run across. This easy, fast recipe is great for a light lunch when you're in a hurry but still want to have something healthy.

2 large whole-wheat flour tortillas, preferably fat-free
4 slices soy cheese (or thinly sliced low-fat cheddar cheese)

½ cup salsa
Topping vegetables, such as shredded lettuce, sliced tomato, and chopped jalapeños or onions

Place a tortilla in a large heated skillet on high heat, and spread ¼ cup salsa and 2 slices cheese (or half the amount of cheddar you prepared) over half the tortilla. Heat for 1 minute or until the cheese starts melting.

Top with your favorite vegetables, fold the other half of the tortilla over the cheese and salsa, then slide the quesadilla onto a serving plate. Cut into halves.

Make another quesadilla with the remaining tortilla, cheese, salsa, and vegetables. Serve warm.

NUTRITION FACTS: 1 SERVING WITH ¼ cup chopped tomato and 2 tablespoons chopped onion; Caloric Density 1.0; Calories (Kcal) 151; Protein (g) 6; Carbohydrate (g) 23; Total Fat (g) 4; Saturated Fat (g) 1.1; Monounsaturated Fat (g) 1.8; Polyunsaturated Fat (g) 0.6; Dietary Fiber (g) 10.1; Flavonoid and Other Phyto (mg) 10.1; Cholesterol (mg) 0; Sodium (mg) 446; Vitamin A (IU) 784; Vitamin C (mg) 12; Calcium (mg) 202; Iron (mg) 0.6; PERCENTAGE (%) Protein 16.0; Carbohydrate 62.2; Fat 21.7

Nuts 'n' Seeds Bread

MAKES 2 MEDIUM LOAVES OR 1 LARGE LOAF; 28 SLICES

Despite the fact that two-thirds of the world's walnuts are produced in California, they're adored in Okinawa, where they're commonly coated in a raw sugar or soybean paste and served with a fragrant jasmine tea. Here they add extra healthy monounsaturated fats to an already incredibly nutritious bread.

2 cups warm water (100 to 115°F)
2 packages (¼ ounce each) active dry
    yeast
2 tablespoons turbinado or brown sugar
5 cups whole-wheat flour
2¼ cups all-purpose unbleached flour
1 teaspoon sea salt
1 cup soymilk, plain

½ cup honey
2 tablespoons canola oil
Canola oil spray
¼ cup roasted, unseasoned pine nuts
¼ cup roasted, unseasoned chopped
    walnuts
¼ cup flax seeds
3 tablespoons white sesame seeds

Pour ½ cup warm water in a small mixing bowl and stir in the yeast and turbinado sugar. Dissolve and let stand for 4 to 5 minutes or until foamy, to make sure the yeast is active.

In a large bowl, place both flours and the salt and stir well to mix evenly. Add the remaining warm water, the soymilk, and the honey and mix. Add the yeast mixture and mix well. Add the 2 tablespoons canola oil and mix well.

Transfer the dough to a lightly floured working surface and knead until the dough is smooth and elastic, approximately 10 to 12 minutes.

Spray a large mixing bowl with canola oil and place the dough in the bowl. Turn over the dough once to grease the upper half. Cover and let rise in warm place (about 90°F) until the dough doubles in size, about 1½ hours.

Punch down dough to remove air bubbles. Knead in the nuts and seeds. Divide the dough in half. Shape each piece into a loaf. Spray two 9 × 5 × 3-inch loaf pans with canola spray. Place the loaves in the pans. Cover and let rise in warm place (about 90°F) until the dough doubles in size, about 1 hour.

Preheat the oven to 425°F.

Bake the loaves for 10 minutes, then reduce the heat to 350°F and bake an additional 25 to 30 minutes, or until the temperature inside the bread is 190° to 200°F.

Remove the loaves from pans and let cool on a rack. Cut each loaf into 14 slices, each approximately ⅝ inch thick.

NUTRITION FACTS: 1 SLICE; Caloric Density 2.3; Calories (Kcal) 162; Protein (g) 5; Carbohydrate (g) 30; Total Fat (g) 3; Saturated Fat (g) 0.4; Monounsaturated Fat (g) 0.8; Polyunsaturated Fat (g) 1.6; Dietary Fiber (g) 3.9; Flavonoid and Other Phyto (mg) 4.3; Cholesterol (mg) 0; Sodium (mg) 14; Vitamin A (IU) 3; Vitamin C (mg) 0; Calcium (mg) 25; Iron (mg) 1.9; PERCENTAGE (%) Protein 12.6; Carbohydrate 71.3; Fat 16.1

Healthy Tip: Use walnuts and other nuts sparingly, as in the preceding recipe, because although they're healthy, most nuts are very high in fat—good fat, but fat nonetheless. It's best to sprinkle them in with vegetables, salads, or fruits, or to use nut butters on breads instead of regular butter or margarine.

Banana-Vanilla French Toast

SERVES 4

French toast is called poor knight's pudding in England and *pain perdu* ("lost bread") in French. These somewhat lowly names reflect its origins—a tasty way to make use of stale bread. Although high-calorie French toast can still conjure up unhealthy images (saturated fat, cholesterol, and sugar), this recipe shows that a little imagination and the right ingredients can go a long way toward making a healthy alternative without sacrificing taste.

1 ripe banana
1 cup light soymilk, vanilla
¼ teaspoon ground cinnamon

Canola oil spray
8 slices whole-wheat bread

Process the banana, soymilk, and cinnamon in a blender until smooth. Pour into a shallow bowl.

Coat a skillet or griddle with nonstick canola spray and heat it over medium-high heat.

Dip the bread slices into the banana batter and cook them 30 to 45 seconds per side, or until lightly browned.

NUTRITION FACTS: 1 SERVING, 2 SLICES; Caloric Density 1.4; Calories (Kcal) 211; Protein (g) 6; Carbohydrate (g) 41; Total Fat (g) 4; Saturated Fat (g) 0.6; Monounsaturated Fat (g) 0.8; Polyunsaturated Fat (g) 1.9; Dietary Fiber (g) 4.1; Flavonoid and Other Phyto (mg) 2.6; Cholesterol (mg) 0; Sodium (mg) 224; Vitamin A (IU) 24; Vitamin C (mg) 3; Calcium (mg) 27; Iron (mg) 2.0; PERCENTAGE (%) Protein 10.4; Carbohydrate 74; Fat 15.6

Sweet Potato Orange Muffins

SIX 2½-INCH MUFFIN CUPS

This recipe mingles the wonderful tastes of three of our favorite foods: the subtle flavor of almond butter, the earthiness of sweet potato, and the citrus zing of orange. The combination makes for a wonderfully intriguing taste. The almond butter also gives you an additional hit of nutrition. The monounsaturated fat in almonds makes them extremely heart-healthy, and they pack a good amount of calcium too (248 mg per 100 g). No wonder they're such a popular snack throughout Japan.

⅓ cup all-purpose unbleached flour
⅓ cup whole-wheat flour
1 teaspoon baking powder
½ pound peeled, cubed sweet potato
½ cup calcium-fortified orange juice
2 teaspoons canola oil

2½ tablespoons almond butter, chunky (if not available, use unsalted peanut butter)
2 tablespoons canola oil
⅓ cup turbinado or brown sugar
1 free-range, omega-3 egg or ¼ cup egg substitute or egg white

Combine both flours and the baking powder in a small bowl.

Preheat the oven to 375°F.

In a microwavable container, place the sweet potato, the orange juice, and 2 teaspoons canola oil and cook on high for 8 minutes. Transfer to a blender and process until smoothly blended.

In a large mixing bowl, combine the almond butter, the 2 tablespoons canola oil, and the turbinado sugar. Whisk vigorously until smooth. Add the egg and whisk again until smooth. Add the sweet potato mixture and mix well. Add the dry ingredients to the sweet potato bowl and stir with a wooden spoon, about 20 times, just until mixed evenly.

Pour the batter into the muffin cups (if they are not nonstick, use canola spray). Bake for 18 to 20 minutes, or until the muffins turn golden brown and a toothpick inserted in the center comes out clean.

NUTRITION FACTS: 1 MUFFIN; Caloric Density 2.3; Calories (Kcal) 236; Protein (g) 4; Carbohydrate (g) 32; Total Fat (g) 11; Saturated Fat (g) 1.1; Monounsaturated Fat (g) 6.5; Polyunsaturated Fat (g) 2.9; Dietary Fiber (g) 2.4; Flavonoid and Other Phyto (mg) 0.0; Cholesterol (mg) 35; Sodium (mg) 80; Vitamin A (IU) 7653; Vitamin C (mg) 15; Calcium (mg) 127; Iron (mg) 1.4; PERCENTAGE (%) Protein 7.3; Carbohydrate 51.6; Fat 41.1

Easy, Hearty Vegetarian Pancakes
SERVES 4

With hardly any effort, you can turn another of North America's favorite high-calorie breakfasts into a delicious, calorie-busting alternative. This cholesterol-free, low-fat oatmeal pancake is not only a delight to the taste buds but is also chock-full of healthy ingredients, including rich amounts of cholesterol-fighting soluble fiber. Compare the nutritional differences: Regular buttermilk pancakes are 638 calories per serving and have only 3.1 grams of fiber; while our pancakes contain 267 calories and have 8.4 grams of fiber per serving. Now, that's our kind of pancake!

2 small very ripe bananas, mashed
1 tablespoon turbinado or brown sugar
1 cup light soymilk, vanilla
½ cup instant oatmeal
1½ cups whole-wheat flour
2 teaspoons baking powder

⅓ teaspoon ground cinnamon
Pinch of sea salt
Canola oil spray (optional)
1 cup fruits, such as berries, kiwi, or banana

In a large bowl, mix together the bananas and the turbinado sugar. Add the soymilk and ⅔ cup water and mix well.

Combine the oatmeal, flour, baking powder, cinnamon, and salt in a separate bowl. Fold into the wet ingredients, using a wooden spoon. Do not overmix—the mixture can have some lumps.

Heat a griddle or a frying pan over medium heat. Spray with canola oil if the pan is not nonstick.

When the pan is hot, pour in ½ cup batter. Cook for 2 minutes, or until bubbles rise through the center of the pancake. Flip and cook another 2 minutes, or until set. Transfer to a plate. Repeat to make 3 more pancakes.

Serve with the fruits on top of or beside the pancakes.

NUTRITION FACTS: 1 SERVING, 1 PANCAKE; Caloric Density 1.4; Calories (Kcal) 267; Protein (g) 9; Carbohydrate (g) 57; Total Fat (g) 2; Saturated Fat (g) 0.4; Monounsaturated Fat (g) 0.5; Polyunsaturated Fat (g) 0.9; Dietary Fiber (g) 8.4; Flavonoid and Other Phyto (mg) 3.3; Cholesterol (mg) 0; Sodium (mg) 284; Vitamin A (IU) 46; Vitamin C (mg) 26; Calcium (mg) 208; Iron (mg) 2.9; PERCENTAGE (%) Protein 12.6; Carbohydrate 79.9; Fat 7.5

Buckwheat Flax Pancakes

SERVES 4

Buckwheat is one of the great traditional grains of Japan—and it is still much revered. Because of its ability to grow and flourish in poor soil, buckwheat proved a lifesaver to many Japanese over the centuries. Its red-bottomed stems have long been celebrated in Japanese folklore, and most folktales are as colorful as the stems themselves. According to one story, an evil witch tried to climb to heaven on a long buckwheat plant, but her athletic abilities didn't match her aspirations and she tumbled from the sky into a field of buckwheat. To purify the site and bring luck to others, the gods dyed the buckwheat stems red. So perhaps these buckwheat pancakes will bring you luck as well as a healthy, hearty meal. You never know.

1 cup buckwheat flour
½ cup all-purpose unbleached flour
2 teaspoons baking powder
Pinch of sea salt
4 tablespoons flax seeds
1 free-range, omega-3 egg or ¼ cup egg substitute or egg white

2 tablespoons canola oil
2 tablespoons turbinado or brown sugar
1¼ cups light soymilk, vanilla
Canola oil spray

In a large mixing bowl, combine both flours, the baking powder, the sea salt, and the flax seeds.

In another large mixing bowl, whisk the egg well. Add the canola oil and sugar and stir, then add the soymilk and mix well. Fold the flour mixture into the egg mixture. Mix gently with a wooden spatula. Do not mix vigorously; mixture can have some lumps.

Heat a skillet over medium heat and spray with canola oil.

Pour ¼ cup batter into the skillet. Cook for 1 minute, or until the top is covered with bubbles. Turn over the pancake and cook another minute, or until set. Makes twelve 3-inch pancakes.

NUTRITION FACTS: 1 SERVING, 3 PANCAKES; Caloric Density 2.1; Calories (Kcal) 339; Protein (g) 11; Carbohydrate (g) 44; Total Fat (g) 15; Saturated Fat (g) 1.6; Monounsaturated Fat (g) 5.9; Polyunsaturated Fat (g) 5.9; Dietary Fiber (g) 7.7; Flavonoid and Other Phyto (mg) 30.2; Cholesterol (mg) 53; Sodium (mg) 283; Vitamin A (IU) 103; Vitamin C (mg) 0; Calcium (mg) 222; Iron (mg) 3.7; PERCENTAGE (%) Protein 12.9; Carbohydrate 49.7; Fat 37.4

Salads

In *The Dictionary of American Food and Drink* by John F. Mariani, *salad* is defined as "a dish of leafy green vegetables dressed with various seasonings, sauces, and other vegetables or fruits." But we think salads have a much broader definition these days. Chicken salad, macaroni salad, egg salad, tuna salad, and so on, are a far cry from the green leafy kind—and they can be much higher in calories. A typical leafy green salad has a CD of less than 0.2, but a typical macaroni salad has a CD of 1.5, and a chicken or tuna salad could be up to 2.3! In keeping with our goal of bringing salads back to their healthier origins, here are our three principles for a sensible salad:

1. At least 90 percent of the salad should be made up of low-CD vegetables or whole grains.

2. The caloric density of the salad should be under 1.0.

3. The salad should be colorful—five colors are ideal for optimal health and appeal. (This is an easy principle to follow, as vegetables and fruits are among the most colorful foods on the planet.)

❧

Garden Greens with Balsamic Vinaigrette

Wakame Asparagusu

Asian Okra and Tomato

Ryukyu Swiss Chard (Nsunaba Usachi)

Shima Tofu and Vegetable Terrine

Daikon Shrimp Som Tam Salad

Stuffed Summer Tomato

Sweet Potato Salad

Soba Salad

Fava Bean and Tomato Salad

Warm Tofu Salad of Wilted Greens and Macadamia Nuts

Garden Greens with Balsamic Vinaigrette

SERVES 4

This is great, quick, hassle-free side dish. Just grab a bagful of greens from the grocery (organic, if available), wash them well under cold running water, and toss them into a salad bowl. *Quick Tip:* If the greens look a bit withered, wrap them in dampened paper towels after washing, place them in a plastic bag, fill the bag with air (you can blow it in), close the bag tight, and refrigerate for ten minutes. Amazingly, the greens will be reborn!

½ tablespoon balsamic vinegar
½ teaspoon minced garlic
1 teaspoon fresh lemon juice
⅓ tablespoon olive oil
1 teaspoon Dijon mustard

4 cups baby green salad mix, baby spinach, baby arugula, or any combination of these
⅔ cup halved grape tomatoes or cherry tomatoes

Place the vinegar, garlic, lemon juice, olive oil, and mustard in a small bowl or jar and stir well.

Place the greens and tomatoes in a large salad bowl. Drizzle with the vinaigrette and toss. Serve on salad plates—and perhaps you'd like to add your favorite vegetables on top.

NUTRITION FACTS: 1 SERVING; Caloric Density 0.4; Calories (Kcal) 26; Protein (g) 1; Carbohydrate (g) 3; Total Fat (g) 1; Saturated Fat (g) 0.2; Monounsaturated Fat (g) 0.9; Polyunsaturated Fat (g) 0.2; Dietary Fiber (g) 1.2; Flavonoid and Other Phyto (mg) 0.0; Cholesterol (mg) 0; Sodium (mg) 55; Vitamin A (IU) 2202; Vitamin C (mg) 15; Calcium (mg) 32; Iron (mg) 1.0; PERCENTAGE (%) Protein 16.2; Carbohydrate 41.5; Fat 42.4

Wakame Asparagusu

SERVES 4

There's a Japanese cucumber salad called *su-no-mono* ("food with vinaigrette") that's usually served in a tiny porcelain bowl as refreshment between other courses. Our recipe is close to traditional Japanese *su-no-mono* salad, except we use asparagus instead of the usual finely sliced Japanese cucumber. We've made the substitution because asparagus is more filling, which helps cut the caloric density of the meal, and it's generally more readily available than Japanese cucumber. Asparagus also has five times more vitamin C (25 mg per 100) and ten times more folate (119 mg per 100) than cucumber. The wakame seaweed in the recipe provides a beneficial hit of calcium.

6 tablespoons dried wakame seaweed
1⅓ cups asparagus, peeled and cut into ⅓-inch pieces

2 tablespoons low-sodium soy sauce
2 tablespoons rice vinegar
2 teaspoons turbinado or brown sugar

In a large bowl, rehydrate the wakame in plenty of water for 15 minutes. Drain.

Boil or steam the asparagus until crisp-tender.

In a large bowl, combine the soy sauce, vinegar, and turbinado sugar. Stir until the sugar is dissolved. Add the asparagus and wakame to the dressing bowl and toss to coat evenly. Chill and serve.

NUTRITION FACTS: 1 SERVING; Caloric Density 0.5; Calories (Kcal) 29; Protein (g) 2; Carbohydrate (g) 5; Total Fat (g) 0; Saturated Fat (g) 0.0; Monounsaturated Fat (g) 0.0; Polyunsaturated Fat (g) 0.0; Dietary Fiber (g) 1.8; Flavonoid and Other Phyto (mg) 0.0; Cholesterol (mg) 0; Sodium (mg) 426; Vitamin A (IU) 323; Vitamin C (mg) 6; Calcium (mg) 27; Iron (mg) 0.9; PERCENTAGE (%) Protein 25.0; Carbohydrate 72.2; Fat 2.9

Asian Okra and Tomato
SERVES 4

Although okra is originally from Africa, it's now a favorite in Okinawa vegetable gardens. Okinawans and other Japanese use it to create many distinctive dishes and are fascinated by its special sticky texture. The stickiness comes from a substance called mucilage that has been used for centuries to treat intestinal disorders and, more recently, to reduce cholesterol levels. Okra is also high in vitamins A and C as well as folate and potassium.

20 small okras	1 tablespoon low-sodium soy sauce
3 tomatoes, peeled and diced	Olive oil spray
2 tablespoons lemon juice	½ cup dried bonito flakes
Pinch of turbinado or brown sugar	

Cook okras in a pot of boiling water for 2 minutes. Drain and rinse with cold water. Remove the hard tops. Cut into horizontal halves.

In a mixing bowl, combine the tomatoes and okra.

In a small bowl or a bottle with a lid, combine the lemon juice, turbinado sugar, soy sauce, and 2 sprays of olive oil and mix well.

Place the vegetables on a large plate or 4 salad plates and top with the bonito flakes. Pour 2 teaspoons dressing over each plate and serve. Use all the dressing if you are serving the entire mixture in a large plate.

NUTRITION FACTS: 1 SERVING; Caloric Density 0.3; Calories (Kcal) 50; Protein (g) 3; Carbohydrate (g) 10; Total Fat (g) 1; Saturated Fat (g) 0.1; Monounsaturated Fat (g) 0.1; Polyunsaturated Fat (g) 0.1; Dietary Fiber (g) 3.0; Flavonoid and Other Phyto (mg) 0.0; Cholesterol (mg) 0; Sodium (mg) 165; Vitamin A (IU) 970; Vitamin C (mg) 34; Calcium (mg) 55; Iron (mg) 1.1; PERCENTAGE (%) Protein 23.1; Carbohydrate 68.2; Fat 8.6

Ryukyu Swiss Chard (Nsunaba Usachi)

SERVES 4

Recipe from *Okinawan Mixed Plate: Generous Servings of Culture, Customs and Cuisine*, published by Hui O Laulima, August 2000. To order, call Bobbi Kuba at (808) 523-5858 or e-mail emkuba@yahoo.com / thelma@hawaii.rr.com.

Nsunaba, or Swiss chard, is grown in Okinawa year-round, but its tastiest season is from spring into summer. Interestingly, this tangy vegetable is not sold in groceries in Okinawa but rather grown mostly in home gardens. In this traditional Okinawan recipe, the tart, dark green leaves are combined with milder-tasting, creamy pureed tofu in a delicious mixture that is the exemplar of a true home-cooked Okinawan meal.

10 ounces water-packed firm light tofu	Pinch of sea salt
5 cups Swiss chard leaves	1 tablespoon white sesame seeds,
⅔ tablespoon white miso	toasted and ground
1 tablespoon turbinado or brown sugar	1 tablespoon almond butter (optional)

Cut the tofu in thirds. Drain and place the slices on a single layer on a microwavable plate, lined with a double thickness of paper towel. Cover and microwave on low for 3 minutes.

Cook the Swiss chard in boiling water for 2 minutes. Drain and rinse with cold water. Squeeze out the water and cut the chard into 1-inch slices.

Process the tofu, miso, turbinado sugar, salt, sesame seeds, and almond butter in a blender until smooth. In a mixing bowl, gently toss the sauce and the chard. Sprinkle with sesame seeds. Serve chilled.

NUTRITION FACTS: 1 SERVING; Caloric Density 0.6; Calories (Kcal) 68; Protein (g) 8; Carbohydrate (g) 5; Total Fat (g) 2; Saturated Fat (g) 0.1; Monounsaturated Fat (g) 0.3; Polyunsaturated Fat (g) 1.2; Dietary Fiber (g) 1.0; Flavonoid and Other Phyto (mg) 17.2; Cholesterol (mg) 0; Sodium (mg) 274; Vitamin A (IU) 1488; Vitamin C (mg) 14; Calcium (mg) 289; Iron (mg) 1.8; PERCENTAGE (%) Protein 44.8; Carbohydrate 31.9; Fat 23.3

Shima Tofu and Vegetable Terrine

SERVES 8

Recipe provided by Chef Tomoaki Oomura at Restaurant Wa no Ichi, Naha, Okinawa, phone: 81.98.869.1557

This recipe comes from Chef Oomura, the main chef at Restaurant Wa no Ichi in Naha, Okinawa, and a renowned tofu expert. Even though Chef Oomura ate tofu a few times a week as a child, he preferred meat. It wasn't until after working as a chef in a Japanese restaurant in Los Angeles and seeing how enthusiastically Americans embraced tofu that he returned to his Okinawan roots to become the tofu aficionado he is today. Now there is no end to Chef Oomura's new and inventive versions of this traditional food. He is a pro at blending East and West.

Canola oil spray
Pinch of sea salt
4 thin green beans
⅓ cup thinly sliced carrot
¼ cup thinly sliced bitter melon
⅓ cup thinly julienned yellow bell pepper
15 ounces water-packed firm light tofu
8 ounces fat-free cream cheese or soy cream cheese
½ cup soymilk, plain
1 tablespoon agar-agar powder (or 1 envelope gelatin powder, unflavored)
2 tablespoons water
½ cup no-salt-added tomato sauce
2 tablespoons apple cider vinegar or white wine vinegar
Freshly ground pepper (preferably white)
½ tablespoon olive oil

Spray a terrine mold (9⅞ × 3⅜ × 2¾ inches) or a similar mold with canola oil, line it with plastic wrap, and place it in the refrigerator.

Bring a large pot of water to a boil and add a pinch of sea salt. Add the green beans and cook for 1 minute, then add the carrot, bitter melon, and yellow pepper. Boil for 2 minutes and drain. Set aside.

Wrap the tofu in 2 paper towels and place on a plate. Microwave on medium for 3 minutes. Place the tofu, cream cheese, and soymilk in a blender and process until smooth. Transfer to a large bowl.

Combine agar-agar powder and water and stir to dissolve; stir into the tofu mixture. Mix in the vegetables and transfer the mixture to the mold. Tap the mold on the counter several times to let the air out from the mixture. Cover with plastic wrap, then with aluminum foil, and refrigerate overnight.

For serving: In a small mixing bowl, combine the tomato sauce, vinegar, pepper, and olive oil. Spoon about 1½ tablespoons sauce onto each salad plate, making a beautiful circle.

On a cutting board, unmold the terrine; on another cutting board, turn it upside down. Remove the plastic wrap carefully. Slice with a serrated knife into 1¼-inch-thick slices and serve on the sauce.

NUTRITION FACTS: 1 SERVING, 1 SLICE; Caloric Density 0.6; Calories (Kcal) 79; Protein (g) 9; Carbohydrate (g) 4; Total Fat (g) 2; Saturated Fat (g) 0.4; Monounsaturated Fat (g) 0.8; Polyunsaturated Fat (g) 0.9; Dietary Fiber (g) 0.8; Flavonoid and Other Phyto (mg) 11.3; Cholesterol (mg) 2; Sodium (mg) 196; Vitamin A (IU) 1895; Vitamin C (mg) 20; Calcium (mg) 248; Iron (mg) 0.9; PERCENTAGE (%) Protein 49.9; Carbohydrate 23.5; Fat 26.6

Daikon Shrimp Som Tam Salad

SERVES 4

This popular spicy Thai salad is traditionally made with green papaya, a favorite fruit in Okinawa that dates back to the great trading days of the old Ryukyu Kingdom. Here we've created a variation on the theme by using daikon, a marvelous long white Asian radish, somewhat milder than the little red ones you're used to. Okinawans love daikon and believe it helps protect against disease. We're crazy about it too; it's highly nutritious, wonderfully tangy, and practically calorie-free—an all-around winner. When you buy daikon, choose a firm and shiny one, as they tend to become wrinkled and soft with age.

1 pound daikon radish, peeled and
    sliced in thin rounds, then julienned
1 cup shredded carrot
1 teaspoon sea salt
½ pound medium shrimp, peeled

Juice from 1 lime
1 tablespoon Thai or Vietnamese fish
    sauce
Pinch of turbinado or brown sugar
½ teaspoon cayenne pepper

In a large colander, place the daikon and carrot. Sprinkle the vegetables with salt and coat evenly. Leave them for 5 minutes or until tender. Rinse under cold water to wash off the salt. Drain.

Cook the shrimp in plenty of boiling water for 3 minutes. Then drain and rinse.

In a large bowl, combine the lime juice, fish sauce, turbinado sugar, and cayenne pepper and whisk together. Add the vegetables and shrimp to the sauce and toss to coat. Chill and serve.

NUTRITION FACTS: 1 SERVING; Caloric Density 0.4; Calories (Kcal) 92; Protein (g) 11; Carbohydrate (g) 10; Total Fat (g) 1; Saturated Fat (g) 0.2; Monounsaturated Fat (g) 0.2; Polyunsaturated Fat (g) 0.4; Dietary Fiber (g) 2.8; Flavonoid and Other Phyto (mg) 0.0; Cholesterol (mg) 75; Sodium (mg) 456; Vitamin A (IU) 8764; Vitamin C (mg) 32; Calcium (mg) 68; Iron (mg) 1.9; PERCENTAGE (%) Protein 48.4; Carbohydrate 41.2; Fat 10.3

Stuffed Summer Tomato

SERVES 4

When tomatoes first reached Japan through Dutch traders around the end of the seventeenth century, they were greatly appreciated—but for their beauty only. While they were the subject of many still-life paintings and widely planted for ornamental purposes, no one would dare eat them. Even though their culinary potential was introduced in the 1890s book, *Edible Plants of Japan,* written by a professor of agricultural science, it wasn't until the postwar period that the Japanese really took to them. Today, tomatoes are a summer garden favorite in Japan and Okinawa.

4 large, ripe tomatoes	Pinch of sea salt
2 cups arugula, finely chopped	4 romaine lettuce leaves
½ cup finely diced cucumber	2 tablespoons balsamic vinegar
½ cup diced avocado	Olive oil spray
1 teaspoon lemon juice	Freshly ground black pepper

Make a shallow, skin-depth cross-cut on the bottom of each tomato; scald in boiling water for 30 seconds and rinse with running cold water as you peel the skins. Cut the top off the tomatoes and scoop out the seeds with a teaspoon. Let stand in the refrigerator for 15 minutes, or while preparing the other ingredients.

In a large mixing bowl, combine the arugula, cucumber, avocado, lemon juice, and salt and toss to mix evenly. Let stand for 3 minutes, or until vegetables are seasoned well.

Evenly divide the vegetable mixture into 4 mounds and fill the tomato cups. Place the stuffed tomatoes on 4 plates lined with the romaine lettuce leaves. Top each tomato with ½ tablespoon with balsamic vinegar. Spray each with olive oil, and top with black pepper. Serve chilled.

NUTRITION FACTS: 1 SERVING; Caloric Density 0.3; Calories (Kcal) 92; Protein (g) 3; Carbohydrate (g) 13; Total Fat (g) 4; Saturated Fat (g) 0.8; Monounsaturated Fat (g) 2.0; Polyunsaturated Fat (g) 0.8; Dietary Fiber (g) 4.5; Flavonoid and Other Phyto (mg) 0.0; Cholesterol (mg) 0; Sodium (mg) 88; Vitamin A (IU) 2843; Vitamin C (mg) 46; Calcium (mg) 57; Iron (mg) 1.7; PERCENTAGE (%) Protein 11.3; Carbohydrate 52.6; Fat 36.1

Sweet Potato Salad

SERVES 4

Although I often cursed the sweet potato as a child, and much preferred rice when we could get it, my grandmother taught me to appreciate the sweet potato through song. We sang the praises of the sweet potato for sustaining us through the best of times and the worst of times. . . . Following the war, as a young husband, I saved my family from starvation by planting a garden of sweet potatoes. It was only then that I realized the wisdom of my grandmother's teaching.

—SOKEI-SAN, A TEACHER AND MUSICIAN FROM SHURI, OKINAWA, 102 YEARS OLD

3 medium sweet potatoes, peeled and cut into 1-inch rounds	**½ tablespoon Dijon mustard**
4 tablespoons low-fat soy (or canola) mayonnaise	**⅓ cup thinly sliced carrot**
	⅓ cup thinly sliced cucumber
	Freshly ground black pepper

Steam the sweet potatoes, tightly covered, for 12 minutes, or until cooked through. Transfer to a large bowl and mash. Let cool.

Combine the mayonnaise and mustard in a small bowl.

Add the carrot, cucumber, and mayonnaise mixture to the sweet potatoes and stir to mix evenly.

Adjust the seasoning with black pepper.

NUTRITION FACTS: 1 SERVING; Caloric Density 1.1; Calories (Kcal) 145; Protein (g) 2; Carbohydrate (g) 26; Total Fat (g) 4; Saturated Fat (g) 0.6; Monounsaturated Fat (g) 0.0; Polyunsaturated Fat (g) 0.1; Dietary Fiber (g) 3.3; Flavonoid and Other Phyto (mg) 0.0; Cholesterol (mg) 0; Sodium (mg) 174; Vitamin A (IU) 22,425; Vitamin C (mg) 23; Calcium (mg) 26; Iron (mg) 0.7; PERCENTAGE (%) Protein 4.9; Carbohydrate 71.4; Fat 23.7

Soba Salad

SERVES 4

Soba are Japanese buckwheat noodles. Buckwheat's been eaten in Japan for over 6,000 years. In ancient times the grain was steamed or boiled, as grinders had yet to be invented. Noodles are a relatively new kid on the block—only about 1,600 years old. Because buckwheat is hardier and more easily grown than rice in Japan and Okinawa, the poor and rich in both regions benefited immensely from this grain when rice crops failed, which happened frequently throughout history. Even in modern, affluent Japan, buckwheat remains a favorite—and it's one of ours too.

6 ounces dried soba noodles
3 tablespoons low-sodium soy sauce
2 tablespoons sake rice wine
¼ teaspoon cayenne pepper

5 cups arugula
1 cup dried white wood-ear mushrooms
   (can be found in Chinese groceries)
2 cups julienned cucumber

Cook soba noodles according to the instructions on the package. Drain and rinse under cold running water until the noodles are cold.

In a mixing bowl, combine the soy sauce, sake, cayenne pepper, and ⅓ cup water. Add the soba and the arugula to the sauce, reserving a bit to drizzle over the top, and toss to evenly coat.

In a large bowl of water, rehydrate the wood-ear mushrooms for 5 minutes. Drain.

On the center of 4 salad plates, form small mountains with the soba mixture. Arrange the wood ears around the soba and place the cucumber on top. Pour the remaining sauce over the salad. Serve.

NUTRITION FACTS: 1 SERVING; Caloric Density 1.0; Calories (Kcal) 179; Protein (g) 8; Carbohydrate (g) 37; Total Fat (g) 1; Saturated Fat (g) 0.1; Monounsaturated Fat (g) 0.1; Polyunsaturated Fat (g) 0.2; Dietary Fiber (g) 3.6; Flavonoid and Other Phyto (mg) 0.0; Cholesterol (mg) 0; Sodium (mg) 797; Vitamin A (IU) 684; Vitamin C (mg) 5; Calcium (mg) 66; Iron (mg) 2.3; PERCENTAGE (%) Protein 16.3; Carbohydrate 76.7; Fat 2.8; Alcohol 4.2

Fava Bean and Tomato Salad

SERVES 4

The fava bean, also called the *broad bean,* is an ancient vegetable. It was the *only* bean Europeans ate until the discovery of the New World, and records indicate it was used in Chinese cooking as far back as 5,000 years ago. Fava beans are very low in calories—only 58 calories in ¾ cup beans (80 grams)—and have more fiber than cereal grains, a nice combination for the weight-conscious. Fresh fava beans exude the scent of summer sunshine, and when combined with tomatoes they yield an exceptional summer salad that fulfills all our salad principles.

1 cup fava beans, outer skin removed, inner skins cut vertically to the black part	⅓ cup fresh basil leaves Pinch of sea salt 4 large ripe red tomatoes
2 cloves garlic, minced	6 ounces mozzarella substitute or
1 tablespoon olive oil	low-fat mozzarella cheese, cut into
2 tablespoons apple cider vinegar or white wine vinegar	16 slices

Boil the fava beans in plenty of water for 4 to 5 minutes, or until tender. Drain. Remove inner skins and set the beans aside.

Process the garlic, olive oil, vinegar, basil, and salt in a food processor until smooth. Transfer to a small container and set aside.

Slice each tomato into 4 slices.

On 4 salad plates, arrange 4 tomato slices in a circle. Top each tomato slice with 1 slice mozzarella and some fava beans. Pour 1 tablespoon of dressing onto each plate. Chill in the refrigerator if you like, and serve.

NUTRITION FACTS: 1 SERVING; Caloric Density 0.8; Calories (Kcal) 193; Protein (g) 8; Carbohydrate (g) 21; Total Fat (g) 9; Saturated Fat (g) 2.1; Monounsaturated Fat (g) 5.2; Polyunsaturated Fat (g) 1.3; Dietary Fiber (g) 3.0; Flavonoid and Other Phyto (mg) 1.4; Cholesterol (mg) 0; Sodium (mg) 388; Vitamin A (IU) 1810; Vitamin C (mg) 40; Calcium (mg) 283; Iron (mg) 40; PERCENTAGE (%) Protein 15.9; Carbohydrate 42.3; Fat 41.8

Warm Tofu Salad of Wilted Greens and Macadamia Nuts

SERVES 4

This recipe was provided by Roy Yamaguchi, who is a well-known chef in Hawaii and host of a PBS show, *Hawaii Cooks with Roy Yamaguchi*. His restaurants can be found not only in Hawaii but also in many other parts of the United States, including California and New York. Try this great recipe, which is also introduced in his new book, *Hawaii Cooks: Flavors from Roy's Pacific Rim Kitchen.*

20 ounces firm tofu
½ teaspoon salt
½ teaspoon shichimi seven-spice powder (see page 158)
2 tablespoons macadamia nut oil
1 tablespoon sesame oil
2 teaspoons minced fresh garlic
2 teaspoons minced fresh ginger
1 ounce fresh shiitake mushrooms, sliced (about ½ cup)
1 cup chopped mustard greens
½ cup sugar snap peas

½ cup bean sprouts
½ cup spinach leaves
½ cup radicchio
1 cup watercress, leaves and stems
¾ ounces mung bean noodles (about ½ cup dry), soaked in water
2 tablespoons moromiso or regular miso
2 tablespoons fish sauce
2 cups mesclun, for garnish
¼ cup chopped macadamia nuts, for garnish

Cut the tofu into triangle-shaped pieces about ½ inch thick. Lay the pieces on paper towels and press gently with more paper towels to remove excess moisture. Season each piece with salt and shichimi.

Heat a nonstick sauté pan over high heat and add 1½ tablespoons of the macadamia nut oil. Sear the tofu for 2 to 3 minutes on each side, until golden brown. Drain on paper towels and keep warm.

Place a wok over high heat and add the remaining ½ tablespoon macadamia nut oil and the sesame oil. Add the garlic and ginger and stir-fry for 20 to 30 seconds, until barely light golden brown. Add the mushrooms, mustard greens, snap peas, bean sprouts, spinach, radicchio, and watercress and stir-fry for 2 minutes, or until the vegetables begin to wilt. Add the noodles, moromiso, and fish sauce, mix well, and stir-fry for a minute to blend the seasonings. Remove from the heat.

To serve, divide the fried tofu among 4 plates. Top each with mesclun and stir-fried vegetables. Sprinkle with the macadamia nuts and serve immediately.

NUTRITION FACTS: 1 SERVING; Caloric Density 1.0; Calories (Kcal) 284; Protein (g) 15;Carbohydrate (g) 13; Total Fat (g) 19; Saturated Fat (g) 2.0; Monounsaturated Fat (g) 10.4; Polyunsaturated Fat (g) 5.4; Dietary Fiber (g) 3.1; Flavonoid and Other Phyto (mg) 32.3; Cholesterol (mg) 0; Sodium (mg) 1043; Vitamin A (IU) 1790; Vitamin C (mg) 28; Calcium (mg) 571; Iron (mg) 2.9; PERCENTAGE (%); Protein 21.9; Carbohydrate 18.3; Fat 59.8

Soups and Stews

In Okinawa, they like to say, *"Shiru du kusui yaru"*—"Soups are medicines" —and indeed they are often chock-full of healing herbs and spices. Further, most soups fill you up with relatively few calories, so they make terrific weight-sensible meals. Soup is literally liquid food, made from cooking different kinds of solid food in a liquid base. The term *stew* is most often applied to blended dishes that contain meat, fish, or vegetables in a thick broth made from stewing liquid and the natural juices of the stewed foods. Both are an ancient tradition. Archeologists have uncovered evidence of pots made from bamboo, turtle shells, and even the stomachs of animals that were used for boiling meat or fish and vegetables in water; some date back 10,000 years. We're all for keeping up the tradition— although we recommend steel pots in lieu of reptile shells and animal parts.

Bonito Broth

Kelp Broth

Basic Miso Soup

Slimming Tomato Cabbage Soup

Hearty Vegetable Soup

Sweet Potato Miso Soup

Chicken Tom Yummy Goong

Sea Bass Fennel Soup

Toppuccino Soup

Healthiest Cream of Broccoli Soup

Traditional Tsumire Soup

Salmon Miso Soup

Creamy Split Pea and Sweet Potato Soup

Fragrant Soy Go Vegetable Soup

Okinawan Fish and Vegetarian Broths (Dashi)

Dashi is an all-purpose soup broth and seasoning used in most Okinawan and Japanese soups, dips, sauces, and dishes that call for simmering vegetables, fish, or meat (among other ingredients). Dashi provides a good part of the characteristic flavor of these cuisines. There are two main kinds: *katsuo-dashi* (bonito broth), prepared with dried bonito flakes, and a vegetarian broth called *kombu-dashi* (kelp broth), made from dried kelp seaweed. (Kelp's natural white powder covering delivers considerable flavor and should be lightly wiped off, not washed off entirely.) Making dashi is quick and easy, but you can buy instant bonito or kelp broth powders too. Both are available in most Asian markets and the international food section of large grocery stores (look for the MSG-free variety). Use whichever broth you prefer when a recipe calls for "bonito or kelp broth."

Bonito Broth

3 CUPS

3¼ cups water   **1 cup dried bonito flakes (or 1 teaspoon bonito broth powder)**

Bring the water to a boil, then turn off the heat and stir in the bonito flakes. Let stand for 3 to 5 minutes. Remove the flakes with a slotted spoon or a strainer and discard. The remaining liquid is bonito broth.

If you are using bonito broth powder, simply stir the powder into boiling water and the broth is ready.

Kelp Broth

3 CUPS

3¼ cups water, room temperature   **Two 2 × 3-inch dried kelp strips (or 1 teaspoon kelp broth powder)**

Place the water and the kelp strips in a pot. Let stand for 15 to 20 minutes. Bring the water to a boil over medium heat. Immediately remove kelp strips. The remaining liquid is kelp broth. Discard the kelp or slice it for a low-calorie salad.

If you are using kelp broth powder, simply boil the water, stir in the powder, and the broth is ready.

Basic Miso Soup

SERVES 4

Once you learn how to make a basic miso soup, a new world opens up to you. That's because for this dish, there are no right or wrong additional ingredients—just put in whatever you think is good and tasty (see suggestions below). But choosing the right miso is important. You'll find miso in three colors in most Asian markets: yellowish-white (*shiro,* or white), light brown (*awase,* or mixed), and dark reddish-brown (*aka,* or red). White miso usually has the sweetest and mildest taste. The darker the miso, the saltier it is, but low-sodium versions of all three are often available. Eastern Japanese prefer redder miso; Western Japanese, including Okinawans, prefer white miso. We like the white better too because it has considerably less sodium at the outset. When making your soup, always remember not to bring it to a boil after putting miso paste in the broth. Okinawan cooks say that boiling miso kills the flavor. So make sure all the ingredients are cooked to your liking and *then* put in your miso. Simmer over low heat if you want the miso taste to permeate the ingredients.

3 cups bonito or kelp broth (see page 229)
1 tablespoon white miso

Your choice of vegetables, tofu, or seaweeds

Warm the broth over medium heat—do not bring it to a boil—and dissolve the miso in the broth.

Add your favorite vegetables, tofu, or seaweed. If the ingredients must be cooked, simmer over low heat until they are ready.

SUGGESTED INGREDIENTS
1 tablespoon dried wakame seaweed and 1 ounce tofu cubes
1 cup spinach
1 cup thinly sliced daikon radish quarter-rounds

1 cup mustard greens
1 cup chopped zucchini
1 tablespoon dried wakame seaweed and ½ cup diced red potatoes
½ cup thinly sliced konnyaku and ½ cup thinly sliced carrot

NUTRITION FACTS: 1 SERVING WITH 1 TABLESPOON DRIED WAKAME SEAWEED AND 1 OUNCE FIRM LIGHT TOFU CUBES; Caloric Density 0.9; Calories (Kcal) 17; Protein (g) 2; Carbohydrate (g) 1; Total Fat (g) <1; Saturated Fat (g) 0.0; Monounsaturated Fat (g) 0.0; Polyunsaturated Fat (g) 0.2; Dietary Fiber (g) 0.4; Flavonoid and Other Phyto (mg) 5.4; Cholesterol (mg) 0; Sodium (mg) 191; Vitamin A (IU) 18; Vitamin C (mg) 0; Calcium (mg) 35; Iron (mg) 0.3; PERCENTAGE (%) Protein 42.9; Carbohydrate 33.8; Fat 23.3

Slimming Tomato Cabbage Soup

SERVES 4

Cabbage (*tamanaa,* or "ball vegetable") is loaded with vitamin C and is wonderfully low in caloric density. It's cherished throughout Okinawa—and apparently has been highly considered in other cultures for thousands of years. Here, for instance, is what the Roman politician and general Cato (Marcus Porcius) had to say about this superveggie in the second century B.C.:

The cabbage surpasses all other vegetables. If, at a banquet, you wish to dine a lot and enjoy your dinner, then eat as much cabbage as you wish, seasoned with vinegar, before dinner, and likewise after dinner eat some half-dozen leaves. It will make you feel as if you had not eaten, and you can drink as much as you like.

2 cups low-sodium vegetable broth	1 dried bay leaf
1 cup ripe tomato, chopped	Pinch of sea salt
2 cups cabbage, shredded	Freshly ground black pepper

Bring 1 cup water and the vegetable broth to a boil. Add the tomato, cabbage, and bay leaf and return to a boil. Simmer over low heat for 4 minutes or until the cabbage is tender.

Season with the salt and pepper, remove the bay leaf, and serve hot.

NUTRITION FACTS: 1 SERVING; Caloric Density 0.1; Calories (Kcal) 33; Protein (g) 2; Carbohydrate (g) 8; Total Fat (g) 0; Saturated Fat (g) <1; Monounsaturated Fat (g) 0.0; Polyunsaturated Fat (g) 0.1; Dietary Fiber (g) 2.0; Flavonoid and Other Phyto (mg) 0.0; Cholesterol (mg) 0; Sodium (mg) 167; Vitamin A (IU) 1465; Vitamin C (mg) 26; Calcium (mg) 36; Iron (mg) 0.9; PERCENTAGE (%) Protein 15.8; Carbohydrate 77.9; Fat 6.3

Hearty Vegetable Soup

SERVES 4

This amazing low-CD soup contains ten full servings of vegetables (that's 2½ servings per person) and gives you half the amount of daily vegetables recommended by the National Institutes of Health. It is great with a slice of whole-grain bread for lunch or served as an appetizer or even a main meal. Double the recipe and refrigerate the extra for a good low-cal anytime energy booster.

2 cups low-sodium vegetable broth	**2 dried bay leaves**
2 cups water	**Pinch of sea salt**
1 cup diced carrots	**Freshly ground black pepper**
2 cups diced daikon radish	**3 cups shredded romaine lettuce**
1 cup diced celery	

In a large pot, place the vegetable broth, water, carrots, and radish and bring to a boil. Reduce the heat to low and cook for 8 minutes or until the daikon is semitransparent. Add the celery, bay leaves, salt, and black pepper and cook for 10 minutes. Add the romaine lettuce, increase the heat to high, and cook for 2 minutes, or just until the lettuce is tender. Serve hot.

NUTRITION FACTS: 1 SERVING; Caloric Density 0.1; Calories (Kcal) 41; Protein (g) 2; Carbohydrate (g) 9; Total Fat (g) <1; Saturated Fat (g) 0.0; Monounsaturated Fat (g) 0.0; Polyunsaturated Fat (g) 0.1; Dietary Fiber (g) 3.1; Flavonoid and Other Phyto (mg) 3.4; Cholesterol (mg) 0; Sodium (mg) 134; Vitamin A (IU) 10,837; Vitamin C (mg) 24; Calcium (mg) 55; Iron (mg) 1.2; PERCENTAGE (%) Protein 16.2; Carbohydrate 79.7; Fat 4.1

Sweet Potato Miso Soup

SERVES 4

This soup uses three of Okinawa's most popular ingredients: sweet potato, miso, and kelp. Kelp is, in fact, a very important food in Okinawa—and amazingly rich in potassium, calcium, iodine, and carotene. It thrives in the cold waters of northern Japan. When Japan traded with China in the old days of the Ryukyu Kingdom, the ships always made a stop at Naha (Okinawa's capital) and unloaded wilted kelp at bargain prices. Sharp business folks, the Uchinanchu (Okinawans) never failed to snap up all the excess kelp. Okinawa is still the number-one kelp-eating prefecture in Japan. Simmered and seasoned kelp is a must in local New Year dishes and is beautifully served in delicate lacquerware boxes.

Three 1-inch-long dried kelp strips
1 cup dried bonito flakes
1 cup diced sweet potato, soaked in
    water for 5 minutes
⅔ cup thinly sliced and quartered
    daikon radish

½ cup thinly sliced and quartered
    carrot
1¼ tablespoons white miso
¼ cup finely chopped green onion

In a stew pot, place 4 cups water and the kelp. Bring to a boil. Immediately turn off the heat and add the bonito flakes. Stir. Let stand for 5 to 10 minutes. Remove the kelp and bonito with a slotted spoon and discard. Add the sweet potato, daikon, and carrot to the broth and bring to a boil. Reduce the heat to low and cook for 15 minutes, or until the vegetables are tender.

In a small mixing bowl, combine the miso and a ladleful of soup. Dissolve the miso in the broth and return it to the stew pot.

Serve hot topped with the green onion.

NUTRITION FACTS: 1 SERVING; Caloric Density 0.2; Calories (Kcal) 58; Protein (g) 2; Carbohydrate (g) 12; Total Fat (g) 1; Saturated Fat (g) 0.1; Monounsaturated Fat (g) 0.1; Polyunsaturated Fat (g) 0.3; Dietary Fiber (g) 2.0; Flavonoid and Other Phyto (mg) 7.4; Cholesterol (mg) 0; Sodium (mg) 265; Vitamin A (IU) 10,978; Vitamin C (mg) 11; Calcium (mg) 25; Iron (mg) 0.6; PERCENTAGE (%) Protein 10.8; Carbohydrate 80.9; Fat 8.3

Chicken Tom Yummy Goong

SERVES 4

They say in Okinawa, *"Kaagee kaaru yaru"*—"Beauty is skin deep." That's certainly the case when it comes to lemongrass, one of this soup's main ingredients and a staple of Asian cooking. Lemongrass, with its long, thin, gray-green leaves and scallionlike base, looks more like a drab weed than the fragrant, magical plant it is. (Its fresh lemony scent is from an essential oil called *citral,* also found in lemon peel.) Dried lemongrass stalks are available in most groceries, natural food stores, and Asian food stores. As you're cooking this recipe, try steeping a teaspoon of chopped, dried lemongrass in hot water for a soothing herbal tea.

3 ounces boneless, skinless chicken breast	1 bundle (1 ounce) mung bean threads (optional)
2 cloves garlic, halved	1 teaspoon oyster sauce
2 tablespoons sliced ginger	2 tablespoons lemon juice
Two 3-inch-long lemongrass stalks	½ teaspoon cayenne pepper
½ cup chopped celery	Pinch of sea salt
⅓ cup sliced daikon radish	Freshly ground black pepper
⅓ cup chopped carrot	

In a large stockpot, bring 4 cups water to a boil. Add the chicken, garlic, ginger, and lemongrass and return to a boil. Reduce the heat to low, cover, and cook for 10 to 15 minutes. Occasionally remove scum with a spoon.

Remove the garlic, ginger, and lemongrass with a slotted spoon and add the celery, daikon, and carrot. Bring to a boil over high heat and reduce heat to low. Cook for 5 to 7 minutes, or until the vegetables are cooked.

In the meantime, cook the mung bean threads in a pot of boiling water for 3 to 5 minutes. Transfer to a colander, rinse under cold water, and drain well. Transfer the threads to a cutting board and chop them several times.

Add the oyster sauce, lemon juice, and cayenne pepper to the stockpot. Cook for 4 minutes, or until ingredients are seasoned well. Adjust the seasoning with the salt and pepper.

Divide the mung bean threads evenly among 4 soup bowls. Pour the soup over them. Serve hot.

NUTRITION FACTS: 1 SERVING; Caloric Density 1.1; Calories (Kcal) 82; Protein (g) 5; Carbohydrate (g) 14; Total Fat (g) 0; Saturated Fat (g) 0.1; Monounsaturated Fat (g) 0.1; Polyunsaturated Fat (g) 0.1; Dietary Fiber (g) 0.9; Flavonoid and Other Phyto (mg) 1.7; Cholesterol (mg) 12; Sodium (mg) 138; Vitamin A (IU) 2977; Vitamin C (mg) 8; Calcium (mg) 21; Iron (mg) 0.5; PERCENTAGE (%) Protein 26.1; Carbohydrate 69.2; Fat 4.8

Sea Bass Fennel Soup

SERVES 4

Fennel (*ichoba*) is one of the most popular herbs in Okinawa. It's thought to help digestion and strengthen the stomach, and many Okinawan elders, including our friend, 101-year-old Ushi Okushima, raise it in their gardens for medicinal purposes. They also love that it's practically maintenance-free. Its strong scent drives plant-eating bugs away, so essentially you just plant it and forget it—until you're ready to cook, that is. It's especially good with seafood.

Four 3-ounce sea bass fillets with skin
⅔ cup thinly sliced daikon radish, each
**   slice cut into 6 wedges**
1 tablespoon sake rice wine

½ teaspoon sea salt
½ teaspoon low-sodium soy sauce
½ cup fresh fennel leaves, in small
**   stalks**

Preheat the broiler.

Place the sea bass fillets on a baking dish lined with baking paper and broil for 4 minutes on each side.

In the meantime, bring 4 cups water to a boil and cook the daikon over medium heat for 5 to 7 minutes, or until transparent.

Transfer the sea bass carefully to the radish pot; then add the sake, salt, and soy sauce. Reduce the heat to low and simmer for 15 minutes, covered. Add the fennel leaves and turn off the heat. Let stand for 2 minutes.

Serve hot with a fillet in each bowl.

NUTRITION FACTS: 1 SERVING; Caloric Density 0.2; Calories (Kcal) 82; Protein (g) 17; Carbohydrate (g) 1; Total Fat (g) 0; Saturated Fat (g) 0.0; Monounsaturated Fat (g) 0.0; Polyunsaturated Fat (g) 0.0; Dietary Fiber (g) 0.1; Flavonoid and Other Phyto (mg) 0.0; Cholesterol (mg) 0; Sodium (mg) 324; Vitamin A (IU) 210; Vitamin C (mg) 4; Calcium (mg) 34; Iron (mg) 0.2; PERCENTAGE (%) Protein 88.8; Carbohydrate 4.6; Fat 1.4; Alcohol 5.2

Toppuccino Soup

SERVES 4

This is another interesting way to eat healthy tofu. In this soup, the smoothly blended tofu and egg float on the surface. It looks, in fact, a bit like a cup of cappuccino—especially when served in small Japanese lacquer soup bowls or handleless French café-au-lait cups. It's perfectly appropriate to forgo the spoon and drink directly from the bowl.

10 ounces water-packed light silken tofu, excess water squeezed out in cheesecloth
3 free-range, omega-3 eggs or ¾ cup egg substitute or egg white
4 cups water or 2 cups low-sodium vegetable broth and 2 cups water

2 cubes low-sodium vegetable bouillon (if not using vegetable broth)
Freshly ground black pepper
4 tablespoons chopped parsley

Process the tofu and eggs in a blender until smooth. Transfer to a mixing bowl and whisk vigorously to add air.

Bring water or vegetable broth mixture to a boil. Reduce the heat to medium and add the bouillon cubes (if not using vegetable broth). Pour in the tofu mixture. When the tofu mixture becomes foamy, remove the pot from the heat.

Ladle the soup into 4 soup bowls and top each with 1 tablespoon parsley. Serve hot.

NUTRITION FACTS: 1 SERVING; Caloric Density 0.3; Calories (Kcal) 93; Protein (g) 9; Carbohydrate (g) 4; Total Fat (g) 5; Saturated Fat (g) 1.2; Monounsaturated Fat (g) 1.4; Polyunsaturated Fat (g) 0.5; Dietary Fiber (g) 0.7; Flavonoid and Other Phyto (mg) 14.6; Cholesterol (mg) 159; Sodium (mg) 189; Vitamin A (IU) 2729; Vitamin C (mg) 8; Calcium (mg) 270; Iron (mg) 1.8; PERCENTAGE (%) Protein 39.6; Carbohydrate 16.2; Fat 44.2

Healthiest Cream of Broccoli Soup

SERVES 4

You can buy cream of broccoli soup at most local grocery stores—but take a look at the calorie information on the can. One serving of condensed cream of broccoli soup, when prepared with a cup of whole milk, has 248 calories and a CD of 0.68. Our healthier homemade version with soymilk and fresh broccoli has under 100 calories and a CD of 0.3—a true featherweight, and much more delicious than the store-bought kind.

Canola oil spray
2 cloves garlic, minced
½ cup thinly sliced white onion
3 cups broccoli florets

½ cup chopped celery
1½ cups low-sodium vegetable broth
1½ cups soymilk, plain
¼ cup all-purpose unbleached flour

Spray the bottom of medium stockpot with canola oil and heat over medium heat. Cook the garlic and onion for 5 minutes, or until the onion is tender and half transparent. Add the broccoli and celery, stir, and add the vegetable broth. Cover and cook for 8 minutes, or until all the vegetables are tender. Transfer to the blender and process until pureed. Return the soup to the stockpot and add the soymilk. Simmer over low heat for 5 minutes. Do not boil.

In the meantime, combine the flour and ⅓ cup water and mix until smooth. Add this to the soup and stir. Simmer for additional 1 to 2 minutes, or until the soup is thickened. Serve warm.

NUTRITION FACTS: 1 SERVING; Caloric Density 0.3; Calories (Kcal) 99; Protein (g) 6; Carbohydrate (g) 16; Total Fat (g) 2; Saturated Fat (g) 0.3; Monounsaturated Fat (g) 0.4; Polyunsaturated Fat (g) 0.9; Dietary Fiber (g) 4.4; Flavonoid and Other Phyto (mg) 17.3; Cholesterol (mg) 0; Sodium (mg) 107; Vitamin A (IU) 1910; Vitamin C (mg) 67; Calcium (mg) 57; Iron (mg) 1.9; PERCENTAGE (%) Protein 22.5; Carbohydrate 59.6; Fat 17.9

Traditional Tsumire Soup

SERVES 4

In the old days, making sardine balls (*tsumire*) was a time-consuming process in Okinawa. Cooks used to remove the skin, tails, and large bones, then meticulously extract the thin bones of this tiny omega-3-rich fish with tweezers. Then they'd grind the fish and spices together for what seemed like an eternity, until the ingredients were completely smooth. Nowadays, most people just buy prepared, vacuum-packed *tsumire* at the grocery store. Our special recipe hearkens back to the spirit of old but introduces a new technology—the blender. Thanks to this miracle invention, you now can grind and eat every part of the fish (except the head, stomach, and tail) in an instant. These fresh ingredients make this soup wonderfully tasty and fresh—and the fish bones are an excellent source of calcium.

18 ounces (4 to 6) fresh raw sardines
2 teaspoons ginger, minced
⅓ cup finely chopped leek, white part only

2 tablespoons kudzu powder or
1½ tablespoons arrowroot powder
1 tablespoon sake rice wine
1 cup sliced fresh shiitake mushrooms
1 tablespoon white miso

Hold a sardine's caudal fin with one hand; using a small knife, scrape the scales off the sardine, from head to tail. Chop the head off as well as the caudal and dorsal fins. Make a cut along the belly (do not cut through to the back) and open the fish. Remove the abdomen and wash the dark red flesh with cold running water. Repeat with the remaining sardines. Wipe off the excess water with paper towels. You can also simply ask the fishmonger to clean them.

In a blender, process the sardines and the ginger until smooth. Transfer to a medium mixing bowl. Add the leek, kudzu, and sake and knead by hand for 1 minute, or until the mixture sticks together when compressed. Divide the mixture into 12 balls. Flatten them slightly.

Bring 3 cups water to a boil and add the sardine balls. Cook over medium-high heat for 7 minutes, or until all the balls float to the surface. Add the shiitake mushrooms and cook for another 3 minutes.

In the meantime, in a small cup, dissolve the miso in some liquid taken from the pot. Return to the pot and stir once. Serve hot.

NUTRITION FACTS: 1 SERVING; Caloric Density 0.4; Calories (Kcal) 132; Protein (g) 18; Carbohydrate (g) 7; Total Fat (g) 3; Saturated Fat (g) 0.4; Monounsaturated Fat (g) 1.1; Polyunsaturated Fat (g) 1.6; Dietary Fiber (g) 1.3; Flavonoid and Other Phyto (mg) 12.3; Cholesterol (mg) 111; Sodium (mg) 247; Vitamin A (IU) 73; Vitamin C (mg) 1; Calcium (mg) 74; Iron (mg) 1.4; PERCENTAGE (%) Protein 53.8; Carbohydrate 22.1; Fat 21.0; Alcohol 3.1

Salmon Miso Soup

SERVES 4

Although all this soup's ingredients are available throughout the year, it's a perfect winter soup. Its ethereal color combination—the creamy custard yellow of the miso, the pink of the salmon, and the gold of the squash—is guaranteed to brighten up any cold, dreary winter day. And salmon's heart-healthy omega-3 fatty acids help hold the temperature of the soup, so it warms your bones and your heart at the same time.

Canola oil spray
2 cups thinly sliced white onion
8 ounces salmon with skin, sliced into
    1 × 1-inch squares
1 cup diced carrot
2 dried bay leaves
2 cups diced potatoes

1 cup winter squash with skin
    (preferably green-skin kabocha
    pumpkin), cut into 1 × 1-inch
    squares
1½ cups soymilk, plain
1½ tablespoons white miso

Spray the bottom of a stew pot with canola oil and cook the onion over medium heat for 5 minutes, or until tender. Add the salmon and carrot. Stir. Add 2½ cups water and the bay leaves. Cover and bring to a boil. Reduce heat to very low and simmer covered for 7 minutes.

Increase the heat to medium and add the potatoes, squash, and soymilk. Cook for 3 minutes and reduce heat to low. Do not boil. Continue to simmer for another 7 minutes.

In a small mixing bowl, combine the miso and ⅓ cup liquid from the stew pot and dissolve well. Return the mixture to the pot and stir once. Simmer for another 15 minutes. Serve warm.

NUTRITION FACTS: 1 SERVING; Caloric Density 0.4; Calories (Kcal) 179; Protein (g) 16; Carbohydrate (g) 16; Total Fat (g) 6; Saturated Fat (g) 0.9; Monounsaturated Fat (g) 1.6; Polyunsaturated Fat (g) 2.5; Dietary Fiber (g) 4.4; Flavonoid and Other Phyto (mg) 43.3; Cholesterol (mg) 31; Sodium (mg) 301; Vitamin A (IU) 9100; Vitamin C (mg) 13; Calcium (mg) 50; Iron (mg) 1.9; PERCENTAGE (%) Protein 35.5; Carbohydrate 35.1; Fat 29.4

Creamy Split Pea and Sweet Potato Soup

SERVES 4

Split pea is a variety of the green or yellow field pea that is specifically grown for drying. After it's dried, the pea splits along the natural seam, which makes for quicker cooking— and, as you've probably deduced, gives the pea its name. Neither split peas nor lentils, which are both very thin and small, need to be soaked for rehydration like other dried beans. Serve this thick, tasty soup as a filling low-calorie lunch or light dinner. If you prefer thinner soup, add water or low-fat, low-sodium vegetable broth.

3 cups peeled sweet potato, cut into ½-inch slices	2 dried bay leaves
½ tablespoon olive oil	1 cube low-sodium vegetable bouillon
⅔ cup thinly sliced yellow onion	½ teaspoon dried cumin seeds
½ cup split peas, rinsed	Salt and freshly ground black pepper

Steam the sweet potatoes in a tightly covered steamer for 15 to 18 minutes, or until tender.

In the meantime, coat a medium stew pot with the olive oil and cook the onion over medium heat for 5 minutes, or until it is tender and transparent. Stir continuously. Add the split peas and stir. Pour in 4 cups water, add the bay leaves, and cook over high heat until boiling. Reduce the heat to low and cook covered for 20 minutes or until the peas are tender.

When the sweet potatoes are cooked, transfer them to a blender and add ½ cup liquid from the stew pot. Process until smooth. Set aside.

When the peas are done, remove the bay leaves and add the bouillon cube and dissolve it. Then add the sweet potato mixture to the stew pot. Mix well. Stir in the cumin. Adjust the seasonings with salt and pepper to taste. Serve warm.

NUTRITION FACTS: 1 SERVING; Caloric Density 0.6; Calories (Kcal) 218; Protein (g) 8; Carbohydrate (g) 43; Total Fat (g) 2; Saturated Fat (g) 0.3; Monounsaturated Fat (g) 1.4; Polyunsaturated Fat (g) 0.4; Dietary Fiber (g) 9.8; Flavonoid and Other Phyto (mg) 11.9; Cholesterol (mg) 0; Sodium (mg) 66; Vitamin A (IU) 20,614; Vitamin C (mg) 26; Calcium (mg) 52; Iron (mg) 2.1; PERCENTAGE (%) Protein 14.4; Carbohydrate 76.0; Fat 9.5

Fragrant Soy Go Vegetable Soup

SERVES 4

Cooked and ground soybeans are called *go* in Japan. *Go,* one of the healthy by-products of making tofu, adds a flavonoid-rich thick texture and distinctive flavor to simple miso soup. In this recipe, we don't attempt to make tofu; we just go with the *go.*

1½ cups thinly sliced daikon radish, each slice cut into 6 wedges

1 cup thinly sliced carrot

4 ounces konnyaku yam cake, thinly sliced (see page 304), or 1 cup diced eggplant

1 cup thinly sliced burdock root, soaked in plenty of water with 1 teaspoon any vinegar for 5 to 10 minutes, drained

6 ounces water-packed firm light tofu, cut into small cubes

2 cups boiled soybeans or canned soybeans

2 tablespoons white miso

Bring 3 cups water to a boil. Add the daikon, carrot, konnyaku, and burdock and cook for 10 minutes over medium-high heat, or until the daikon is transparent. Add the tofu and reduce heat to low.

In a food processor, process the soybeans for a few seconds; the beans' shapes should still be visible. Add the soybeans to the vegetables and stir.

Add the miso and dissolve it. Cook over low heat for 5 minutes. Serve hot.

NUTRITION FACTS: 1 SERVING; Caloric Density 0.5; Calories (Kcal) 230; Protein (g) 20; Carbohydrate (g) 21; Total Fat (g) 9; Saturated Fat (g) 1.2; Monounsaturated Fat (g) 1.8; Polyunsaturated Fat (g) 5.2; Dietary Fiber (g) 8.5; Flavonoid and Other Phyto (mg) 54.9; Cholesterol (mg) 0; Sodium (mg) 353; Vitamin A (IU) 8594; Vitamin C (mg) 9; Calcium (mg) 285; Iron (mg) 5.7; PERCENTAGE (%) Protein 32.7; Carbohydrate 34.2; Fat 33.1

Chicken

In the old days, chicken was a luxury few people in Okinawa could afford. Most felt lucky to get meat once or twice a month. Since the 1960s, though, chicken has been gaining in popularity, and it is fast becoming second only to the traditional meat, pork. After sampling a few of these outstanding chicken recipes, you will definitely understand why.

Poached Chicken with Herb Dressing

Chilled Chicken Wontons

Okinawan Coq au Vin

Winter Soy Chicken with Vegetables

Chicken and Peanut Stir-Fry in Oyster Sauce

Spicy Stewed Chicken

Nasi Goreng Ayam (Chicken Rice)

Walnut-Dressed Chicken

Simple and Easy Tandoori Chicken

Chicken Asparagus Cordon Bleu

Chicken and Mushroom Linguine

Chicken Edamame Curry

Poached Chicken with Herb Dressing

SERVES 4

Like boiling, poaching is a great low-fat cooking technique. It's akin to boiling, but the ingredients being poached are just barely covered with liquid. And while the liquid bubbles in boiling, it just quivers a bit in poaching. The green herb sauce here is a perfect complement to the blanched white chicken breasts. Think about serving this dish on bright yellow or red plates if you have some. Remember, beautiful presentation is part and parcel of the Okinawa way.

2 cups (10 ounces) asparagus, tough stems snapped off
7 ounces boneless, skinless chicken breast, diced
1 tablespoon olive oil
1 tablespoon apple cider vinegar or white wine vinegar

Pinch of sea salt
Freshly ground black pepper
Pinch of turbinado or brown sugar
1 teaspoon fresh rosemary
1 teaspoon fresh thyme

In a pot of boiling water, cook the asparagus for 2 minutes, or until crisp-tender. Drain and let cool.

In the same pot, poach the chicken for 4 to 5 minutes or until cooked thoroughly. Drain and let cool.

In a large mixing bowl, combine olive oil, vinegar, salt, pepper, sugar, rosemary, and thyme. Add the asparagus and chicken and toss to coat evenly. Serve.

NUTRITION FACTS: 1 SERVING; Caloric Density 0.8; Calories (Kcal) 103; Protein (g) 13; Carbohydrate (g) 4; Total Fat (g) 4; Saturated Fat (g) 0.7; Monounsaturated Fat (g) 2.6; Polyunsaturated Fat (g) 0.5; Dietary Fiber (g) 1.5; Flavonoid and Other Phyto (mg) 0.0; Cholesterol (mg) 29; Sodium (mg) 102; Vitamin A (IU) 414; Vitamin C (mg) 10; Calcium (mg) 22; Iron (mg) 1.1; PERCENTAGE (%) Protein 50.3; Carbohydrate 13.7; Fat 36.0

Chilled Chicken Wontons

SERVES 4

The wonton—finely chopped vegetables (and often meat) in a thin flour wrapping—is alive and well in Okinawa, and we're not surprised. Wontons originated in China, and Okinawan cuisine has long been influenced by China because it was a tributary nation of that country from the fourteenth to the late nineteenth century. Wontons have a slick and shiny skin after boiling and are irresistible to many Asians. Make a bunch and float them in a large bowl of water with a few flowers when entertaining.

2 dried shiitake mushrooms	Pinch of sea salt
3 large cabbage leaves	16 wonton wrappers
½ cup finely chopped green onion	1 tablespoon low-sodium soy sauce
3 ounces ground skinless chicken	½ tablespoon rice vinegar
½ tablespoon sake rice wine	Pinch of chili powder
½ teaspoon sesame oil	⅓ cup fresh cilantro leaves
½ teaspoon grated ginger	

In a small mixing bowl, soak the shiitake mushrooms in some water to rehydrate for 15 minutes, or until tender. Squeeze out the excess water and chop finely.

Boil the cabbage leaves in a large pot of water for 3 minutes, or until soft. Drain and rinse under cold water, squeezing out excess water. Chop very finely and squeeze water out again.

In a large mixing bowl, place the shiitake mushrooms, cabbage, green onion, chicken, sake, sesame oil, ginger, and salt and knead well by hand until the mixture sticks together.

Spoon ½ tablespoon chicken mixture into the center of a wonton wrapper. Wet half of the edge, fold, and pinch the edges together. Repeat with the rest of the wrappers.

Combine the soy sauce, vinegar, and chili powder and divide the mixture among 4 small sauce plates.

Bring a large pot of water to boil. Boil the wontons for 3 minutes, or until the wrappers are half-clear and float on the surface. Remove the wontons from the pot with a slotted spoon and transfer them to a large mixing bowl of cold water.

In a large serving bowl, put cold water and ice cubes. Float the wontons and cilantro in the water. At the table, diners should pick up the wontons with chopsticks and dip them in the sauce to eat.

NUTRITION FACTS: 1 SERVING; Caloric Density 1.4; Calories (Kcal) 139; Protein (g) 7; Carbohydrate (g) 19; Total Fat (g) 4; Saturated Fat (g) 0.2; Monounsaturated Fat (g) 0.2; Polyunsaturated Fat (g) 0.3; Dietary Fiber (g) 1.6; Flavonoid and Other Phyto (mg) 2.8; Cholesterol (mg) 3; Sodium (mg) 314; Vitamin A (IU) 201; Vitamin C (mg) 17; Calcium (mg) 39; Iron (mg) 1.1; PERCENTAGE (%) Protein 19.3; Carbohydrate 54.2; Fat 25.0; Alcohol 1.4

Okinawan Coq au Vin

SERVES 4

This is one of the recipes we highly recommend as an ideal meat dish because of its large number and wide variety of low–caloric density vegetables. White wine, like sake, is a great meat tenderizer and gives the chicken a rich, juicy taste. Use a dry wine instead of rich sweet wine to avoid a perfumelike scent and to maximize the flavor of the ingredients. Avoid cooking wines, as most have a rather high sodium content.

Four 3-ounce boneless, skinless chicken breasts	**⅓ cup sliced white onion**
Pinch of sea salt	**⅓ cup sliced carrot**
Freshly ground black pepper	**½ cup sliced celery**
Canola oil spray	**1 cup halved ½-inch zucchini slices**
¼ cup white wine	**3 tablespoons apple cider vinegar or white wine vinegar**
½ tablespoon olive oil	**1 tablespoon low-sodium soy sauce**
1 clove garlic, minced	

Pat the chicken breasts with salt and pepper. Refrigerate for 10 minutes.

Spray a large skillet with canola oil and heat it over medium-high. Place the chicken in the skillet and cook for 2 minutes on each side, or until golden. Reduce the heat to low and add the white wine. Cover and cook for 8 to 10 minutes, or until the chicken is cooked thoroughly.

In the meantime, heat another skillet over medium heat and cook the olive oil and garlic for 45 seconds to 1 minute, or until golden. Increase the heat to medium-high and add the onion, carrot, celery, and zucchini and cook for 5 minutes, continuously stirring. When the vegetables are tender, season with the vinegar, soy sauce, and pepper.

Put a breast on each of 4 dinner plates and top with evenly divided vegetables.

NUTRITION FACTS: 1 SERVING; Caloric Density 0.8; Calories (Kcal) 140; Protein (g) 21; Carbohydrate (g) 4; Total Fat (g) 3; Saturated Fat (g) 0.5; Monounsaturated Fat (g) 1.5; Polyunsaturated Fat (g) 0.4; Dietary Fiber (g) 1.2; Flavonoid and Other Phyto (mg) 7.7; Cholesterol (mg) 49; Sodium (mg) 292; Vitamin A (IU) 2991; Vitamin C (mg) 7; Calcium (mg) 30; Iron (mg) 1.1; PERCENTAGE (%) Protein 60.7; Carbohydrate 13.0; Fat 19.3

Winter Soy Chicken with Vegetables

SERVES 4

We find this a wonderfully comforting dish on a cold winter's night. But a couple of quick tips: When using soymilk in cooking, be careful not to boil it too long, as it will separate. Make sure to get low-sodium, low-fat chicken broth. Do a little comparison shopping and check the labels. Several brands claim "low-sodium, low-fat," but the amounts vary. The research time is worth it. Once you find "your" chicken broth, you can stick to it—kind of like a good financial stock.

Canola oil spray
Four 3-ounce boneless, skinless chicken
   breasts
1 shallot, minced
2 cloves garlic, minced
½ cup sliced carrot
½ cup sliced zucchini
½ cup sliced button mushrooms
½ cup white wine

⅓ cup low-sodium, low-fat chicken
   broth
½ cup soymilk, plain
Pinch of sea salt
Freshly ground black pepper
2 tablespoons all-purpose unbleached
   flour, mixed well with ¼ cup water
4 tablespoons minced Italian parsley

Spray a large skillet with canola oil and cook the chicken over medium-high heat for 2 minutes each side, or until golden. Set aside.

In the same skillet, spray canola oil again and sauté the shallot, garlic, carrot, zucchini, and mushrooms over medium heat for 2 to 3 minutes, or until the flavors of the vegetables blend. Return the chicken to the skillet. Add the white wine and cover. Simmer over medium heat for 3 minutes, or until the wine is reduced by half. Stir in the chicken broth. Cover and simmer over low heat for 8 to 10 minutes, or until the chicken and vegetables are cooked thoroughly. Transfer the chicken and vegetables to a plate and set aside. Reserve the liquid in the pan.

Add the soymilk, salt, and pepper to the skillet and simmer over low heat for 2 minutes. Add the flour-water mixture and whisk until the liquid is thick. Return the chicken and vegetables to the skillet and stir.

Evenly divide the chicken and vegetables on individual plates. Sprinkle with parsley.

NUTRITION FACTS: 1 SERVING; Caloric Density 0.7; Calories (Kcal) 143; Protein (g) 22; Carbohydrate (g) 5; Total Fat (g) 2; Saturated Fat (g) 0.4; Monounsaturated Fat (g) 0.4; Polyunsaturated Fat (g) 0.6; Dietary Fiber (g) 1.3; Flavonoid and Other Phyto (mg) 0.5; Cholesterol (mg) 49; Sodium (mg) 142; Vitamin A (IU) 4625; Vitamin C (mg) 10; Calcium (mg) 32; Iron (mg) 1.5; PERCENTAGE (%) Protein 61.3; Carbohydrate 13.5; Fat 11.6; Alcohol 13.6

Chicken and Peanut Stir-Fry in Oyster Sauce

SERVES 4

Note the kudzu powder in the ingredients—it's a very interesting compound. The kudzu plant (*Pueraria lobata* or *Thunbergiana*) is native to Japan and has been cultivated in Asian countries for centuries for its edible tubers and hemplike fiber. It's also long been used as a treatment for inflammation, injuries, burns, cuts, and infections. This plant contains rich amounts of a powerful flavonoid called *daidzin,* and it's high in fiber, protein, and vitamins A and D. A real power plant! Okinawans and Japanese use the powder (made of the dried tuber) as a culinary thickener. *Arrowroot* is a common name for many tuberous plants, including kudzu, so check the label to see if a product really uses kudzu or not. If not, it's almost always available in Asian groceries or health food stores.

²⁄₃ cup low-sodium, low-fat chicken broth
1 tablespoon oyster sauce
½ tablespoon turbinado or brown sugar
½ tablespoon low-sodium soy sauce
1 teaspoon minced garlic
1 teaspoon minced ginger
1 tablespoon kudzu powder or 2 teaspoons arrowroot powder
1 tablespoon water, room temperature

Canola oil spray
½ cup sliced yellow onion
6 ounces chicken breast, skinless, boneless, diced
⅓ cup peanuts, unsalted, preferably raw
½ cup diced green bell pepper
½ cup diced red bell pepper
Dash of sesame oil

In a small mixing bowl, combine the broth, oyster sauce, turbinado sugar, soy sauce, garlic, and ginger and whisk to mix well.

In another small mixing bowl, combine the kudzu powder and the water and stir to mix well.

Spray a large skillet with canola oil. Cook the onion over medium heat for 4 minutes, or until slightly tender. Increase the heat to medium-high. Add the chicken and peanuts and cook for 4 minutes, or until chicken is thoroughly cooked. Add the green and red bell peppers and sauté for 3 minutes, or until the peppers are slightly tender.

Stir the seasoning mixture and pour it into the skillet. Increase the heat to high and cook for 4 minutes, or until liquid is reduced by a third.

Stir the kudzu mixture and add it to the skillet. Cook for 1 minute, or until the liquid is thickened. Stir in a dash of sesame oil. Serve warm.

NUTRITION FACTS: 1 SERVING; Caloric Density 0.9; Calories (Kcal) 152; Protein (g) 14; Carbohydrate (g) 10; Total Fat (g) 7; Saturated Fat (g) 1.0; Monounsaturated Fat (g) 3.2; Polyunsaturated Fat (g) 2.1; Dietary Fiber (g) 2.2; Flavonoid and Other Phyto (mg) 13.5; Cholesterol (mg) 25; Sodium (mg) 226; Vitamin A (IU) 1195; Vitamin C (mg) 54; Calcium (mg) 29; Iron (mg) 1.2; PERCENTAGE (%) Protein 35.8; Carbohydrate 25.1; Fat 39.1

Spicy Stewed Chicken

SERVES 4

The tomatoes in this dish give you a nice hit of lycopene, a bright red natural pigment also found in watermelon, red grapefruit, and balsam pear, which has been linked to lower risk for prostate and breast cancer. This antioxidant is reputed to pack a heavier free-radical quenching punch than many others, including vitamin E and beta-carotene. The canola oil will not only help improve your cholesterol profile but also will boost lycopene absorption and increase its overall health benefits.

Freshly ground black pepper
5 tablespoons whole-wheat flour
Four 3-ounce boneless, skinless chicken thighs
Canola oil spray
2 cloves garlic, minced
⅓ teaspoon dried cumin seeds
1 cup thinly sliced white onion
½ teaspoon dried oregano
¼ teaspoon ground turmeric
1 can (14.5-ounce) low-sodium stewed tomatoes
2 cups chopped chard

In a plastic bag, combine the pepper and the flour. Put the chicken in the bag and shake to coat it evenly. Remove the chicken and reserve 2 tablespoons of the flour.

Spray a large skillet with canola oil and heat it over medium-high heat. Place the chicken in the skillet and sauté on each side for 2 minutes, or until golden. Transfer to a plate.

Spray the same pan with canola oil again and cook the garlic over medium heat for 45 seconds to 1 minute, or until golden. Add the cumin and onion and cook for 5 minutes, or until onion is tender and half transparent. Stir in the oregano and turmeric. Add the stewed tomatoes and bring to a boil over medium-high heat.

Return the chicken to the pan and reduce the heat to low; simmer for 10 minutes, stirring occasionally.

Add the chard and cook for another 8 minutes. Stir in the reserved flour little by little, and then simmer for 2 minutes, or until the liquid is thickened. Serve warm.

NUTRITION FACTS: 1 SERVING; Caloric Density 0.7; Calories (Kcal) 185; Protein (g) 20; Carbohydrate (g) 18; Total Fat (g) 4; Saturated Fat (g) 0.9; Monounsaturated Fat (g) 1.1; Polyunsaturated Fat (g) 1.0; Dietary Fiber (g) 3.7; Flavonoid and Other Phyto (mg) 17.9; Cholesterol (mg) 71; Sodium (mg) 141; Vitamin A (IU) 990; Vitamin C (mg) 18; Calcium (mg) 68; Iron (mg) 2.9; PERCENTAGE (%) Protein 42.4; Carbohydrate 38.4; Fat 19.1

Nasi Goreng Ayam (Chicken Rice)

SERVES 4

Portuguese accounts of Okinawan traders whom they regularly encountered in Malacca and other trading centers of Southeast Asia in the early 1500s describe them as "truthful men . . . who bring porcelain, damask, onions and many vegetables." The Okinawan traders brought something back too. *Nasi goreng* is an Indonesian dish that's enhanced by the fish sauce commonly used in Thailand (*nam pla* in Thai) and Vietnam (*nuoc mam* in Vietnamese). This lively sauce (found in Asian food stores) gives a special Asian zing to almost any dish you flavor with it. If you find its aroma a bit strong, substitute a mixture of 1 teaspoon low-sodium soy sauce and ½ teaspoon water.

Canola oil spray
2 cloves garlic, minced
¼ teaspoon red chili flakes
½ cup finely chopped yellow onion
8 ounces boneless, skinless chicken breast, diced
⅓ cup chopped green bell pepper
⅓ cup chopped red bell pepper

1½ teaspoons Thai or Vietnamese fish sauce
1 tablespoon Asian sweet-and-hot chili sauce
2 cups cooked brown rice
1 cup sliced cucumber
8 thin tomato wedges
2 tablespoons chopped fresh cilantro

Spray a large skillet with canola oil and cook the garlic and chili flakes over medium heat for 45 seconds to 1 minute, or until the garlic is golden. Add the onion and cook for 5 minutes, or until transparent. Add the chicken and cook for 3 minutes, or until golden. Add the green and red bell peppers and cook for 4 minutes, or until the chicken and peppers are cooked thoroughly. Add the fish sauce and chili sauce, then stir to coat evenly. Add the rice and quickly stir with a wooden spatula, shaking the skillet back and forth.

Divide the chicken rice among plates and garnish each with ¼ cup cucumber slices, 2 tomato wedges, and ½ tablespoon cilantro. Serve.

NUTRITION FACTS: 1 SERVING; Caloric Density 0.8; Calories (Kcal) 206; Protein (g) 17; Carbohydrate (g) 29; Total Fat (g) 2; Saturated Fat (g) 0.4; Monounsaturated Fat (g) 0.5; Polyunsaturated Fat (g) 0.6; Dietary Fiber (g) 3.2; Flavonoid and Other Phyto (mg) 9.2; Cholesterol (mg) 33; Sodium (mg) 275; Vitamin A (IU) 1067; Vitamin C (mg) 44; Calcium (mg) 34; Iron (mg) 1.4; PERCENTAGE (%) Protein 32.4; Carbohydrate 57.1; Fat 10.5

Walnut-Dressed Chicken

SERVES 4

Boiling meat is a popular and healthy cooking style in Okinawa. It removes excess oil from the meat, which lowers the fat content up to 80 percent. That's a great way of turning a CD heavyweight into a lightweight. Walnuts, although high in caloric density, are also high in omega-3 fatty acids, so in small amounts, as in this recipe, they're a healthy—and tasty—addition.

10 ounces skinless, boneless chicken
    breast
1 cup chopped watercress
1 cup bonito or kelp broth (see
    page 229)
2 teaspoons low-sodium soy sauce
2 tablespoons mirin sweet rice wine

1 cup fresh, julienned bamboo shoots
    (if fresh is not available, use canned,
    drained bamboo shoots)
⅓ cup raw walnuts
½ tablespoon low-sodium soy sauce
3 tablespoons turbinado or brown sugar

Boil the chicken in plenty of water for 7 minutes, or until cooked through. Rinse the chicken with cold water and tear it into small pieces.

Put the watercress in a colander and pour 2 cups boiling water over it. Let cool, then squeeze out the excess water.

In a pot, bring the broth, soy sauce, and mirin to a boil. Add the bamboo shoots, return to the boil, and then remove the pot from heat.

Roast the walnuts in a nongreased skillet over low heat for 4 minutes, stirring continuously. In a food processor, process the walnuts, soy sauce, and turbinado sugar until smooth.

In a mixing bowl, combine the chicken, watercress, bamboo shoots, and walnut dressing. Divide evenly among 4 plates to serve.

NUTRITION FACTS: 1 SERVING; Caloric Density 1.1; Calories (Kcal) 229; Protein (g) 20; Carbohydrate (g) 18; Total Fat (g) 9; Saturated Fat (g) 1.0; Monounsaturated Fat (g) 2.0; Polyunsaturated Fat (g) 5.3; Dietary Fiber (g) 1.6; Flavonoid and Other Phyto (mg) 0.0; Cholesterol (mg) 41; Sodium (mg) 489; Vitamin A (IU) 422; Vitamin C (mg) 8; Calcium (mg) 47; Iron (mg) 1.6; PERCENTAGE (%) Protein 35.0; Carbohydrate 31.1; Fat 33.9

Simple and Easy Tandoori Chicken

SERVES 4

Indian food has influenced Okinawan taste since the Middle Ages; chili, turmeric, and bitter melon, now among Okinawa's most revered "traditional" foods and spices, came from India during the great trading days of the old Ryukyu Kingdom in the fourteenth to sixteenth centuries. Here we've given the traditional Northern Indian tandoori chicken an Okinawan twist, turning it into an easier and healthier version. If you like spices, you will love this dish!

1 cup low-fat yogurt, plain	**1 teaspoon poultry seasoning**
5 tablespoons ground paprika	**½ teaspoon garlic powder**
½ teaspoon ground allspice	**½ teaspoon sea salt**
1 teaspoon ground turmeric	**4 chicken legs, skin and visible fat**
⅔ teaspoon cayenne pepper	**removed**

Prepare the broiler.

In a large mixing bowl, combine the yogurt, paprika, allspice, turmeric, cayenne pepper, poultry seasoning, garlic, and salt. Place the chicken in the spice mixture, coat it well, and let stand in the refrigerator for at least 30 minutes.

Cook the chicken in the broiler for 20 to 30 minutes, or until it is cooked through.

NUTRITION FACTS: 1 SERVING; Caloric Density 1.2; Calories (Kcal) 235; Protein (g) 31.; Carbohydrate (g) 11.; Total Fat (g) 8; Saturated Fat (g) 1.8; Monounsaturated Fat (g) 1.5; Polyunsaturated Fat (g) 1.3; Dietary Fiber (g) 3.3; Flavonoid and Other Phyto (mg) 0.0; Cholesterol (mg) 109; Sodium (mg) 443; Vitamin A (IU) 3734; Vitamin C (mg) 6; Calcium (mg) 132; Iron (mg) 3.1; PERCENTAGE (%) Protein 52.8; Carbohydrate 17.9; Fat 29.3

Chicken Asparagus Cordon Bleu

SERVES 4

Chicken Cordon Bleu is pounded chicken rolled up to enclose other ingredients. In this healthy variation, we use asparagus as a core ingredient because it allows you to roll the chicken more easily. When you get used to the rolling technique, your only limitation is your imagination. Try ingredients with interesting color combinations, such as carrot and zucchini or yellow and red bell pepper. Make a large quantity, slice the rolls into bite-size pieces, and arrange on a large plate over a mound of shredded cucumber. Garnish with watercress or decorate with raspberry sauce. This presentation is great for parties.

4 asparagus spears, tough stems snapped off, halved
Four 3-ounce boneless, skinless chicken breasts
4 soy cheese slices

¼ cup whole-wheat flour
⅓ cup egg white
⅔ cup bread crumbs
Canola oil spray

Preheat the oven to 400°F.

Boil the asparagus for 3 minutes, or until crisp-tender.

Pound the chicken breasts to about ⅛ inch thick. Place 1 soy cheese slice and 2 asparagus pieces in the center of a chicken piece and roll up; secure the roll with a toothpick. Repeat with each chicken breast.

Place the flour in a medium bowl. Whisk the egg white and 2 tablespoons water in another bowl. Place the bread crumbs in a third bowl.

Dredge the chicken rolls in the flour and remove the excess. Then dip the rolls in the egg white and, finally, in the bread crumbs.

Spray a baking dish with canola oil, place the rolls in it, and bake for 10 to 15 minutes or until the top bread crumbs are golden brown. Turn over the rolls and bake for another 10 to 15 minutes, or until golden brown and cooked thoroughly. Remove the toothpicks and serve warm.

NUTRITION FACTS: 1 SERVING; Caloric Density 1.5; Calories (Kcal) 267; Protein (g) 27; Carbohydrate (g) 26; Total Fat (g) 6; Saturated Fat (g) 1.6; Monounsaturated Fat (g) 2.5; Polyunsaturated Fat (g) 1.0; Dietary Fiber (g) 1.7; Flavonoid and Other Phyto (mg) 1.1; Cholesterol (mg) 49; Sodium (mg) 417; Vitamin A (IU) 519; Vitamin C (mg) 3; Calcium (mg) 227; Iron (mg) 2.3; PERCENTAGE (%) Protein 41.5; Carbohydrate 39.3; Fat 19.2

Chicken and Mushroom Linguine

SERVES 4

Most mushrooms have less than 15 calories per half-cup, which means they always lower the overall caloric density of a dish. They also easily absorb the flavor of the other ingredients. Here, that means you'll feel like you're eating more chicken than you actually are. Strangely, although raw mushrooms don't have a significant scent, when they are cooked they produce a great aroma that permeates the entire dish. *Quick Tip:* If you can't find whole-wheat linguine in your local grocery store, use whole-wheat spaghetti or any kind of short whole-wheat pasta.

Olive or canola oil spray	1 can (14.5 ounces) low-sodium stewed
2 cloves garlic, minced	tomatoes
½ cup minced yellow onion	⅓ cup white wine
6 ounces boneless, skinless chicken	1 dried bay leaf
breast, diced	Pinch of sea salt
1½ cups quartered button	Freshly ground black pepper
mushrooms	8 ounces whole-wheat dry linguine

Spray a skillet with olive oil and cook the garlic and onion over medium heat for 4 minutes, or until the onion is tender and half transparent. Add the chicken and cook over medium-high heat for 2 minutes, or until golden. Add the mushrooms and cook for another 3 minutes, or the mushrooms are tender. Stir continuously. Add the tomatoes, white wine, bay leaf, salt, and pepper and bring to a boil. Reduce the heat to low and simmer for 10 minutes.

In the meantime, cook the linguine per the package directions. Drain the linguine, add it to the chicken, and toss. Remove the bay leaf before serving.

NUTRITION FACTS: 1 SERVING; Caloric Density 0.8; Calories (Kcal) 308; Protein (g) 20; Carbohydrate (g) 53; Total Fat (g) 2; Saturated Fat (g) 0.3; Monounsaturated Fat (g) 0.3; Polyunsaturated Fat (g) 0.5; Dietary Fiber (g) 11.1; Flavonoid and Other Phyto (mg) 9.0; Cholesterol (mg) 25; Sodium (mg) 130; Vitamin A (IU) 551; Vitamin C (mg) 9; Calcium (mg) 92; Iron (mg) 3.3; PERCENTAGE (%) Protein 25.1; Carbohydrate 65.8; Fat 5.1; Alcohol 4.0

Chicken Edamame Curry

SERVES 4

Edamame (literally, "beans on branches") are soybeans that are harvested early, before ripening, when they're still green, fresh, and soft—and they're extremely rich in isoflavones. Edamame are especially beloved in Okinawa, where they're frequently used in cooking and eaten as an everyday snack—Okinawans love to pop them from the pod directly into their mouths. Now edamame have found their way across the ocean and are becoming popular in North America as well. They're now available in the frozen food section of most supermarkets (both with and without pods).

1 teaspoon canola oil	1 tablespoon curry powder
3 cloves garlic	½ teaspoon ground nutmeg
¼ teaspoon red chili flakes (or more to taste)	½ teaspoon ground cloves
	1 teaspoon ground turmeric
8 ounces boneless, skinless chicken breast, cut into 1-inch dice	Pinch of sea salt
	2⅔ cups cooked brown rice or wild rice, warm
8 cups chopped cabbage	
1½ cups frozen edamame green soybeans (*not* in the pod)	

Heat the canola oil, garlic, and chili flakes in a skillet over medium heat for 45 seconds to 1 minute, or until the garlic is golden. Add the chicken and sauté over high heat for 3 minutes, or until the surface is golden. Add the cabbage and sauté for 4 minutes, or until cabbage is tender. Add the edamame, curry powder, nutmeg, cloves, turmeric, and salt and stir. Add 1 cup water and bring to a boil. Reduce the heat to low and simmer for 5 minutes.

Divide the rice among 4 plates. Evenly divide the curry over the rice.

NUTRITION FACTS: 1 SERVING; Caloric Density 0.7; Calories (Kcal) 367; Protein (g) 27; Carbohydrate (g) 50; Total Fat (g) 8; Saturated Fat (g) 1.2; Monounsaturated Fat (g) 2.1; Polyunsaturated Fat (g) 3.1; Dietary Fiber (g) 10.0; Flavonoid and Other Phyto (mg) 29.0; Cholesterol (mg) 33; Sodium (mg) 150; Vitamin A (IU) 378; Vitamin C (mg) 70; Calcium (mg) 213; Iron (mg) 4.5; PERCENTAGE (%) Protein 28.6; Carbohydrate 52.5; Fat 18.9

Fish and Seafood

Surrounded by the ocean and its abundant resources, Okinawans have always respected it, and fishing has been a big part of their lives. In many small villages, people still believe the ocean gods provide them with fish, shellfish, and seaweed. After a good catch, the men in these villages make a circle on the beach and offer fish to the gods before bringing their share home. There's even an annual first-fishing ceremony day, when boys just turned thirteen leave school in the middle of the day and are initiated into the village fishing activities. At other ritual occasions, fish is offered to the gods on a sacred lacquer tray, along with Okinawan rice wine and a bowl of seaweed, vegetables, and rice. Because the Okinawan waters are warm and the fish don't need to store cold-protecting fat, most local fish have white, flaky flesh that is relatively low in calories and cholesterol. Many Japanese mainlanders, who are used to seeing silver-gray fish at home, are amazed at the astounding array of beautiful bright red, blue, and yellow fish in the Okinawan markets. Fish in Okinawa are indeed a visual as well as a culinary sensation.

Sea Bream Carpaccio with
Turmeric Sauce

Garlic Mussels with
White Wine Sauce

Poached White Fish
with Honey-Lime Sauce

Cod Wa no Ichi

Ryukyu Fish Curry

Hawaiian Lemon-Ahi Poke

Grilled Fish with Grated Radish

Baked Salmon Mousse

Cheesy Scallops and Potatoes

Spicy Garlic Shrimp

Papaya and Shrimp Spring Roll

Miso Salmon with Vegetables

Teriyaki Yellowtail with Rice

Shrimp and Broccoli Penne

Salmon with Nuts and Rice

Sea Bream Carpaccio with Turmeric Sauce

SERVES 4

Recipe provided by Chef Masayoshi Miyazato at Restaurant Wa no Ichi, Naha, Okinawa, phone: 81.98.869.1557

Carpaccio, originally a raw beef dish, was named after the fifteenth-century Italian painter Vittore Carpaccio, whose doctor advised him to eat only uncooked meat. These days one sees lots of carpaccio variations, most using fish, such as this recipe. Chef Miyazato highly recommends you try it at his restaurant in Naha. But for those of you who can't make it to Okinawa, he's generously allowed us to bring his superb recipe direct to your kitchen.

¼ cup lime juice
1 teaspoon ground turmeric
1 clove garlic, minced
1½ teaspoons olive oil
½ teaspoon turbinado or brown sugar
Pinch of sea salt
Freshly ground black pepper
4 ounces very fresh sea bream or similar fish, such as pollock or perch; salmon is fine, too (look for crisp edges, shiny skin, no unclear juice)

⅔ cup thinly sliced white onion or red onion, soaked in a bowl of water for 5 minutes and then squeezed out
⅓ cup matchstick-cut nori laver seaweed
2 tablespoons minced green onion
2 tablespoons minced red bell pepper
2 tablespoons minced yellow bell pepper

In a small mixing bowl, combine the lime juice, turmeric, garlic, olive oil, turbinado sugar, salt, and pepper. Blend until smooth. Chill in the refrigerator.

Slice the sea bream into very thin, almost see-through, rectangular sashimi slices. Place the onion in the center of a large platter. Arrange the sea bream slices in a circle around the onion. Top the onion with the nori and sprinkle the green onion and the red and yellow bell peppers on the sea bream.

Drizzle the chilled sauce over the sea bream and serve as soon as possible. Alternatively, the entire dish can be refrigerated until chilled through, then served.

NUTRITION FACTS: 1 SERVING; Caloric Density 0.8; Calories (Kcal) 66; Protein (g) 6; Carbohydrate (g) 6; Total Fat (g) 2; Saturated Fat (g) 0.3; Monounsaturated Fat (g) 1.3; Polyunsaturated Fat (g) 0.2; Dietary Fiber (g) 1.0; Flavonoid and Other Phyto (mg) 12.6; Cholesterol (mg) 0; Sodium (mg) 140; Vitamin A (IU) 281; Vitamin C (mg) 17; Calcium (mg) 30; Iron (mg) 0.7; PERCENTAGE (%) Protein 34.9; Carbohydrate 33.7; Fat 31.4

Garlic Mussels with White Wine Sauce

SERVES 4

Mussels have been used as food for over 20,000 years in Europe, and even played a part in politics. In ancient Greece, the names of candidates were scratched inside mussel shells—no hanging chads there. Mussels, with their creamy, juicy, sweet-flavored meat, are believed to be brain food in Japan because of their omega-3 fat, which is required for a healthy nervous system. Mussels have much less cholesterol than other shellfish, including oysters and shrimp. Another bonus: Because this dish is cooked with the shells intact, you'll eat it more slowly over a longer period, which means your appetite will be slowed as you eat—an excellent weight management strategy.

Healthy Tip: When you buy the mussels, choose ones with tightly closed shells or those that snap shut when tapped—an indication of freshness. Never buy mussels with broken shells or that feel light and loose when shaken.

1½ pounds blue mussels in their shells
2 teaspoons olive oil
4 large cloves garlic, minced

⅔ cup white wine
⅓ teaspoon sea salt

Wash the mussels thoroughly under running cold water and remove the beards. Discard any mussels that are open.

Heat a large skillet over medium heat and cook the olive oil and garlic for 45 seconds to 1 minute, or until the garlic is golden. Add the mussels and coat with the oil. Pour the wine into the skillet and immediately cover it tightly. When you see steam coming out from under the lid, reduce the heat to low. Simmer for 5 minutes.

When all the shells are opened, add the salt and simmer for another 2 minutes, stirring occasionally. Serve hot.

NUTRITION FACTS: 1 SERVING; Caloric Density 0.9; Calories (Kcal) 99; Protein (g) 7; Carbohydrate (g) 3; Total Fat (g) 4; Saturated Fat (g) 0.5; Monounsaturated Fat (g) 1.9; Polyunsaturated Fat (g) 0.5; Dietary Fiber (g) 0.1; Flavonoid and Other Phyto (mg) 0.0; Cholesterol (mg) 16; Sodium (mg) 551; Vitamin A (IU) 91; Vitamin C (mg) 6; Calcium (mg) 29; Iron (mg) 2.4; PERCENTAGE (%) Protein 28.2; Carbohydrate 13.7; Fat 32.2; Alcohol 25.9

Poached White Fish with Honey-Lime Sauce

SERVES 4

Flaky white-fleshed fish are common in Okinawa's warm waters. They're lower in calories than cold-water, red-fleshed fish, which need the fat to protect them from the cold. As you've seen on the Okinawa Caloric Density pyramid, white fish is a lightweight (CD 1.0), while red fish is a middleweight (CD1.8.), making white fish a great choice when watching calories. If you dislike fish because of its "fishy" smell, try this little secret—add some lime juice. Okinawans use a similar type of citrus fruit called *shikwasa,* which eliminates any fishy aroma and enhances flavor at the same time.

1 teaspoon dried thyme
Four 3-ounce white flaky fish fillets,
　　such as orange roughy, haddock,
　　char, or pollock
1 tablespoon honey
2 tablespoons lime juice
Pinch of sea salt
1 teaspoon olive oil

1 tablespoon kudzu powder or
　1 teaspoon arrowroot powder
1 tablespoon water, room temperature
½ cup white wine
1 tablespoon ground paprika or
　4 tablespoons minced Italian parsley
　for garnish

In a large skillet, bring 1 to 1½ cups water to a boil. Stir in the thyme. Carefully place the fish fillets in the skillet and poach over medium heat for 3 minutes. Turn over carefully and cook for another 2 minutes, or until cooked thoroughly. Remove the fish from the water and set aside.

Combine the honey, lime juice, salt, and olive oil in a small mixing bowl.

Dissolve the kudzu powder in the tepid water.

In a small pan, bring the white wine to a boil and reduce the heat to low. Stir the honey mixture and the kudzu mixture into the white wine. Stir until the liquid thickens.

Spoon 2 tablespoons sauce on each of 4 plates and place the fish in the center. Sprinkle with ¼ tablespoon paprika or 1 tablespoon Italian parsley.

NUTRITION FACTS: 1 SERVING; Caloric Density 0.9; Calories (Kcal) 121; Protein (g) 13; Carbohydrate (g) 7; Total Fat (g) 2; Saturated Fat (g) 0.2; Monounsaturated Fat (g) 1.2; Polyunsaturated Fat (g) 0.1; Dietary Fiber (g) 0.8; Flavonoid and Other Phyto (mg) 2.1; Cholesterol (mg) 17; Sodium (mg) 125; Vitamin A (IU) 839; Vitamin C (mg) 3; Calcium (mg) 38; Iron (mg) 0.8; PERCENTAGE (%) Protein 43.7; Carbohydrate 29.5; Fat 15.5; Alcohol 16.3

Cod Wa no Ichi

SERVES 4

Recipe provided by Chef Tomoaki Oomura at Restaurant Wa no Ichi, Naha, Okinawa,
phone: 81.98.869.1557

This recipe comes from Restaurant Wa no Ichi, one of the most inventive restaurants in
Okinawa. Their mantra is *"Oishii ishoku dogen"*—"Food should heal and taste good at
the same time." This recipe absolutely exemplifies that sentiment. The cod provides
lean protein, the garlic is heart-healthy, and the tomato soup is full of the antioxidant
lycopene—and that's just for starters.

6 ounces water-packed light silken tofu	1½ tablespoons kudzu powder or
4 large cabbage leaves	1 tablespoon arrowroot powder
½ pound skinless, boneless cod, diced	⅓ cup minced carrot
1 clove garlic	½ cup minced celery
Pinch of sea salt	⅓ cup chopped dill weed
Freshly ground black pepper	1 cup fat-free tomato soup

Wrap the tofu in a paper towel, set it on a plate, and microwave on high for
2 minutes.

Steam the cabbage leaves in a tightly covered steamer for 3 minutes, or until
tender.

In a food processor, process the cod, tofu, garlic, salt, and pepper until
smooth. Place the cod mixture in a medium mixing bowl. Add the kudzu powder,
carrot, celery, and dill weed and combine until the mixture holds together when
compressed.

Place a cabbage leaf on a flat board. Spoon 4 to 5 tablespoons cod mixture on
the front end of the leaf and roll up. Tuck the sides as you roll. Repeat with the
remaining three cabbage leaves.

Place the rolled cabbage in a pot and add the tomato soup. Cook over high
heat for about 3 minutes, or until just before the soup boils. Reduce the heat to
low and cook for another 10 minutes.

NUTRITION FACTS: 1 SERVING; Caloric Density 0.4; Calories (Kcal) 122; Protein (g) 16; Carbohydrate (g) 14; Total Fat (g) 1;
Saturated Fat (g) 0.1; Monounsaturated Fat (g) 0.1; Polyunsaturated Fat (g) 0.3; Dietary Fiber (g) 4.0; Flavonoid and Other
Phyto (mg) 16.7; Cholesterol (mg) 24; Sodium (mg) 222; Vitamin A (IU) 6277; Vitamin C (mg) 34; Calcium (mg) 215;
Iron (mg) 2.7; PERCENTAGE (%) Protein 48.9; Carbohydrate 43.0; Fat 8.1

Ryukyu Fish Curry

SERVES 4

Curry, originally from India, is very popular in Okinawa. As so many other foods did, it reached Okinawa during the ancient trading days when the Ryukyu Kingdom was a dynamo of foreign trade because of its industrious people and fortunate location. At the hub of Asian commerce, Okinawa was *the* link between India, Siam (Thailand), Java, and Malacca (Indonesia) in the southeast, Korea and Japan to the north, and China to the west. *Quick Tip:* It's very important to choose fresh fish. Remember that fresh fish fillets are clear and shiny, show no excess juice, and have crisp edges.

3 tablespoons whole-wheat flour	⅔ cup chopped leeks
1 tablespoon curry powder	⅔ cup low-sodium vegetable broth
Four 3-ounce white flaky fish fillets,	4 cups chopped spinach
such as orange roughy, haddock,	⅓ cup soymilk, plain
char, or pollock	Pinch of sea salt
Canola oil spray	Freshly ground black pepper

In a small mixing bowl, combine the flour and curry powder. Evenly coat the fish fillets with the flour mixture. Pat off excess.

Spray a large skillet with canola oil. Over medium-high heat, sauté the fillets for 2 minutes on each side, or until golden brown. Add the leeks and vegetable broth and bring to a boil. Reduce the heat to low and gently simmer for 7 minutes.

In the meantime, place the spinach in a microwavable container and sprinkle with water. Cover and microwave on medium for 3 minutes.

Add the spinach and the soymilk, salt, and pepper to the skillet and simmer on low heat for 5 minutes.

NUTRITION FACTS: 1 SERVING; Caloric Density 0.6; Calories (Kcal) 123; Protein (g) 15; Carbohydrate (g) 10; Total Fat (g) 3; Saturated Fat (g) 0.2; Monounsaturated Fat (g) 1.5; Polyunsaturated Fat (g) 0.8; Dietary Fiber (g) 2.7; Flavonoid and Other Phyto (mg) 0.4; Cholesterol (mg) 17; Sodium (mg) 179; Vitamin A (IU) 2485; Vitamin C (mg) 11; Calcium (mg) 79; Iron (mg) 2.2; PERCENTAGE (%) Protein 48.2; Carbohydrate 29.9; Fat 21.8

Hawaiian Lemon-Ahi Poke

SERVES 4

Poke, essentially marinated raw fish, is a prize-winning Hawaiian dish with strong Japanese overtones. The fish used in poke range from tuna and salmon to mussels or shrimp, and it can be combined with all sorts of exotic goodies, such as the crunchy Hawaiian seaweed called *limu,* flying fish roe, green onions, wasabi horseradish, or laver seaweed. Poke can be found in most Hawaiian restaurants and grocery stores, and is so popular that the half-dozen or so huge poke containers in the supermarkets are usually empty by evening;

sometimes there are even gentlemanly or ladylike scuffles over the last scoop. It pays to know how to make your own!

3 tablespoons fresh lemon juice
1 teaspoon sesame oil
1 teaspoon canola oil
1 tablespoon low-sodium soy sauce
1 teaspoon minced garlic
1 teaspoon minced ginger

½ cup thinly sliced white onion
12 ounces very fresh tuna or bonito
    block, diced into
    1-inch cubes
¼ cup chopped green onion

In a mixing bowl, combine the lemon juice, sesame oil, canola oil, soy sauce, garlic, ginger, and onion.

Add the bonito cubes and toss. Place in the refrigerator for at least 5 to 10 minutes, and up to 1 hour.

Divide the bonito evenly among 4 plates and sprinkle with the green onion.

NUTRITION FACTS: 1 SERVING; Caloric Density 1.0; Calories (Kcal) 135; Protein (g) 20; Carbohydrate (g) 4; Total Fat (g) 5; Saturated Fat (g) 0.3; Monounsaturated Fat (g) 1.1; Polyunsaturated Fat (g) 0.8; Dietary Fiber (g) 0.5; Flavonoid and Other Phyto (mg) 10.3; Cholesterol (mg) 0; Sodium (mg) 194; Vitamin A (IU) 51; Vitamin C (mg) 7; Calcium (mg) 26; Iron (mg) 1.6; PERCENTAGE (%) Protein 59.3; Carbohydrate 10.4; Fat 30.2

Grilled Fish with Grated Radish

SERVES 4

A recent survey of Japanese housewives and househusbands (a rare breed in Japan) asked the question "What is the easiest dinner to make in your house?" More than 70 percent answered *yaki-zakana*—"grilled fish." Every Okinawan and Japanese household has a special gridiron specially made for grilling fish. The cook simply puts a fish fillet on the gridiron for each member of the family and quickly whips up some steamed spinach and wakame seaweed miso soup while the fish grills. It's the most popular home dinner menu in Japan—and might be yours soon too.

Four 3-ounce fish fillets, preferably with
    skin, such as mackerel, pacific saury,
    trout, or salmon

⅓ teaspoon sea salt
One 6-inch-long piece of daikon radish,
    peeled and grated

Sprinkle the fish with salt and refrigerate for 10 minutes.

Prepare a grill.

Grill the fish for 4 to 5 minutes on each side, or until thoroughly cooked.

Serve on individual plates with a small mound of grated daikon on the side.

NUTRITION FACTS: 1 SERVING; Caloric Density 1.1; Calories (Kcal) 190; Protein (g) 16; Carbohydrate (g) 4; Total Fat (g) 12; Saturated Fat (g) 2.8; Monounsaturated Fat (g) 4.7; Polyunsaturated Fat (g) 2.9; Dietary Fiber (g) 1.4; Flavonoid and Other Phyto (mg) 0.0; Cholesterol (mg) 59; Sodium (mg) 287; Vitamin A (IU) 140; Vitamin C (mg) 19; Calcium (mg) 36; Iron (mg) 1.7; PERCENTAGE (%) Protein 35.1; Carbohydrate 7.5; Fat 57.5

Baked Salmon Mousse

SERVES 4

I use this recipe as a great appetizer for a special, elegant dinner or party.
On the other hand, it's a perfect baby food, too. You decide!

—MRS. SHIMABUKURO, AGE 102, OF OKINAWA CITY, OKINAWA

Canola oil spray
10 ounces fresh raw salmon, skinless,
   boneless
2 tablespoons white wine
1 egg white

2 tablespoons half-and-half or cream
   substitute
¼ cup plus 3 tablespoons soymilk, plain
Pinch of sea salt
Freshly ground black pepper

Preheat the oven to 350°F.

Spray a small loaf pan or 4 small ramekins (1½ inches deep × 3 inches in diameter) with canola oil.

In a blender, process the salmon, wine, egg white, half-and-half, soymilk, salt, and pepper until smooth. Transfer the mixture into the mold.

Pour water into a baking pan that is at least 2 inches deep until it is two-thirds full. Place the mold in the water. For a single large mold, bake for 20 to 25 minutes. For 4 small molds, bake for 15 to 20 minutes. The mousse is done when a toothpick inserted in the center comes out clean. Serve warm or chilled.

NUTRITION FACTS: 1 SERVING; Caloric Density 1.2; Calories (Kcal) 142; Protein (g) 16; Carbohydrate (g) 1; Total Fat (g) 7; Saturated Fat (g) 1.3; Monounsaturated Fat (g) 2.8; Polyunsaturated Fat (g) 2.5; Dietary Fiber (g) 0.4; Flavonoid and Other Phyto (mg) 0.5; Cholesterol (mg) 41; Sodium (mg) 119; Vitamin A (IU) 65; Vitamin C (mg) 0; Calcium (mg) 20; Iron (mg) 0.8; PERCENTAGE (%) Protein 45.8; Carbohydrate 2.9; Fat 47.8; Alcohol 3.5

Cheesy Scallops and Potatoes

SERVES 4

Small, red new potatoes are lower on the glycemic index and thus are better for your blood sugar than the bigger white russet potatoes. They're also more flavorful and more beautiful. When cooked unpeeled, their rich red skins have a glorious shine.

Canola oil spray
8 ounces medium scallops
2 cloves garlic
1 teaspoon canola oil
3 cups halved red-skinned potatoes
1 cup soymilk, plain
1 teaspoon curry powder

¼ cup low-sodium grated Parmesan
   cheese
Pinch of sea salt
½ teaspoon red chili flakes or cayenne
   pepper (optional)
2 cups halved snow peas

Spray a skillet with canola oil and heat it over medium-high heat. Sauté the scallops for 1 minute on each side, or until golden. Set aside.

In the same skillet, increase the heat to high and cook the garlic in the canola oil for 20 seconds or until it sizzles. Add the potatoes and cook for 4 minutes. Keep stirring. Pour in 2 cups water. Bring to a boil and reduce the heat to low. Cook for 10 minutes, or until potatoes are cooked but firm.

Increase the heat to high and stir in the soymilk, curry powder, Parmesan cheese, salt, red chili flakes, snow peas, and scallops. When the liquid is about to boil, immediately reduce the heat to low. Cook for 4 more minutes, stirring occasionally.

NUTRITION FACTS: 1 SERVING; Caloric Density 0.5; Calories (Kcal) 147; Protein (g) 15; Carbohydrate (g) 8; Total Fat (g) 6; Saturated Fat (g) 1.4; Monounsaturated Fat (g) 2.3; Polyunsaturated Fat (g) 1.6; Dietary Fiber (g) 2.8; Flavonoid and Other Phyto (mg) 5.7; Cholesterol (mg) 23; Sodium (mg) 176; Vitamin A (IU) 157; Vitamin C (mg) 35; Calcium (mg) 117; Iron (mg) 2.0; PERCENTAGE (%) Protein 41.2; Carbohydrate 22.2; Fat 36.6

Spicy Garlic Shrimp

SERVES 4

Garlic is among the oldest cultivated food plants. Its culinary, ritual, and medicinal uses date back more than 6,000 years. Researchers are now backing up old anecdotal claims with evidence that garlic can bolster the immune system, lower blood pressure, and prevent heart disease; some people even believe garlic can ward off vampires, although we've been unable to uncover any scientific support for that one. In Okinawa, garlic has long been considered an energy booster, and garlic bulbs, along with red chili peppers, are found in mixtures of local *awamori* (Okinawan sake) and sprinkled into soups and noodles.

2 teaspoons canola oil	3 cups sugar snap peas
4 cloves garlic, minced	Pinch of sea salt
Red chili flakes to taste	Freshly ground black pepper
1 pound shrimp, peeled and deveined	½ cup chopped Italian parsley

Heat the canola oil in a large skillet over medium heat. Cook the garlic and red chili flakes for 45 seconds to 1 minute, or until golden.

Increase the heat to high. Add the shrimp and cook for 1 minute, stirring continuously. Add the sugar peas and cook for 2 more minutes. Season with salt and pepper.

Turn off the heat and add the Italian parsley. Stir until parsley is tender.

NUTRITION FACTS: 1 SERVING; Caloric Density 0.9; Calories (Kcal) 179; Protein (g) 26; Carbohydrate (g) 8; Total Fat (g) 5; Saturated Fat (g) 0.6; Monounsaturated Fat (g) 1.7; Polyunsaturated Fat (g) 1.5; Dietary Fiber (g) 2.4; Flavonoid and Other Phyto (mg) 6.9; Cholesterol (mg) 172; Sodium (mg) 243; Vitamin A (IU) 731; Vitamin C (mg) 57; Calcium (mg) 108; Iron (mg) 4.8; PERCENTAGE (%) Protein 58.1; Carbohydrate 18.8; Fat 23.0

Papaya and Shrimp Spring Roll

SERVES 4

Green papaya (immature papaya) is one of the most popular foods in Okinawa. Every house used to have a few papaya trees planted outside—usually one in full sun and others in the shade, as temperature alters the flavor of the fruit. Today, shredded green papaya is available in groceries for Okinawans who do not have papaya trees in their garden. People who want whole green papayas go to the open markets to bargain with the *obaas* ("grand-mothers") who sell fresh fruit and vegetables.

16 medium shrimp, peeled
1 cup mung bean sprouts
2 tablespoons soy mayonnaise
1 teaspoon Dijon mustard
Sea salt
Freshly ground black pepper
1 cup julienned green, young papaya
    (matchstick thin)

1 cup julienned cucumber (matchstick thin)
1 tablespoon smooth low-sodium peanut butter
⅓ cup soymilk, plain
½ teaspoon cayenne pepper
8 rice paper wrappers (8½ inches in diameter, available at most Asian groceries)

Cook the shrimp in a pot of boiling water for 2 to 3 minutes, or until cooked.

Drain and let cool on ice.

Cook the mung bean sprouts in a pot of boiling water for 1 to 2 minutes, or until crisp-tender. Drain and rinse under cold running water.

In a medium mixing bowl, combine the mayonnaise, mustard, a pinch of salt, and pepper until blended. Add the papaya, cucumber, and bean sprouts and toss to coat evenly.

In a small mixing bowl, combine the peanut butter, soymilk, cayenne pepper, and a pinch of salt. Transfer to a dip bowl and set aside.

Place 1 or 2 kitchen towels on your work surface. Fill a pan with lukewarm water to a depth of about 1 to 2 inches. Soak a rice wrapper for 5 to 10 seconds. Do not soak until too soft. Gently transfer the wrapper to the work surface. Quickly arrange 2 shrimps on the front edge of the wrapper and top with ⅓ cup papaya mixture. Roll up the wrapper tightly but gently, tucking in the sides. Repeat with remaining wrappers.

Serve with the peanut sauce.

If the spring rolls are not eaten immediately, cover them with a damp paper towel or cloth and plastic wrap and refrigerate.

NUTRITION FACTS: 1 SERVING; Caloric Density 1.1; Calories (Kcal) 184; Protein (g) 10; Carbohydrate (g) 26; Total Fat (g) 5; Saturated Fat (g) 0.8; Monounsaturated Fat (g) 1.1; Polyunsaturated Fat (g) 1.0; Dietary Fiber (g) 2.7; Flavonoid and Other Phyto (mg) 0.4; Cholesterol (mg) 43; Sodium (mg) 277; Vitamin A (IU) 277; Vitamin C (mg) 27; Calcium (mg) 39; Iron (mg) 1.7; PERCENTAGE (%) Protein 20.7; Carbohydrate 56.0; Fat 23.3

Miso Salmon with Vegetables

SERVES 4

The French gastronome James de Coquet once declared, "Salmon are like men; too soft a life is not good for them." We agree. There's a world of difference in taste between the wild salmon (CD 1.4) that fight an upstream battle to return to their place of birth to spawn and those that lounge around salmon farms (CD 1.8), living the easy life. Go for wild salmon whenever you can; it's almost always worth the extra cost, and it's lower in caloric density due to its lower fat content.

½ teaspoon sesame oil
½ teaspoon canola oil
1 clove garlic, minced
1 tablespoon chopped ginger
½ pound boneless fresh salmon, diced into 1-inch cubes
½ teaspoon red chili powder or cayenne pepper (optional)
2 cups diced carrots
3 cups cauliflower florets
1½ cups diced celery
¼ cup sake rice wine
1½ tablespoons white miso

In a large skillet, heat the sesame oil, canola oil, garlic, and ginger over medium heat for 45 seconds to 1 minute, or until the garlic and ginger are golden.

Increase the heat to medium-high and add the salmon. Sauté for approximately 3 minutes per side, or until golden. If using chili powder or cayenne pepper, add it here. Stir in the carrots, cauliflower, and celery.

Increase the heat to high. Add the sake and 1 cup water, bring to a boil, and then reduce the heat to low. Cook for 5 minutes, or until the carrots are cooked through.

Dissolve the miso using a ladle of boiling water. Add to the skillet. Cook an additional 2 minutes.

NUTRITION FACTS: 1 SERVING; Caloric Density 0.6; Calories (Kcal) 188; Protein (g) 16; Carbohydrate (g) 15; Total Fat (g) 6; Saturated Fat (g) 0.9; Monounsaturated Fat (g) 2.0; Polyunsaturated Fat (g) 2.4; Dietary Fiber (g) 4.9; Flavonoid and Other Phyto (mg) 11.0; Cholesterol (mg) 35; Sodium (mg) 359; Vitamin A (IU) 17,264; Vitamin C (mg) 44; Calcium (mg) 67; Iron (mg) 1.6; PERCENTAGE (%) Protein 33.2; Carbohydrate 30.7; Fat 27.7; Alcohol 8.5

Teriyaki Yellowtail with Rice

SERVES 4

One important ingredient in this recipe—rice wine—has a special place in Okinawan and Japanese cuisine. Sake and mirin are both rice wines, but sake is dry and transparent and has a watery consistency, while mirin is sweeter, light yellow, and thicker. Further, while sake is primarily a drinking beverage, mirin is strictly for cooking and seasoning. It adds a shine to ingredients—*teriyaki* actually means "shiny bake." Because of its low alcohol content, mirin must be stored in the refrigerator after opening. Okinawan sake (*awamori*), incidentally, is said to be one of the secrets to the elders' remarkable longevity (consumed in moderation, of course), and 115-year-old Kamato Hongo from Amami Island, currently the world's oldest living person, is proud to say she still enjoys a glass now and then.

2 tablespoons low-sodium soy sauce	2 tablespoons whole-wheat flour
3 tablespoons mirin sweet rice wine	Canola oil spray
2 tablespoons sake rice wine	2 cups cooked brown rice
Four 3-ounce yellowtail or regular tuna fillets	¼ cup finely chopped green onion
	1 teaspoon grated ginger

In a large resealable plastic bag, place the soy sauce, mirin, sake, and 1 tablespoon water and mix well. Place the fish fillets in the bag and toss to coat. Place in refrigerator for 15 to 20 minutes.

Remove the fish from the bag; reserve the liquid. On a plate, sprinkle the flour over the fish to coat it slightly.

Spray a large skillet with canola oil and heat it over medium heat. Cook the fish for 3 minutes on each side. Reduce the heat to low and cook 2 more minutes on each side. Transfer to the plate and set aside.

Place the saved marinade in the same skillet and boil it over medium heat for 5 minutes, or until thickened. Turn off the heat and return the fish to the pan. Season by turning once.

Divide the rice among 4 individual plates and top with the fish. Any marinade remaining in the skillet can be evenly divided and poured over the fish. Garnish with the green onion and ginger.

NUTRITION FACTS: 1 SERVING; Caloric Density 1.2; Calories (Kcal) 260; Protein (g) 21; Carbohydrate (g) 35; Total Fat (g) 3; Saturated Fat (g) 0.3; Monounsaturated Fat (g) 1.3; Polyunsaturated Fat (g) 0.8; Dietary Fiber (g) 2.4; Flavonoid and Other Phyto (mg) 1.4; Cholesterol (mg) 0; Sodium (mg) 353; Vitamin A (IU) 66; Vitamin C (mg) 1; Calcium (mg) 43; Iron (mg) 1.2; PERCENTAGE (%) Protein 32.7; Carbohydrate 53.0; Fat 11.1; Alcohol 3.1

Shrimp and Broccoli Penne

SERVES 4

For this recipe we recommend fresh shrimp, as they have springier texture than the pre-cooked kind. Removing the shells is easy—just pluck off the legs first and then peel back the shell. We like leaving the tail on, because it's a better look (and less work), but taking the tails off works fine too. Deveining is not necessary when using medium shrimp or smaller, but it is suggested for bigger shrimp because the intestinal vein of larger shrimp contains grit. The high ratio of vegetables to shrimp in this recipe makes it a tasty treat for seafood beginners and aficionados alike—and when it comes to health, this dish is heads and tails above deep-fried shrimp, which can have more than double the calorie count.

20 medium shrimp	**1 shallot, minced**
2 cups broccoli florets	**½ teaspoon red chili flakes**
9 ounces whole-wheat dried penne or ziti pasta	**½ teaspoon dried oregano**
2 tablespoons olive oil	**Pinch of sea salt**
2 cloves garlic, minced	**Freshly ground black pepper**

Peel the shrimp, except the tails, and wash them gently under cold running water. Set aside.

Steam the broccoli, tightly covered, until bright green and just tender.

Cook the pasta per the directions on package. Drain, saving ¼ cup cooking water.

While the pasta cooks, heat the olive oil, garlic, shallot, and red chili flakes in a large skillet over medium heat for 60 to 90 seconds, or until the garlic is golden. Add the shrimp to skillet and cook over high heat, stirring continuously with a wooden spatula, for 2 minutes, or until the shrimp is bright red. Stir in the broccoli. Stir in the oregano, salt, and pepper. Stir in the ¼ cup saved water.

In a large mixing bowl toss the pasta with the shrimp mixture.

NUTRITION FACTS: 1 SERVING; Caloric Density 1.2; Calories (Kcal) 335; Protein (g) 18; Carbohydrate (g) 51; Total Fat (g) 9; Saturated Fat (g) 1.2; Monounsaturated Fat (g) 5.2; Polyunsaturated Fat (g) 1.3; Dietary Fiber (g) 9.4; Flavonoid and Other Phyto (mg) 3.4; Cholesterol (mg) 53; Sodium (mg) 138; Vitamin A (IU) 868; Vitamin C (mg) 43; Calcium (mg) 76; Iron (mg) 3.0; PERCENTAGE (%) Protein 20.5; Carbohydrate 57.8; Fat 21.8

Salmon with Nuts and Rice

SERVES 4

I remember when I was a child we couldn't afford white rice. Brown rice was much cheaper. Now I can afford the white, but only eat brown. Sometimes I mix it with other grains like millet. It's better and healthier. I love its nutty flavor . . . and it goes so beautifully with salmon.

—Mrs. Kinjo, ninety-nine years old, Naha City

Canola oil spray
⅔ cup finely chopped yellow onion
1 cup raw brown rice
⅓ cup chopped raw, unsalted nuts, such
   as almonds, pine nuts, cashews, or
   any combination of these
1 cup low-sodium vegetable broth
12 ounces skinless salmon, cut into
   1-inch cubes

Freshly ground black pepper
2 tablespoons whole-wheat flour
1 teaspoon sesame oil
1 tablespoon chopped ginger
4 cups bok choy, cut into 2-inch lengths
2 tablespoons sake rice wine
1 tablespoon low-sodium soy sauce

Spray a large skillet with canola oil and cook the onion over medium heat for 5 minutes, or until tender and transparent. Add the rice and nuts and toss to mix evenly.

Transfer the mixture to a rice cooker. Add the vegetable broth and 1 cup water. Turn the rice cooker on and cook until the rice is done. If you don't own a rice cooker, place the same ingredients in a medium pot and bring to a boil. Cover and simmer over very low heat for 10 to 18 minutes, or until the liquid is evaporated and the rice is cooked.

In a medium mixing bowl, coat the salmon with the pepper and flour.

In a large skillet, heat the sesame oil and ginger over medium heat for 45 seconds to 1 minute, or until golden. Add the salmon to the skillet and cook for 5 to 7 minutes, or until cooked through, turning occasionally. Raise the heat to high and add the bok choy; cook 1 to 2 minutes or until tender. Add the sake and soy sauce and cook another 1 minute.

Evenly divide the rice among 4 individual plates and top it with the salmon-vegetable mixture.

NUTRITION FACTS: 1 SERVING; Caloric Density 1.1; Calories (Kcal) 418; Protein (g) 25; Carbohydrate (g) 47; Total Fat (g) 14; Saturated Fat (g) 1.7; Monounsaturated Fat (g) 6.3; Polyunsaturated Fat (g) 4.6; Dietary Fiber (g) 4.9; Flavonoid and Other Phyto (mg) 12.0; Cholesterol (mg) 47; Sodium (mg) 280; Vitamin A (IU) 2697; Vitamin C (mg) 35; Calcium (mg) 140; Iron (mg) 3.1; PERCENTAGE (%) Protein 23.9; Carbohydrate 45.0; Fat 29.2; Alcohol 1.9

Lean Meats

The traditional Okinawan diet included lean meats like boiled pork and goat, but only on special occasions. The main protein sources were always soy, vegetables, and fish. Considerable research suggests that vegetarians or semivegetarians like the Okinawans and Seventh-Day Adventists outlive people who eat a lot of meat because vegetables are usually low in calories and rich in antioxidants. Meat is not and can be heavy in saturated fat and methionine, which raises artery-toxic cholesterol and homocysteine levels. Still, eating limited amounts of meat can be consistent with good health—if you eat it in a healthy way. A few tips:

1. Choose lean meat. Always get the butcher to trim the fat off the meat as much as possible. When it comes to pork, fat-trimmed loin is the best choice. For beef, extra-lean (less than 17 percent fat) ground beef, top sirloin with fat removed, and tenderloin are good choices.

2. Eat meat with lots of veggies. Try to cook meat with vegetables. Instead of having a 10-ounce steak, have 3 ounces of beef cooked with 7 ounces of vegetables. That reduces the caloric density of the dish considerably. The CD of 10 ounces of lean top sirloin is 1.3, but if you cook 3 ounces of lean top sirloin with 7 ounces of, say, broccoli, the caloric density is only 0.6—less than half.

3. Try boiling. In Okinawa, pork is a delicacy that often appears at celebratory meals. Okinawans traditionally boil the pork for hours before cooking and then discard the greasy boiling water. That transforms the pork into reasonably lean meat. Boiling results in fewer calories than sautéing, grilling, and barbecuing, which not only raise calories but also are associated with a higher risk for colon cancer.

Beef in Oyster Sauce

Balsamic Pork with Mushrooms

Pork Daikon

Nsunaba Sukiyaki

Shabu Shabu Pork with Herb Sauce

Sloppy Tofu with Beef

Veggieful Beef Stew

Veggie Pork Pita

Beef à la Crème

Bambou Short Ribs

Beef in Oyster Sauce

SERVES 4

Oyster sauce is widely used in Okinawa and Japan—mostly for stir-fries. It's a smooth, thick, dark-brown liquid with a very rich flavor. Traditional oyster sauce is made of boiled oysters seasoned with soy sauce and other Chinese spices. After months of preservation, the liquid on the surface is skimmed off and becomes the oyster sauce. Commercial oyster sauces that read "oyster-flavored sauce" on the label are most likely oyster extract combined with water. Both kinds are high in sodium, so limit the amount you use. Also, don't forget to compare the amount of sodium in various brands of oyster sauces when shopping for the product. The lower the better.

Canola oil spray
1 teaspoon sesame oil
1 teaspoon minced ginger
1 teaspoon minced garlic
9 ounces lean beef, preferably top sirloin or tenderloin, cut into 1/2-inch pieces
1 cup chopped green bell pepper

5 cups chopped Chinese napa cabbage, green and white parts separated
1/2 cup chopped leek
1 tablespoon oyster sauce
1 tablespoon sake rice wine
1/2 tablespoon mirin sweet rice wine
1 teaspoon low-sodium soy sauce
1/2 teaspoon cayenne pepper

Spray a wok or skillet with canola oil and add the sesame oil. Cook the ginger and garlic over medium heat for 45 seconds to 1 minute, or until golden. Add the beef and cook over medium-high heat for 3 minutes, or until browned.

Raise the heat to high and add the green bell pepper, the white part of the Chinese cabbage, and the leek. Cook for 2 to 3 minutes, or until the green pepper is tender and the cabbage is half transparent. Add the green part of the Chinese cabbage. Stir frequently and cook for 3 minutes, or until the cabbage is tender and the liquid is almost evaporated.

Quickly add the oyster sauce, sake, mirin, soy sauce, and cayenne pepper. Frequently shake the wok and, when the beef is seasoned evenly, transfer it with the vegetables to a large plate and serve.

NUTRITION FACTS: 1 SERVING; Caloric Density 0.6; Calories (Kcal) 140; Protein (g) 15; Carbohydrate (g) 9; Total Fat (g) 4; Saturated Fat (g) 1.2; Monounsaturated Fat (g) 1.7; Polyunsaturated Fat (g) 0.8; Dietary Fiber (g) 3.9; Flavonoid and Other Phyto (mg) 0.8; Cholesterol (mg) 39; Sodium (mg) 210; Vitamin A (IU) 1481; Vitamin C (mg) 61; Calcium (mg) 90; Iron (mg) 2.5; PERCENTAGE (%) Protein 43.1; Carbohydrate 26.2; Fat 27.8; Alcohol 2.9

Balsamic Pork with Mushrooms

SERVES 4

This recipe combines the thick, sweet flavor of pork with the refreshing tartness of balsamic vinegar—a new taste experience for most of us. Maitake mushrooms look like hands waving to the sky, which is totally apt, as *maitake* means "dancing mushroom" in Japanese. If you have difficulty finding maitake, substitute sliced shiitake or button mushrooms.

½ tablespoon olive oil
Four 3-ounce portions lean pork loin
2 cups maitake mushrooms, divided into
  small pieces
2 cups sliced fresh shiitake mushrooms

3 tablespoons white wine
½ cup chopped Italian parsley
1 teaspoon low-sodium soy sauce
2 tablespoons balsamic vinegar

Coat a large skillet with the olive oil and cook the pork over medium-high heat for 3 minutes on each side, or until brown on all sides and thoroughly cooked. Transfer to 4 dinner plates.

In the same skillet, add the maitake and shiitake mushrooms and cook over medium heat for 1 minute, stirring continuously. Add the white wine, parsley, soy sauce, and vinegar. Cook another 3 minutes, or until the mushrooms are tender.

Evenly distribute the mushrooms over the pork.

NUTRITION FACTS: 1 SERVING; Caloric Density 0.8; Calories (Kcal) 155; Protein (g) 20; Carbohydrate (g) 5; Total Fat (g) 5; Saturated Fat (g) 1.3; Monounsaturated Fat (g) 2.6; Polyunsaturated Fat (g) 0.5; Dietary Fiber (g) 2.2; Flavonoid and Other Phyto (mg) 0.0; Cholesterol (mg) 55; Sodium (mg) 75; Vitamin A (IU) 400; Vitamin C (mg) 12; Calcium (mg) 19; Iron (mg) 2.1; PERCENTAGE (%) Protein 52.3; Carbohydrate 14.2; Fat 28.8; Alcohol 4.7

Pork Daikon

SERVES 4

Besides being a great cancer-fighter, the low-calorie daikon is also believed to help digestion and improve the tone of one's voice in Japan. This vitamin C–rich vegetable has just a trace of pungency when raw, but when cooked, it becomes unbelievably sweet and mild, absorbing the flavorful taste of other ingredients cooked with it. In this recipe, the flavor of pork, one of the most popular and beloved tastes of Okinawa, transforms the daikon and gives it a brand-new dimension.

12 large or 16 small dried shiitake
   mushrooms
6 ounces lean pork loin, cut into 1-inch
   cubes
Canola oil spray
1 tablespoon minced ginger

2 pounds daikon radish, peeled and cut
   into 1-inch cubes
2 tablespoons sake rice wine
½ teaspoon turbinado or brown sugar
2 tablespoons white miso
15 ounces water-packed light firm tofu,
   cut into 1-inch cubes (optional)

Soak the shiitake mushrooms in plenty of lukewarm water for 15 to 20 minutes or until tender. Drain, saving the soaking liquid.

In a stockpot, bring 4 cups water to a boil and cook the pork cubes for 10 minutes. Drain and rinse the meat with warm water to remove scum and fat.

Clean the stockpot and spray the bottom with canola oil. Heat the pot over medium heat and cook the ginger for 45 seconds to 1 minute, or until golden. Add the pork and cook for 2 minutes, stirring continuously. Add the daikon and stir, tossing to mix well. Pour in 2 cups of the reserved shiitake soaking liquid. Raise the heat to high and bring to a boil. Add the sake and turbinado sugar. Cook for 10 minutes, or until the daikon is half transparent.

Ladle a bit of liquid from the pot, dissolve the miso in it, and stir it back in. Stir in the tofu and cook for another 5 to 10 minutes, or until the daikon is cooked.

NUTRITION FACTS: 1 SERVING; Caloric Density 0.5; Calories (Kcal) 156; Protein (g) 12; Carbohydrate (g) 21; Total Fat (g) 2; Saturated Fat (g) 0.7; Monounsaturated Fat (g) 0.9; Polyunsaturated Fat (g) 0.6; Dietary Fiber (g) 5.4; Flavonoid and Other Phyto (mg) 8.0; Cholesterol (mg) 28; Sodium (mg) 399; Vitamin A (IU) 10; Vitamin C (mg) 51; Calcium (mg) 71; Iron (mg) 1.9; PERCENTAGE (%) Protein 30.4; Carbohydrate 51.1; Fat 13.5; Alcohol 5.0

Nsunaba Sukiyaki

SERVES 4

Eating sukiyaki is a big family event in Japan, especially since beef used to be rare and considered a luxury of sorts. The sukiyaki pot (a shallow, clay pot similar to a Dutch oven) is placed on a tabletop stove, and everyone picks their favorite items out of the pot with chopsticks and drops them into their own bowls. We Okinawanized this classic Japanese recipe by using Swiss chard, which is called *nsunaba* and is commonly used in Okinawa. (You can go all veggie too—check out our Nsunaba Sukiyaki Vegetarian recipe on page 293.)

2½ tablespoons low-sodium soy sauce
2 tablespoons turbinado or brown sugar
¼ cup sake rice wine
Canola oil spray
6 ounces lean beef, preferably top sirloin or tenderloin, thinly sliced
10 ounces konnyaku yam noodles (shirataki), cut into 2-inch lengths

2 cups chopped green onion
4 cups chopped Swiss chard, stems and center ribs removed
4 cups chopped Chinese napa cabbage
7 ounces water-packed firm light tofu, cut into rectangles

In a small saucepan, bring 1½ cups water and the soy sauce, turbinado sugar, and sake to a boil. Turn off the heat and set aside.

Spray a large skillet with canola oil and cook the beef over medium-high heat for 2 minutes or until thoroughly cooked. Drain away fat from meat and wipe off the grease from the skillet with a paper towel.

Add the sauce, the konnyaku, the green onions, and the Swiss chard to the skillet, and cook over medium heat for 5 minutes, or until green onions and Swiss chard are tender. Add the cabbage and tofu. Cover and cook for 5 minutes, or until cabbage has shrunk and is tender and the tofu is darker in color.

Serve with rice in a separate bowl.

NUTRITION FACTS: 1 SERVING; Caloric Density 0.4; Calories (Kcal) 160; Protein (g) 16; Carbohydrate (g) 14; Total Fat (g) 3; Saturated Fat (g) 0.7; Monounsaturated Fat (g) 0.9; Polyunsaturated Fat (g) 0.8; Dietary Fiber (g) 5.2; Flavonoid and Other Phyto (mg) 21.4; Cholesterol (mg) 26; Sodium (mg) 499; Vitamin A (IU) 2,196; Vitamin C (mg) 36; Calcium (mg) 312; Iron (mg) 3.5; PERCENTAGE (%) Protein 39.7; Carbohydrate 34.1; Fat 16.1; Alcohol 10.2

Shabu Shabu Pork with Herb Sauce

SERVES 4

Shabu shabu is a popular Japanese *nabemono*—hearty soup pot. (The other most common *nabemono* are sukiyaki and *mizutaki*.) Chinese napa cabbage (*hakusai,* in Japanese) is an essential ingredient in these kinds of dishes. This low-calorie, hearty cabbage is long (usually about 8 to 12 inches) rather than round and has crinkly, thickly veined leaves that are white on the bottom, light green in the middle, and bright green at the top. The arrival of *hakusai* cabbage in the market signals the beginning of winter for most Japanese—it's rarely consumed in the summer.

12 ounces lean pork, thinly sliced	1 clove garlic, pressed
6 cups chopped Chinese napa cabbage	⅓ teaspoon dried thyme
4 cups chopped spinach	½ teaspoon dried rosemary
1 tablespoon canola oil	3 tablespoons apple cider vinegar or
1 tablespoon olive oil	white wine vinegar

In a medium pot, bring 3 quarts water to a boil. Place the pork slices in the water and cook over high heat for 1 minute, or until thoroughly cooked. Avoid letting the pork slices stick together. Transfer the pork to a colander and rinse under cold water.

Steam the Chinese cabbage for 3 minutes in a steamer, tightly covered. Add the spinach to the steamer and steam for 2 minutes. Squeeze excess water from the vegetables. Place one-quarter of the Chinese cabbage on each of 4 dinner plates, making a circle. Place one-quarter of the spinach on the cabbage and top with the pork slices.

In a small pot, cook the canola oil, olive oil, and garlic over low heat for 2 minutes, or until the garlic is golden. Remove and discard the garlic. Add the thyme and rosemary and cook for 1 minute. Slowly add the vinegar.

Spoon 1 tablespoon of the sauce over each pork portion.

NUTRITION FACTS: 1 SERVING; Caloric Density 0.7; Calories (Kcal) 165; Protein (g) 20; Carbohydrate (g) 5; Total Fat (g) 7; Saturated Fat (g) 1.4; Monounsaturated Fat (g) 3.6; Polyunsaturated Fat (g) 1.1; Dietary Fiber (g) 4.5; Flavonoid and Other Phyto (mg) 0.0; Cholesterol (mg) 55; Sodium (mg) 77; Vitamin A (IU) 3419; Vitamin C (mg) 40; Calcium (mg) 126; Iron (mg) 2.4; PERCENTAGE (%) Protein 49.6; Carbohydrate 13.5; Fat 36.9

Sloppy Tofu with Beef

SERVES 4

This is a variation of a Chinese dish called Ma Bo Tofu, and it's packed with heart-healthy flavonoids. The American Heart Association tells us "twenty-five grams of soy (2½ Tbs. dry soybeans) in conjunction with a low saturated fat diet lowers blood cholesterol." This dish will definitely help you on your way. It is fabulous when served with brown rice.

2 tablespoons white miso	¾ cup minced green onion
½ teaspoon cayenne pepper	5 ounces extra-lean ground beef
2 tablespoons sake rice wine	12 ounces water-packed silken light tofu
1 teaspoon canola oil	2 tablespoons kudzu powder or
2 tablespoons minced ginger	1½ tablespoons arrowroot powder
2 cloves minced garlic	

In a small mixing cup or bowl, combine the miso, cayenne pepper, and sake. Set aside.

In a large wok, heat the canola oil over high heat and cook the ginger and garlic for 20 seconds, or until golden. Add the green onion and ground beef. Cook for 5 minutes or until the beef is cooked through. Stir in the miso mixture. Add 1 cup water and the tofu. Crumble the tofu with a spatula and cook for 4 minutes, or until the liquid is reduced by half.

In a small mixing bowl, dissolve the kudzu powder in 2 tablespoons room-temperature water. Stir in the kudzu mixture and stir continuously until the liquid is thickened.

NUTRITION FACTS: 1 SERVING; Caloric Density 0.8; Calories (Kcal) 170; Protein (g) 13; Carbohydrate (g) 8; Total Fat (g) 9; Saturated Fat (g) 2.6; Monounsaturated Fat (g) 3.4; Polyunsaturated Fat (g) 0.9; Dietary Fiber (g) 1.0; Flavonoid and Other Phyto (mg) 37; Cholesterol (mg) 24; Sodium (mg) 416; Vitamin A (IU) 1530; Vitamin C (mg) 2; Calcium (mg) 300; Iron (mg) 1.9; PERCENTAGE (%) Protein 30.0; Carbohydrate 18.8; Fat 46.6; Alcohol 4.8

Veggieful Beef Stew

SERVES 4

Beef stew is a classic Western dish, and many people have their own family recipes for it. Now you can add this vegetable-rich, low-calorie, healthy beef stew to your family collection. One of the great things about stew is its low-maintenance nature. Once it's prepared you can just let it cook while you take care of other business. Make double the amount and freeze (without the broccoli) for quick, easy meals over the next few days. When you thaw and reheat the stew, add fresh broccoli or any of your favorite vegetables.

½ teaspoon ground nutmeg
½ teaspoon ground allspice
½ teaspoon dried thyme
1 tablespoon whole-wheat flour
12 ounces lean beef, preferably top sirloin or tenderloin, cut into ½-inch cubes
Pinch of sea salt
⅓ teaspoon freshly ground black pepper

Canola oil spray
1 cup thinly sliced yellow onion
1 cup diced carrot
1½ cups halved red-skinned new potatoes
1 cup diced celery
1 cup button mushrooms, cut in half
2 cups low-sodium, low-fat beef broth
2 dried bay leaves
1 cup broccoli florets

In a medium bowl, combine the nutmeg, allspice, thyme, and flour. Add the beef and toss to coat evenly. Season with the salt and pepper.

Spray a large stew pot with canola oil and cook the beef over medium-high heat for 6 minutes, or until entirely cooked. Set aside.

Using the same pot, cook the onion over medium heat for 5 minutes, or until tender and transparent. Add the carrot, potatoes, celery, and mushrooms and cook over high heat for 3 minutes, or until the vegetables are coated evenly with the juices.

Place the beef back in the pot and pour in the beef broth. If the beef and vegetables are not fully covered by the liquid, add enough water to cover them. Cover the pot and bring to a boil.

Reduce the heat to low and remove any fat from the surface. Add the bay leaves, cover, and cook for 40 minutes, stirring occasionally. Stir in the broccoli. Cook for another 6 minutes. Remove the bay leaves before serving.

NUTRITION FACTS: 1 SERVING; Caloric Density 0.5; Calories (Kcal) 185; Protein (g) 21; Carbohydrate (g) 15; Total Fat (g) 4; Saturated Fat (g) 1.5; Monounsaturated Fat (g) 1.6; Polyunsaturated Fat (g) 0.4; Dietary Fiber (g) 5.7; Flavonoid and Other Phyto (mg) 23.0; Cholesterol (mg) 52; Sodium (mg) 232; Vitamin A (IU) 9216; Vitamin C (mg) 30; Calcium (mg) 78; Iron (mg) 3.4; PERCENTAGE (%) Protein 45.3; Carbohydrate 33.2; Fat 21.3

Veggie Pork Pita

SERVES 4

Okinawa's favorite meat, pork, becomes wonderfully lean when boiled rather than sautéed, and whole-wheat pita is a great alternative to white bread. Introduce some veggies into the mix, and you've got a healthy and filling lunch. If you can't find whole-grain pita, don't go for white pita—think outside the box and use whole-grain flour tortillas to roll up the ingredients.

9 ounces lean pork loin	½ cup sliced cucumber
2 dried bay leaves	1 cup alfalfa sprouts
1 tablespoon lemon juice	½ cup thinly sliced red onion
2 large whole-grain pita breads	4 large, thick slices tomato
4 tablespoons hummus	1 cup shredded romaine lettuce

Bring a medium pot of water to a boil. Add the pork and 1 bay leaf and cook over high heat until boiling. Reduce heat to low and cook for another 6 minutes. Transfer the pork to a colander.

Rinse the pot and bring the same amount of fresh water to a boil. Add the pork again and the remaining bay leaf and bring to a boil. Reduce the heat to low and cook for another 5 minutes.

Transfer the pork to a cutting board and cut it into thick strips. Coat with the lemon juice and cool.

Cut the pita breads into halves and open them up to make 4 pockets. Spread 1 tablespoon hummus in each half. Arrange the vegetables and the pork in the pita bread.

NUTRITION FACTS: 1 SERVING; Caloric Density 0.9; Calories (Kcal) 190; Protein (g) 19; Carbohydrate (g) 22; Total Fat (g) 4; Saturated Fat (g) 1.0; Monounsaturated Fat (g) 1.6; Polyunsaturated Fat (g) 1.0; Dietary Fiber (g) 4.8; Flavonoid and Other Phyto (mg) 9.4; Cholesterol (mg) 41; Sodium (mg) 228; Vitamin A (IU) 694; Vitamin C (mg) 18; Calcium (mg) 58; Iron (mg) 2.1; PERCENTAGE (%) Protein 37.5; Carbohydrate 44.0; Fat 18.6

Beef à la Crème

SERVES 4

If you have been raised on beef dishes in creamy sauces and are longing for that familiar taste—but want to avoid the calories and saturated fat—this is the recipe for you. Substituting canola oil, lean meat, and soymilk for butter, sirloin, and cream while keeping the other ingredients the same as the original French recipe yields a healthy and delicious low-calorie meal. A quick comparison of the two recipes reveals that we have cut our calories practically in half (from 422 to 215), added 45 mg of cancer-fighting flavonoids, and shaved off almost two-thirds of the saturated fat (4 grams to 1.6)—all without sacrificing taste!

1 teaspoon canola oil
2½ cups thinly sliced yellow onion
12 ounces lean beef, preferably top
    sirloin or tenderloin, thinly sliced
4 cups sliced button mushrooms
⅓ cup white wine

⅔ cup soymilk, plain
6 cups chopped spinach
Pinch of sea salt
Freshly ground black pepper
⅓ cup finely chopped parsley

In a large skillet, heat the canola oil over medium heat. Add the onion and cook for 5 minutes, or until tender and golden.

Raise the heat to high and add the beef and mushrooms. Cook for 2 minutes, or until the meat is browned. Add the white wine and cook for 3 minutes. Add the soymilk and cook for 1 minute. Stir in the spinach. Just when the spinach is tender, remove the skillet from the heat and season with salt and pepper. Stir in the parsley.

NUTRITION FACTS: 1 SERVING; Caloric Density 0.6; Calories (Kcal) 215; Protein (g) 24; Carbohydrate (g) 14; Total Fat (g) 6; Saturated Fat (g) 1.6; Monounsaturated Fat (g) 2.3; Polyunsaturated Fat (g) 1.1; Dietary Fiber (g) 4.6; Flavonoid and Other Phyto (mg) 45.4; Cholesterol (mg) 52; Sodium (mg) 167; Vitamin A (IU) 3298; Vitamin C (mg) 27; Calcium (mg) 86; Iron (mg) 5.1; PERCENTAGE (%) Protein 43.0; Carbohydrate 25.9; Fat 25.3; Alcohol 5.8

Bambou Short Ribs

SERVES 4

Recipe provided by Chef Masamitsu Geruma at Café Restaurant Bambou, Naha, Okinawa, phone: 81.98. 861.6056

This recipe comes directly from one of our favorite Okinawan restaurants, and we're not surprised that the chef suggests you also try this dish using Okinawan tofu instead of beef. Chef Geruma's grandmother was a professional tofu maker. In the old days, when Okinawan tofu was made with seawater, Grandma Geruma would scour numerous bays, beaches, and coastlines to find the seawater that provided the best magnesium chloride for solidifying Okinawan-style tofu. (Extra-firm tofu is the closest Western equivalent.) But whether you opt for tofu or go for ribs, this dish guarantees total satisfaction.

1 pound short ribs with the bone in, lean
2 tablespoons low-sodium soy sauce
1/2 cup water
1 teaspoon chili powder
2 cloves garlic, minced
1 teaspoon honey
1 shallot, minced
1 pound peeled wax gourd, zucchini, or winter melon, cut into 1-inch cubes

1 can (8 ounces) no-salt-added tomato sauce
1/3 cup coconut milk
Two 3-inch stalks lemongrass
7 ounces firm light tofu, cut into 9 cubes (optional)
Freshly ground black pepper
2 teaspoons turmeric
Fresh thyme or mint sprigs, for garnish

In a nonstick skillet, cook the short ribs over high heat for 1 minute, or until browned. Turn over and cook for another minute, or until browned.

Transfer the ribs to a large pot of boiling water and cook for 15 minutes, or until cooked. Drain and let cool.

Combine the soy sauce, water, chili powder, garlic, honey, and shallot in a large resealable plastic bag or in a large non-aluminum container with lid. Marinate the ribs in the mixture, refrigerating for 2 hours or overnight.

Place the ribs, wax gourd, tomato sauce, and coconut milk in a large pot and bring to a boil. Reduce the heat to low and add the lemongrass, then cook for 30 to 45 minutes.

Carefully stir in the tofu. Cook for another 2 minutes. Adjust the seasoning with pepper.

Serve the stew in 4 dinner plates. Sprinkle 1/2 teaspoon of turmeric around the edge of each plate. Garnish with fresh thyme or mint on top of the stew.

NUTRITION FACTS: 1 SERVING; Caloric Density 0.8; Calories (Kcal) 298; Protein (g) 29; Carbohydrate (g) 12; Total Fat (g) 15; Saturated Fat (g) 7.2; Monounsaturated Fat (g) 5.1; Polyunsaturated Fat (g) 1.2; Dietary Fiber (g) 4.5; Flavonoid and Other Phyto (mg) 10.2; Cholesterol (mg) 54; Sodium (mg) 539; Vitamin A (IU) 812; Vitamin C (mg) 24; Calcium (mg) 230; Iron (mg) 3.8; PERCENTAGE (%) Protein 38.9; Carbohydrate 15.8; Fat 45.3

Tofu

The Chinese have a saying: "Tofu has the flavor of a hundred different things." And they're right. Tofu goes with almost any dish. It can be eaten fresh, marinated, fried, baked, boiled, or cooked in just about any way you can think of. Its texture ranges from silky, smooth, and creamy to extra-firm or meaty. It goes equally well with vegetables, meats, fish, and beans. It's a winning ingredient in salads, soups, and desserts, and it can be stuffed into pita, sandwiched between hamburger buns, or skewered for shish kabob. Whew! The tofu chef is truly limited only by her or his imagination. Before we get to the recipes, here's a capsule review of everything you need to know about tofu to whet your appetite, and remove any remaining mystery about this incredible food.

SMOOTHNESS AND FIRMNESS OF TOFU

Silken Tofu: This smooth, creamy tofu looks like a very soft white jelly and is the most fragile, delicately textured variety. Most of the time it's eaten as is, warmed in hot soup, or processed into a smooth, creamy thick liquid. Because the percentage of water to soymilk is higher in silken tofu than in other types, it contains a smaller concentration of phytoestrogens, those cancer-fighting soy compounds.

Firm Tofu: This is the most common multipurpose type of tofu. It tastes a little beanier than silken tofu, and is a bit rougher on the surface, and harder—though it still crumbles easily when you handle it. It's rich in phytoestrogens and can be eaten as is, warmed in hot soup, stir-fried, baked, or broiled.

Extra-Firm Tofu: This is the hardest kind of tofu to find—except in Okinawa. It has an even beanier taste and a meaty texture. It's a perfect meat substitute and is great for vegetable stir-fries. This type of tofu is the richest in phytoestrogens.

Silken but Firm Tofu: This admittedly confusing category of tofu was made up by several North American tofu makers. It's smooth like regular silken tofu, but it is less fragile—more like a jelly with extra gelatin. Definitely an in-betweener, this tofu doesn't do much for us.

Ginkgo-Tofu Supreme

Turmeric-Marinated Tofu with Chard

Ryukyu Scrambled Eggs II

Teriyaki Tofu Fingers

Spicy Tofu and Summer Vegetables

Okinawa-Style Refried Beans

Honey Mustard Tofu

Tofu Shish Kabobs

Tofu-Stuffed Mushrooms

Buddhist Temple Tofu

Gumbo à la Okinawa

Nsunaba Sukiyaki Vegetarian

Sloppy Veggie Tofu

Asparagus Tofu Stir-Fry

Fresh Tofu Spring Rolls

Tofu and Veggie Pita Sandwich

Yuki's Indian Tofu Curry

About Tofu

TOFU PACKS

Tofu comes in two types of packaging, *water-packed* and *box-packed*. We recommend the water-packed. You'll find it in the refrigerated section of your grocery store, health food store, or Asian market. Water-packed tofu is packaged in a rectangular white plastic tub with a small amount of water inside and a transparent lid that peels off. It's the kind they use most in Japan, Korea, China, and other countries that know their tofu. It not only tastes best but is also fresher, and you can actually see what the tofu looks like before buying it. Box-packed tofu is found on the grocery shelf. While it might be more convenient because you don't have to keep it refrigerated, its taste and smell are different from authentic tofu found throughout Asia—and not much to our liking. Unless fridge space is a tremendous problem, buy the water-packed. It lasts for one to two months.

LIGHT TOFU

Many grocery stores now carry water-packed light tofu—less fat, same taste. Even though the fat in tofu is the good kind, this is a valuable option as you're whittling away those extra pounds because it's definitely less caloric.

FRESHNESS AND STORAGE

Check the date on the pack before buying. If not opened, most water-packed tofu is good for one to two months in the refrigerator. Some water-packed tofu, especially the kind made by Japanese or Chinese tofu makers who do not add preservatives, should be eaten within three days at most. Read the label. Box-packed tofu is good for a longer time. Whatever type you buy, once you open the pack, cover the unused tofu with water in a container (use the tub, if you purchased water-packed), store it in the fridge, and eat within three days. (If frozen, tofu can last up to six months.)

SEASONED TOFU

We've recently begun seeing seasoned tofu, such as five-spice tofu, garlic-onion tofu, and the like. We have to admit we do enjoy the various flavors and think they make a great substitute for meat. Use them for making hamburgers, barbecues, and stir-fries. And now . . . back to cooking.

Ginkgo-Tofu Supreme

SERVES 4

The ginkgo nut, called "silver plum" in Japanese, has a long history in Asian cuisine. Popular in stir-fries as well as desserts, gingko nuts pair perfectly with tofu and are often found in simmered vegetable dishes in Okinawa and Japan. Ginkgo has recently become popular as an herbal memory-boosting supplement in the West, and popular folklore in Japan has it that eating ginkgo makes you smarter. We can't vouch for ginkgo as a smart pill, but several well-conducted studies support its ability to slow memory decline—and that's a lovely bonus to this delicious meal. Most Asian food stores carry ginkgo nuts with shells. Canned unshelled and peeled nuts are also available, but they can be mealier and less fresh. To shell and peel ginkgo nuts, use a nutcracker to remove the shell; soak the nuts in boiling water for 8 to 10 minutes to soften the skin, then peel the skin off. Because canned nuts are packed in brine, don't forget to rinse them well under running water if you go that route.

2 tablespoons dried hijiki seaweed	1½ cups bonito or kelp broth (see
½ cup shelled and peeled ginkgo nuts	page 229)
10 ounces water-packed firm light tofu	1 tablespoon sake rice wine
2½ tablespoons kudzu powder or	2 tablespoons low-sodium soy sauce
2 tablespoons arrowroot powder	⅓ teaspoon turbinado or brown sugar
Canola oil spray	½ cup finely chopped green onion

In a medium bowl, soak the hijiki in water for 15 minutes, or until tender and rehydrated. Drain. In a small saucepan, boil hijiki in water for 4 minutes. Drain and set aside.

Roast the ginkgo nuts in a dry skillet over low heat for 3 to 4 minutes, or until partly browned. Let cool.

Wrap the tofu with two paper towels and place on a plate; microwave on medium for 3 minutes. Transfer the tofu to a large bowl and mash. Add the hijiki, ginkgo, and ½ tablespoon kudzu powder (or ½ tablespoon arrowroot powder) and mix well by hand. Evenly divide the mixture and make four 1-inch-thick patties.

Spray a large skillet with canola oil and heat over medium heat. Cook the patties for 3 minutes, or until golden brown. Turn over and cook another 2 to 3 minutes, or until golden brown. Transfer the patties to 4 soup bowls.

In a saucepan, bring the broth, sake, soy sauce, and turbinado sugar to a boil. Reduce the heat to low and simmer for 2 minutes.

In a small container, combine the remaining 2 tablespoons kudzu powder (or 1½ tablespoons arrowroot powder) and 2 tablespoons water and mix well. Immediately add the kudzu mixture to the saucepan, along with the green onion. Stir gently until the sauce has thickened and divide evenly over the patties.

NUTRITION FACTS: 1 SERVING; Caloric Density 0.4; Calories (Kcal) 77; Protein (g) 7; Carbohydrate (g) 7; Total Fat (g) 1; Saturated Fat (g) 0.0; Monounsaturated Fat (g) 0.1; Polyunsaturated Fat (g) 0.9; Dietary Fiber (g) 0.3; Flavonoid and Other Phyto (mg) 23.6; Cholesterol (mg) 0; Sodium (mg) 306; Vitamin A (IU) 65; Vitamin C (mg) 2; Calcium (mg) 260; Iron (mg) 1.1; PERCENTAGE (%) Protein 41.2; Carbohydrate 39.2; Fat 13.9; Alcohol 5.7

Turmeric-Marinated Tofu with Chard
SERVES 4

Okinawa is often called the "Treasury of Herbs and Spices," because of its abundance of subtropical flora. Turmeric, or *ucchin,* as it's called in Okinawa, is one of the most popular jewels in the treasury. It's eaten as a spice, imbibed as a tea, and used as a medicinal herb to reduce inflammation; its bright golden color was even used as a dye in the old days—and is a brilliant complement to the deep green chard in this recipe.

7 ounces water-packed firm light tofu
1 teaspoon olive oil
1 tablespoon apple cider vinegar or white wine vinegar
1 teaspoon ground turmeric
1 teaspoon minced ginger

⅓ teaspoon chili powder
Pinch of sea salt
Pinch of turbinado or brown sugar
4 cups chopped green Swiss chard, stems removed

Wrap the tofu with two paper towels and place on a plate; microwave on high for 1½ minutes. Cool and dice.

In a shallow dish, whisk together the olive oil, vinegar, turmeric, ginger, chili powder, salt, turbinado sugar, and 1 tablespoon water. Add the tofu and cover with plastic wrap. Marinate for at least 2 hours in the refrigerator. Remove the tofu from the marinade and set it aside.

Transfer the marinade to a skillet and bring to a boil. Once boiling, stir in the Swiss chard. Reduce the heat to low, cover, and cook for 5 minutes, or until the chard is soft. Stir in the tofu.

NUTRITION FACTS: 1 SERVING; Caloric Density 0.5; Calories (Kcal) 48; Protein (g) 5; Carbohydrate (g) 2; Total Fat (g) 2; Saturated Fat (g) 0.2; Monounsaturated Fat (g) 0.9; Polyunsaturated Fat (g) 0.7; Dietary Fiber (g) 0.8; Flavonoid and Other Phyto (mg) 10.2; Cholesterol (mg) 0; Sodium (mg) 147; Vitamin A (IU) 1256; Vitamin C (mg) 11; Calcium (mg) 197; Iron (mg) 1.4; PERCENTAGE (%) Protein 43.1; Carbohydrate 19.2; Fat 37.7

Ryukyu Scrambled Eggs II

SERVES 4

In *The Okinawa Program,* we offered readers a recipe called Ryukyu Scrambled Eggs. In this new and improved version, we've crumbled the tofu so it blends in with the eggs. This is a great recipe for lowering bad cholesterol levels and raising the good stuff while enjoying eggs at the same time. It's also a great flavonoid booster. Usually two eggs per person are used for a single breakfast, but here we use two eggs to serve four! We also added spinach to increase vitamins, minerals, and fiber, improve taste, and offer a bit of color.

Canola oil spray	**Pinch of sea salt**
10 ounces water-packed firm light tofu,	**Freshly ground black pepper**
drained	**2 free-range, omega-3 eggs or ½ cup**
3 cups chopped spinach	**egg substitute or egg white, beaten**

Spray a large skillet with canola oil. Crumble the tofu and cook over medium-high heat, stirring continuously for 3 minutes, or until dry and golden. Add the spinach and cook for 1 minute, or until tender. Season with salt and pepper. Whisk the eggs and add them to the skillet. Scramble together. Serve.

NUTRITION FACTS: 1 SERVING; Caloric Density 0.7; Calories (Kcal) 81; Protein (g) 10; Carbohydrate (g) 1; Total Fat (g) 3; Saturated Fat (g) 0.8; Monounsaturated Fat (g) 1.0; Polyunsaturated Fat (g) 1.2; Dietary Fiber (g) 0.6; Flavonoid and Other Phyto (mg) 14.6; Cholesterol (mg) 106; Sodium (mg) 117; Vitamin A (IU) 1700; Vitamin C (mg) 6; Calcium (mg) 286; Iron (mg) 1.7; PERCENTAGE (%) Protein 51.7; Carbohydrate 6.2; Fat 42.1

Teriyaki Tofu Fingers

SERVES 4

Teriyaki is one of Japan's most popular cooking styles. *Teri* means "luster;" *yaki* means "roast, broil, or grill." To make a teriyaki dish, you marinate or baste the ingredients in teriyaki sauce, then grill—the teriyaki sauce gives luster to the dish. Serve this vegetarian low-cal, low-GI, and flavonoid-rich variation with brown rice for dinner, and make extra —it's also terrific in a sandwich for lunch.

10 ounces water-packed extra-firm	**3 tablespoons teriyaki sauce,**
light tofu	**low-sodium and low-fat, if available**
1 tablespoon whole-wheat flour	**2 teaspoons dried chives**
	Canola oil spray

Preheat the oven to 350°F.

Wrap the tofu in two paper towels and place on a plate; microwave at medium for 3 minutes.

In a small bowl, whisk together the flour, teriyaki sauce, and chives.

Cut the tofu lengthwise into 4 slices. Dip the tofu into the sauce, coating both sides well.

Spray a baking dish with canola oil. Place the tofu in the dish in a single layer. Bake for 10 minutes, or until golden brown. Turn over. Bake for another 10 minutes, or until golden brown.

NUTRITION FACTS: 1 SERVING; Caloric Density 1.1; Calories (Kcal) 96; Protein (g) 8; Carbohydrate (g) 7; Total Fat (g) 4; Saturated Fat (g) 0.8; Monounsaturated Fat (g) 0.8; Polyunsaturated Fat (g) 2.4; Dietary Fiber (g) 0.2; Flavonoid and Other Phyto (mg) 17; Cholesterol (mg) 0; Sodium (mg) 165; Vitamin A (IU) 28; Vitamin C (mg) 0; Calcium (mg) 49; Iron (mg) 1.2; PERCENTAGE (%) Protein 33.9; Carbohydrate 28.1; Fat 38.0

Spicy Tofu and Summer Vegetables
SERVES 4

Although Szechwan-style hot bean sauce is a Chinese seasoning, people all over Japan love to cook with it—especially the Okinawans. This dish is a perfect illustration of why Okinawan cuisine is often referred to as Japanese food with salsa. The hot bean sauce also adds a wonderful splash of bright red to an already colorful vegetable plate.

1 cup water
1 low-sodium vegetable broth bouillon cube (or 1 cup low-sodium vegetable broth instead of water and bouillon)
½ tablespoon low-sodium soy sauce
1½ teaspoons Szechwan-style hot bean sauce
1 teaspoon sesame oil
1 clove garlic, minced
1 teaspoon ginger, minced
5 ounces water-packed extra-firm light tofu

½ cup bitter melon, sliced into ½-inch-thick pieces
1 cup zucchini, sliced into ½-inch-thick pieces
½ cup diced celery
1 cup broccoli florets
½ cup julienned red bell pepper (½-inch strips)
½ cup julienned yellow bell pepper (½-inch strips)

In a skillet, bring the water, bouillon cube, soy sauce, bean sauce, sesame oil, garlic, and ginger to a boil. Add the tofu, bitter melon, zucchini, celery, broccoli, and bell peppers to the pan, cover, and bring to a boil over medium-high heat. Stir, reduce the heat to low, and cook for 5 minutes.

Cover again and cook for another 3 minutes, or until the vegetables are cooked to the desired texture.

NUTRITION FACTS: 1 SERVING; Caloric Density 0.4; Calories (Kcal) 82; Protein (g) 6; Carbohydrate (g) 8; Total Fat (g) 4; Saturated Fat (g) 0.6; Monounsaturated Fat (g) 0.9; Polyunsaturated Fat (g) 1.7; Dietary Fiber (g) 2.4; Flavonoid and Other Phyto (mg) 12.0; Cholesterol (mg) 0; Sodium (mg) 169; Vitamin A (IU) 2196; Vitamin C (mg) 105; Calcium (mg) 58; Iron (mg) 1.4; PERCENTAGE (%) Protein 25.3; Carbohydrate 37.9; Fat 36.8

Okinawa-Style Refried Beans

SERVES 12 (⅓ CUP)

Frijoles refritos, or refried beans, is a popular Mexican dish, usually made of red or pinto beans that are cooked and mashed, then fried with lard. This multipurpose bean dish is served in burritos or as a side dish. To make this great-tasting staple more Okinawan-style healthy, we use soybeans combined with pinto beans to raise the levels of isoflavones and heart-healthy canola oil rather than high-saturated-fat lard. Presto—Okinawanized and healthy.

¾ cup dried pinto beans, soaked in 2 cups water overnight	⅓ teaspoon ground cumin seeds
⅔ cup dried soybeans, soaked in 2 cups water overnight	1 teaspoon garlic powder
	½ teaspoon chili powder
Canola oil spray	Pinch of sea salt
½ cup thinly sliced yellow onion	½ cup shredded soy cheese (optional)

In a large pot of water, place the pinto beans and soybeans and bring to a boil. Reduce the heat to low and simmer covered for 45 minutes. Check occasionally and if the bottom of the pot is drying, add more water.

In the meantime, spray a skillet with canola oil and cook the onion over medium heat for 5 minutes, or until tender and transparent. Stir in the cumin, garlic powder, chili powder, and salt. Transfer the onion mixture to the bean pot and continue to simmer covered for another 1 to 1½ hours, or until the beans are soft.

While the beans are cooking, preheat the oven to 375°F.

Drain the beans, reserving the bean stock. In batches in a food processor, process the beans and ¼ cup of the bean stock until smooth. If you want softer beans, add more bean stock (or hot water), 2 tablespoons at a time, and process until the desired consistency is achieved.

Coat an 8 × 8-inch baking pan with canola oil spray. Evenly spread the mashed beans in the pan. Sprinkle the soy cheese over the beans. Bake for 4 to 5 minutes, or until the beans are hot.

Serve in or next to burritos, with vegetable sticks or with cooked vegetables.

NUTRITION FACTS: 1 SERVING; Caloric Density 1.7; Calories (Kcal) 84; Protein (g) 6; Carbohydrate (g) 11; Total Fat (g) 2; Saturated Fat (g) 0.3; Monounsaturated Fat (g) 0.5; Polyunsaturated Fat (g) 1.1; Dietary Fiber (g) 3.9; Flavonoid and Other Phyto (mg) 16.0; Cholesterol (mg) 0; Sodium (mg) 26; Vitamin A (IU) 41; Vitamin C (mg) 2; Calcium (mg) 44; Iron (mg) 2.3; PERCENTAGE (%) Protein 27.6; Carbohydrate 51.0; Fat 21.4

Honey Mustard Tofu

SERVES 4

The only reason for being a bee that I know of is making honey . . . and the only reason for making honey is so I can eat it.

—WINNIE-THE-POOH

Winnie-the-Pooh would probably enjoy this recipe. The honey mixed with mustard and curry powder gives a highly unusual taste to this healthy meal.

Healthy Tip: Although honey is not dangerous to adults or older children, never feed it to infants under one year of age, as honey, on rare occasions, can contain spores of the *C. botulinum* toxin and can cause serious illness in babies.

12 ounces water-packed firm light tofu, cut into 4 rectangles	**1½ tablespoons honey or 2 tablespoons turbinado or brown sugar**
1 teaspoon canola oil	**2 tablespoons Dijon mustard**
½ cup minced white onion	**1 teaspoon curry powder**

Preheat the oven to 350°F.

Wrap the tofu with two paper towels and place on a plate; microwave at high for 2 minutes. Let stand.

In a small pot, heat the canola oil over medium heat and cook the onion for 5 minutes, or until tender and half-transparent. Stir in the honey, mustard, and curry powder.

Transfer the sauce to a small baking dish or pie plate. Place the tofu on the sauce. Turn the tofu over once to coat the other sides and bake for 8 minutes. Turn over and bake for another 6 minutes, or until golden.

NUTRITION FACTS: 1 SERVING; Caloric Density 0.8; Calories (Kcal) 96; Protein (g) 7; Carbohydrate (g) 9; Total Fat (g) 2; Saturated Fat (g) 0.1; Monounsaturated Fat (g) 0.7; Polyunsaturated Fat (g) 1.4; Dietary Fiber (g) 0.5; Flavonoid and Other Phyto (mg) 26.5; Cholesterol (mg) 0; Sodium (mg) 174; Vitamin A (IU) 5; Vitamin C (mg) 1; Calcium (mg) 307; Iron (mg) 1.0; PERCENTAGE (%) Protein 35.1; Carbohydrate 40.8; Fat 24.1

Tofu Shish Kabobs

SERVES 4

Tofu originated in China over 2,000 years ago and was introduced to Japan about A.D. 600. It was originally the food of aristocrats, noblemen, and monks, and has long been regarded as "the food for a long, healthy life." This reputation was rooted in the fact that the monks, the healthiest and longest-lived people at that time, ate tofu as part of their vegetarian diets. They were definitely onto something—modern science has been backing up this folk wisdom with evidence of the health properties of the versatile soybean ever since. Making these tofu shish kabobs can be fun too—get the kids into it. Not only will they find it fun, it's also a great way to educate their palate and get them interested in eating tofu and veggies.

7 ounces water-packed extra-firm light tofu
1 tablespoon canola oil
1 tablespoon apple cider vinegar or white wine vinegar
½ tablespoon low-sodium soy sauce
1 teaspoon red wine
½ teaspoon garlic powder

½ teaspoon dried oregano
Freshly ground black pepper
1 cup halved button mushrooms
1 cup sliced green bell pepper, sliced into squares
1 cup diced white onion
1 cup grape or cherry tomatoes
Canola oil spray

Wrap the tofu with two paper towels and place on a plate; microwave at high for 1½ minutes. Let cool.

In a small mixing bowl, whisk together the canola oil, vinegar, soy sauce, wine, garlic powder, oregano, black pepper, and 1 tablespoon water. Transfer to a resealable plastic bag. Place the tofu and mushrooms in the bag, press out all the air, and seal. Refrigerate for 2 to 3 hours.

Preheat the oven to 325°F.

Soak wooden skewers in water for 3 to 5 minutes. Drain. Thread the tofu, mushrooms, bell pepper, onion, and tomatoes on the skewers, alternating ingredients.

Spray a baking dish with canola oil. Place the shish kabobs in the dish and bake for 15 minutes, or until the vegetables are done to your taste. You can also grill them, if you like.

NUTRITION FACTS: 1 SERVING; Caloric Density 0.6; Calories (Kcal) 104; Protein (g) 6; Carbohydrate (g) 10; Total Fat (g) 5; Saturated Fat (g) 0.7; Monounsaturated Fat (g) 1.6; Polyunsaturated Fat (g) 2.3; Dietary Fiber (g) 2.0; Flavonoid and Other Phyto (mg) 30.6; Cholesterol (mg) 0; Sodium (mg) 81; Vitamin A (IU) 529; Vitamin C (mg) 45; Calcium (mg) 51; Iron (mg) 1.4; PERCENTAGE (%) Protein 23.3; Carbohydrate 35.9; Fat 40.0; Alcohol 0.7

Tofu-Stuffed Mushrooms

SERVES 4

One of the most wonderful things about tofu is that you can make it into almost any kind of shape. You can dice it to bake or stir-fry, blend it for drinks, and mash it to make a patty or filling—that's my favorite thing to do.

—MRS. NABE KINJO, NINETY-SEVEN YEARS OLD, URASOE CITY, OKINAWA

We like the idea too. Here we used tofu as a filling for stuffed mushrooms—(*ura chiki chinuku*). This dish can also be made with ground-fish stuffing—a favorite for celebratory dinners in Okinawa. For variety, try using 4 medium portobello mushrooms instead of button mushrooms.

20 large button mushrooms	Pinch of sea salt
7 ounces water-packed firm light tofu	Freshly ground black pepper
⅓ cup finely chopped carrot leaves	⅓ cup bread crumbs
1 tablespoon kudzu powder or	2 tablespoons soy Parmesan cheese
2 teaspoons arrowroot powder	2 teaspoons dried parsley

Preheat the oven to 375°F.

Clean the mushrooms and remove the stems. Finely chop the stems.

Wrap the tofu with two paper towels and place on a plate; microwave at medium for 2 minutes. Transfer the tofu to a large bowl and mash it. When the tofu is cool to the touch, add the chopped mushroom stems, carrot leaves, kudzu powder, salt, and pepper. Mix well by hand.

Spoon about 1 tablespoon of the tofu mixture into each mushroom cap. Place the stuffed mushrooms on a baking dish, tofu side up, and bake for 15 minutes, or until the tofu and mushrooms look slightly dry.

While the mushroom caps are in the oven, in a small mixing bowl combine the bread crumbs, Parmesan cheese, and parsley. Sprinkle the bread crumb mixture over the mushrooms. Return them to the oven and bake for another 5 minutes, or until the bread crumbs are golden.

NUTRITION FACTS: 1 SERVING; Caloric Density 0.7; Calories (Kcal) 105; Protein (g) 10; Carbohydrate (g) 13; Total Fat (g) 2; Saturated Fat (g) 0.2; Monounsaturated Fat (g) 0.2; Polyunsaturated Fat (g) 0.8; Dietary Fiber (g) 1.7; Flavonoid and Other Phyto (mg) 22.1; Cholesterol (mg) 0; Sodium (mg) 217; Vitamin A (IU) 787; Vitamin C (mg) 13; Calcium (mg) 243; Iron (mg) 2.5; PERCENTAGE (%) Protein 35.6; Carbohydrate 49.3; Fat 15.1

Buddhist Temple Tofu

SERVES 4

Yudofu, which literally means "tofu in hot water," has its roots in the Buddhist temples of Kyoto, Japan, where the monks were not allowed to eat meat. *Yudofu* was originally known as *shojin ryori*—"meal of perfect mastery," which referred to the monks' stoic character and preference for simplicity. This dish, though, moved beyond the monasteries a long time ago; it's now a popular winter family meal that graces the table of every Japanese home.

Two 2½-inch pieces of dried kelp strips (kombu)	⅓ cup fresh lemon juice
	1 tablespoon sake rice wine
22 ounces water-packed firm light tofu, sliced lengthwise and then into thirds	3 tablespoons low-sodium soy sauce
	1 cup chopped green onion

Fill a pot a little more than half full of water. Add the kelp strips and let stand for 20 minutes. Cook the kelp strips in the water over medium-high heat for 10 minutes, or until small bubbles rise from the kelp strips.

Put the tofu pieces in the water. Bring to a boil, reduce the heat to low, and cook for 3 minutes. Do not allow the water to boil rapidly.

In the meantime, combine the lemon juice, sake, soy sauce, and ¼ cup of the kelp liquid in a saucepan.

Use a small strainer to lift the tofu onto 4 plates, season with the sauce and green onion, and enjoy your cold winter night with hot *yudofu* tofu!

NUTRITION FACTS: 1 SERVING; Caloric Density 0.5; Calories (Kcal) 105; Protein (g) 13; Carbohydrate (g) 4; Total Fat (g) 2; Saturated Fat (g) 0.0; Monounsaturated Fat (g) 0.0; Polyunsaturated Fat (g) 1.9; Dietary Fiber (g) 0.5; Flavonoid and Other Phyto (mg) 38.4; Cholesterol (mg) 0; Sodium (mg) 452; Vitamin A (IU) 52; Vitamin C (mg) 12; Calcium (mg) 576; Iron (mg) 2.0; PERCENTAGE (%) Protein 60.3; Carbohydrate 17.1; Fat 18.3; Alcohol 4.3

Gumbo à la Okinawa

SERVES 4

Okra's green pointy pods are often used in soups and stews in Okinawa. They are also the main ingredient in the African-inspired dish known as gumbo—practically the lifeblood of New Orleans. Although available fresh year-round in the American South (where it was first introduced by African slaves), okra is in season from about May through October in the rest of the United States. This recipe combines okra and tofu in a rich bonito broth for a flavonoid-rich, low-CD meal with an antioxidant punch.

1 cup bonito or kelp broth (see page 229)

4 cups okra (washed thoroughly, tops removed, cut into half widthwise)

15 ounces water-packed firm light tofu, diced

1 tablespoon sake rice wine

1 tablespoon low-sodium soy sauce

1½ tablespoons kudzu powder or 1 tablespoon arrowroot powder

⅓ cup thinly sliced green onion

In a large pot, bring the broth to a boil. Add the okra and cook for 2 minutes. Stir in the tofu, sake, and soy sauce. Cook for 2 more minutes, or until the liquid is reduced by half.

In a small mixing cup or bowl, combine 1½ tablespoons water and the kudzu powder; stir until dissolved. Add the kudzu mixture to the pot and gently stir until the liquid thickens. Garnish with green onion.

NUTRITION FACTS: 1 SERVING; Caloric Density 0.4; Calories (Kcal) 106; Protein (g) 11; Carbohydrate (g) 11; Total Fat (g) 1; Saturated Fat (g) 0.0; Monounsaturated Fat (g) 0.0; Polyunsaturated Fat (g) 1.3; Dietary Fiber (g) 3.5; Flavonoid and Other Phyto (mg) 31.9; Cholesterol (mg) 0; Sodium (mg) 161; Vitamin A (IU) 693; Vitamin C (mg) 23; Calcium (mg) 465; Iron (mg) 2.0; PERCENTAGE (%) Protein 43.2; Carbohydrate 40.9; Fat 11.9; Alcohol 3.9

Nsunaba Sukiyaki Vegetarian

SERVES 4

Sukiyaki is probably the best-known Japanese beef dish. In Japan, meatless sukiyaki is almost out of question, but vegetarian sukiyaki is surprisingly tasty—and healthier with fewer calories, less saturated fat and cholesterol, and more calcium and flavonoids. We love it.

3 tablespoons low-sodium soy sauce

1 tablespoon turbinado or brown sugar

¼ cup sake rice wine

Canola oil spray

15 ounces water-packed firm light tofu, cut into rectangles

8 ounces konnyaku yam noodles (shirataki), cut into 2-inch lengths

2 cups chopped green onions

16 large fresh shiitake mushrooms

3 cups chopped Swiss chard

8 cups chopped Chinese napa cabbage

In a small saucepan, bring the soy sauce, turbinado sugar, sake, and 1½ cups water to a boil, stirring a few times. Turn off the heat. Set aside.

Spray a large skillet with canola oil and sauté the tofu over medium-high heat for 3 minutes, or until golden. Add the sauce and place the konnyaku noodles and green onions in separate locations in the pot. Cook for 4 minutes, or until the green onions are tender. Add the shiitake mushrooms, Swiss chard, and napa cabbage. Cover and cook for 5 minutes, or until the leafy vegetables are tender.

NUTRITION FACTS: 1 SERVING; Caloric Density 0.3; Calories (Kcal) 140; Protein (g) 13; Carbohydrate (g) 14; Total Fat (g) 2; Saturated Fat (g) 0.1; Monounsaturated Fat (g) 0.1; Polyunsaturated Fat (g) 1.4; Dietary Fiber (g) 7.7; Flavonoid and Other Phyto (mg) 33.1; Cholesterol (mg) 0; Sodium (mg) 535; Vitamin A (IU) 2811; Vitamin C (mg) 54; Calcium (mg) 556; Iron (mg) 3.0; PERCENTAGE (%) Protein 36.3; Carbohydrate 40.6; Fat 11.4; Alcohol 11.7

Sloppy Veggie Tofu

SERVES 4

This is a vegetarian version of Sloppy Tofu with Beef on page 276. Here we use konnyaku, a dense, gelatinous yam cake, instead of beef, to lower the CD and increase the fiber (CD just 0.1, with 2.2 grams of fiber per 100 grams). Konnyaku, available at most Asian groceries, is popular with Japanese women as a diet aid, because it's so filling, fiber-full, and low-cal. (Also see our recipe for Sautéed Shiitake and Konnyaku on page 304.)

8 ounces konnyaku yam cake, thinly
    sliced
2 tablespoons white miso
½ teaspoon chili powder
2 tablespoons sake rice wine
2 teaspoons canola oil
1 tablespoon minced ginger

2 cloves garlic, minced
¾ cup minced green onions
3 cups chopped spinach
2 cups mung bean sprouts
15 ounces water-packed silken light tofu
2 tablespoons kudzu powder or
    1½ tablespoons arrowroot powder

Place the konnyaku in a large colander and pour a pot of boiling water over it to remove tartness. Drain.

In a small mixing cup or bowl, combine the miso, chili powder, and sake. Stir until smooth.

In a large wok, heat the canola oil over high heat. Cook the ginger, garlic, and green onions for 30 seconds, or until the garlic and ginger are golden. Add the spinach, mung bean sprouts, tofu, and 1 cup water. Crumble the tofu with a spatula. Bring to a boil. Reduce the heat to low and add the miso mixture. Stir well to season evenly. Cook for 3 minutes or until liquid is reduced by half.

In the meantime, dissolve the kudzu powder in 2 tablespoons water in a small container. Stir the kudzu mixture into the wok. Stir until liquid thickens.

Serve hot, over rice if you prefer.

NUTRITION FACTS: 1 SERVING; Caloric Density 0.5; Calories (Kcal) 152; Protein (g) 12; Carbohydrate (g) 13; Total Fat (g) 4; Saturated Fat (g) 0.3; Monounsaturated Fat (g) 1.5; Polyunsaturated Fat (g) 2.3; Dietary Fiber (g) 3.8; Flavonoid and Other Phyto (mg) 42.0; Cholesterol (mg) 0; Sodium (mg) 362; Vitamin A (IU) 1679; Vitamin C (mg) 16; Calcium (mg) 448; Iron (mg) 2.8; PERCENTAGE (%) Protein 33.3; Carbohydrate 35.2; Fat 26.0; Alcohol 5.7

Asparagus Tofu Stir-Fry

SERVES 4

Stir-frying vegetables with tofu, called *champuru* or *chample,* is one of the most common cooking methods in Okinawa—and a terrific way to prepare asparagus. This tasty, crisp spring vegetable has one of the lowest caloric densities around—only 0.2, a real feather-weight. It also packs a good amount of vitamin A, as well as iron and vitamins B and C. The most tender stalks are apple green with purple-tinged tips. Asparagus can be stored in the refrigerator for three to four days, if wrapped tightly in a plastic bag. For variety, try making this *chample* with other veggies too—cabbage, bean sprouts, carrots, bitter melon, or zucchini; almost any vegetable will work.

Canola oil spray
4 free-range, omega-3 eggs (optional)
1 teaspoon canola oil
2 cloves garlic, minced
1 tablespoon minced ginger
15 ounces water-packed firm light tofu,
   diced into 1-inch cubes

1 pound asparagus, tough stems
   snapped off, cut into 1-inch lengths
Pinch of sea salt
Freshly ground black pepper

Spray a large skillet with canola oil and heat over high heat.

Crack the eggs into a bowl. Scramble the eggs and cook them for 45 seconds to 1 minute, or until cooked. Set aside on a plate.

Wipe the skillet and heat the canola oil over medium heat. Cook the garlic and ginger for 45 seconds to 1 minute, or until golden. Raise the heat to medium-high. Add the tofu and stir continuously for 4 minutes, or until golden. Add the asparagus and cook for 6 minutes, or until cooked. Add the salt, pepper, and eggs. Toss. Divide evenly among 4 dinner plates and serve.

NUTRITION FACTS: 1 SERVING; Caloric Density 0.5; Calories (Kcal) 205; Protein (g) 29; Carbohydrate (g) 5; Total Fat (g) 5; Saturated Fat (g) 0.1; Monounsaturated Fat (g) 0.7; Polyunsaturated Fat (g) 4.2; Dietary Fiber (g) 2.2; Flavonoid and Other Phyto (mg) 65.6; Cholesterol (mg) 0; Sodium (mg) 70; Vitamin A (IU) 579; Vitamin C (mg) 14; Calcium (mg) 1150; Iron (mg) 3.9; PERCENTAGE (%) Protein 62.9; Carbohydrate 11.6; Fat 25.5

Fresh Tofu Spring Rolls

SERVES 4

The spring roll, *harumaki* in Japanese (*haru* is "spring;" *maki* is "roll"), is a popular simple appetizer in most Asian cuisines. Sizes vary, but they're generally 3 to 5 inches long and 1 to 2 inches thick. Shiitake mushrooms and bamboo shoots are the most common fillings, but lettuce and other vegetables also work well, and even leftover stir-fries are viable ingredients. After the ingredients are rolled up in wheat or rice flour wrappers, spring rolls are either deep-fried or eaten raw, depending on the preparation of the ingredients inside. Ours are the healthier nonfried variety. Once you've tried this low-CD vegetarian recipe a few times, branch out and experiment by adding some of your own favorite veggie fillings. You might just create your own signature dish!

SAUCE
¼ cup peanut butter
2 tablespoons lime juice
½ teaspoon turbinado or brown sugar
½ teaspoon chili powder
½ teaspoon Vietnamese or Thai fish
    sauce or low-sodium soy sauce

1 bundle of Chinese mung bean
    cellophane noodles (a little less than
    2 ounces)
Canola oil spray

7 ounces water-packed firm light tofu,
    cut into 12 rectangles
1 teaspoon ground paprika
1 teaspoon ground turmeric
1 teaspoon low-sodium soy sauce
1 cup soybean sprouts
1 cup julienned red bell pepper
1 cup peeled and thinly sliced cucumber
½ cup fresh cilantro leaves
8 rice paper wrappers (8½ inches
    diameter, available at most Asian
    groceries)

In a small mixing bowl, combine the peanut butter, lime juice, turbinado sugar, chili powder, and fish sauce; mix well. Place in refrigerator.

In a pot of boiling water, cook the cellophane noodles for 2 minutes. Drain and rinse under cold running water. Cut in half. Set aside.

Spray a skillet with canola oil and cook the tofu rectangles gently over medium-high heat for 3 to 5 minutes, or until golden. Add the paprika, turmeric, and soy sauce and toss to evenly coat. Set aside.

Place the soybean sprouts in a colander and pour 4 cups of boiling water over them. Rinse under cold running water. Set aside.

Place the cellophane noodles, tofu, soybean sprouts, bell pepper, cucumber, and cilantro each in a separate plate or bowl and arrange the bowls on your kitchen counter. At the center, place a kitchen cloth. Place 1 or 2 paper towels on your work surface.

In a pie pan or skillet, place lukewarm water about 1 to 2 inches in depth and soak one rice paper for 5 to 10 seconds. Do not oversoak. Gently transfer the wrapper to the work surface and quickly arrange on it some of each filling in this order: 2–3 cilantro leaves, bell pepper, tofu, cellophane noodles, sprouts, and cucumber. Roll up the wrapper tightly but gently. Tuck in the ends if you like. Repeat with remaining wrappers.

Serve with the peanut sauce.

If the spring rolls will not be eaten immediately, cover them with a damp paper towel or cloth.

NUTRITION FACTS: 1 SERVING, 2 ROLLS; Caloric Density 1.3; Calories (Kcal) 290; Protein (g) 13; Carbohydrate (g) 39; Total Fat (g) 10; Saturated Fat (g) 1.0; Monounsaturated Fat (g) 4.2; Polyunsaturated Fat (g) 3.6; Dietary Fiber (g) 3.5; Flavonoid and Other Phyto (mg) 16.8; Cholesterol (mg) 0; Sodium (mg) 129; Vitamin A (IU) 2588; Vitamin C (mg) 82; Calcium (mg) 216; Iron (mg) 2.4; PERCENTAGE (%) Protein 16.8; Carbohydrate 52.1; Fat 31.1

Tofu and Veggie Pita Sandwich

SERVES 4

This is a vegetarian version of our Veggie Pork Pita on page 278. Making it with tofu reduces the cholesterol level of the meal, and helps reduce your blood cholesterol levels. And it's just as scrumptious as the pork version.

6 ounces water-packed five-spice tofu, drained (Nasoya brand)
1 tablespoon whole-wheat flour
2 large whole-wheat pita breads, sliced in half
Olive oil spray
4 soy Swiss cheese slices

1 cup alfalfa sprouts
1/3 cup chopped celery
1 cup baby arugula
1 cup julienned red bell pepper
4 red onion slices
4 tomato slices

Preheat the broiler.

Cut the tofu into 4 slices and coat evenly with the flour. Place on a baking sheet and broil for 4 minutes, turn, and broil an additional 1 minute, or until tofu is golden and dry.

Open the pita pockets and spray olive oil once in each pocket. Evenly arrange the tofu, soy cheese, and vegetables in the pockets.

NUTRITION FACTS: 1 SERVING; Caloric Density 0.9; Calories (Kcal) 205; Protein (g) 12; Carbohydrate (g) 28; Total Fat (g) 6; Saturated Fat (g) 1.3; Monounsaturated Fat (g) 2.4; Polyunsaturated Fat (g) 1.9; Dietary Fiber (g) 4.6; Flavonoid and Other Phyto (mg) 20.4; Cholesterol (mg) 0; Sodium (mg) 472; Vitamin A (IU) 2868; Vitamin C (mg) 80; Calcium (mg) 245; Iron (mg) 1.8; PERCENTAGE (%) Protein 22.4; Carbohydrate 51.7; Fat 25.9

Yuki's Indian Tofu Curry

SERVES 4

Recipe provided by Chef Yukiko Hisano at Yu.Ki.San.Chi (Yuki's House), Yonaguni, Okinawa, phone: 81.9808.2911

This recipe comes from Yuki-san, the chef and owner of a small curry house on Yonaguni, a remote but beautiful island that is the westernmost of the Okinawan archipelago. "I wanted not only to serve food," says Yuki-san, who moved to the island from the big industrial city of Yokohama decades ago, "but also to provide a relaxing, healing place for the community." And indeed she has. Yuki-san's cozy restaurant and hearty curry are a well-known secret throughout Japan. People fly all the way from Tokyo to Yonaguni Island to heal their bodies and their spirits with Yuki-san's food. We think you'll find this delicious and relaxing at your table too.

15 ounces water-packed firm light tofu	1 teaspoon ground allspice
1 tablespoon canola oil	1 tablespoon ground turmeric
2 cloves garlic, minced	½ teaspoon sea salt
½ tablespoon dried cumin seeds	Freshly ground black pepper
2 cups thinly sliced yellow onion	3 tablespoons whole-wheat flour
3 tablespoons paprika	2 cups halved red-skinned new potatoes
½ to 1 tablespoon cayenne pepper	1 cup finely chopped carrot
½ teaspoon ground coriander	1 cup finely chopped celery
½ teaspoon ground cardamom	1 can (28 ounce) crushed tomatoes
½ teaspoon ground cumin	

Wrap the tofu in two paper towels. Microwave at high for 3 minutes. Set aside.

Heat a large pot over low heat. Coat with canola oil and, stirring continuously, cook the garlic, cumin seeds, and onion for 6 to 8 minutes or until the onion starts to caramelize.

Stir in the paprika, cayenne, coriander, cardamom, ground cumin, allspice, turmeric, salt, pepper, and flour. Add the potatoes, carrot, celery, and tomatoes. If the vegetables are not all covered by the tomatoes' liquid, add enough water to cover. Bring to a boil. Reduce the heat to low, cover, and cook for 30 to 40 minutes.

In the meantime, process the tofu in the food processor on low for a few seconds. The tofu should be crumbly. Stir the tofu into the curry mixture. Cook an additional 3 to 4 minutes. Serve over brown rice with Yuki's Yonaguni Pickles (see page 301) or in pita bread.

NUTRITION FACTS: 1 SERVING; Caloric Density 0.5; Calories (Kcal) 222; Protein (g) 15; Carbohydrate (g) 32; Total Fat (g) 5; Saturated Fat (g) 0.3; Monounsaturated Fat (g) 1.3; Polyunsaturated Fat (g) 2.2; Dietary Fiber (g) 9.6; Flavonoid and Other Phyto (mg) 61.1; Cholesterol (mg) 0; Sodium (mg) 601; Vitamin A (IU) 12,218; Vitamin C (mg) 33; Calcium (mg) 516; Iron (mg) 6.6; PERCENTAGE (%) Protein 25.9; Carbohydrate 54.3; Fat 19.9

Vegetables and Grains

If there is one universal bit of wisdom passed down from generation to generation, it has to be the value of veggies. When they were young, today's Okinawan elders worked side by side with their parents in the family fields after school to raise a colorful array of vegetables including *ooha* (green leafy vegetables), *goya* (bitter melon), *oomaami* (green beans), *akamaami* (red adzuki beans), *shima ninjin* (yellow carrots), and more. And who of us growing up in North America wasn't admonished to eat our vegetables? Mom was right. For lifelong health and weight control, there is no better strategy than eating your veggies. They have the lowest caloric density of all foods and are chock-full of vitamins, minerals, fiber, flavonoids, and antioxidants. Color is a useful guide to the vitamin content of vegetables. In general, the deeper and darker the color, the better, as darker leaves indicate a greater quantity of vitamin C and the antioxidant beta-carotene. Deep yellow, orange, and dark green vegetables derive their color from carotenoid pigments (including beta-carotene and lycopene) and the acanthocyanins, a class of flavonoids. These pigments remain stable when cooked and are fat-soluble, so the nutritional content of the veggies is preserved during cooking. Vegetables make it easy to meet the *shojin ryori* goal of having five colors on our table at every meal.

Yuki's Yonaguni Pickles

Cucumber and Wakame Vinaigrette

Shiri-Shiri Carrot and Bitter Melon

Soy-Sake Shiitake Mushroom Steak

Sautéed Shiitake and Konnyaku

Cumin-Chili Cauliflower

Vinegar-Sautéed Shiitake Asparagus

Cumin-Flavored Fava Beans

Genmai Tea, Shiitake, and Potato Medley

Sprouts Stir-Fry (Maamina Chample)

Goya Delight (Goya Nu Nimun)

Baby Bok Choy Stir-Fry

Okinawan Pumpkin Ragout (Nankwa Nbushi)

Mediterranean Ratatouille

Kamato's Modern Herbal Marinade and Dressing

Special Herb Potato Gratin

Millet Brown Rice

Soy Spinach Congee

Creamy Garlic Portobello

Zucchini and Mushroom Pancakes

Herbed Zucchini

Roasted Vegetables with Miso-Sesame Sauce

Nabbie's New-Style Oven-Roasted Vegetables with Herbs

Brilliant Vegetarian Chili

Dandelion Spring Rice

Ogimi Village Sweet Potato Leaf Risotto

Hearty Bean Stroganoff

Goya Sushi Roll

Fresh Garden Quiche

Painted Bean Casserole

Hijiki Brown Rice

Creamed Spinach and Broccoli on Soba

Tomato Broth Soba Noodles

Baked Sweet Potatoes

Bean and Rice Burritos

Edamame Basil Spaghetti

Roasted Tomato Pasta

Yuki's Yonaguni Pickles

SERVES 15

Recipe provided by Chef Yukiko Hisano at Yu.Ki.San.Chi (Yuki's House), Yonaguni, Okinawa, phone: 81.9808.2911

Chef Yuki, who also contributed the recipe for Yuki's Indian Tofu Curry on page 298, makes great low-sodium pickles as well. Her curry house and the laid-back atmosphere of remote Yonaguni Island draw customers from all over Japan—many of whom leave packing a jar or two of Yuki-san's prized pickles. With their sweet and sour taste, these pickles are a wonderful complement to hot curry and other spicy foods.

1 pound pickling cucumbers, ends removed, cut into 1-inch lengths
½ pound baby carrots
½ pound daikon radish, cut to the same size as the carrots

2 teaspoons sea salt
1 tablespoon turbinado or brown sugar
1 cup rice vinegar

In a large container, place the cucumbers, carrots, and daikon. Sprinkle with the sea salt. Let stand for at least 4 hours or overnight, stirring occasionally. Transfer the vegetables to a large colander and drain well.

In a large resealable plastic bag, combine the turbinado sugar, vinegar, and 1 cup water. Add the vegetables. Press the air out of the bag and shake to coat vegetables well. Refrigerate about 6 hours before serving.

NUTRITION FACTS: 1 SERVING; Caloric Density 0.2; Calories (Kcal) 23; Protein (g) 0; Carbohydrate (g) 4; Total Fat (g) 0; Saturated Fat (g) 0.0; Monounsaturated Fat (g) 0.0; Polyunsaturated Fat (g) 0.0; Dietary Fiber (g) 0.9; Flavonoid and Other Phyto (mg) 0.0; Cholesterol (mg) 0; Sodium (mg) 279; Vitamin A (IU) 4275; Vitamin C (mg) 6; Calcium (mg) 13; Iron (mg) 0.3; PERCENTAGE (%) Protein 9.0; Carbohydrate 86.5; Fat 4.5

Cucumber and Wakame Vinaigrette

SERVES 4

Wakame and other seaweeds contain a fiberlike compound called *fucoidan,* known to induce the production of interleukins and interferon, which help the immune system fight infections and cancer. Wakame is popular in Okinawa and is readily available in most Asian groceries and international food sections of grocery stores in the United States. It comes in both wet and dry form. We recommend using the dehydrated type, as the wet variety is usually preserved with heavy amounts of salt. Look for dehydrated wakame flakes rather than long and wide strips, as they're easier to prepare and softer in texture. Wakame goes very well with cucumbers, which are mostly water and a good source of vitamin A and fiber.

¼ cup dried wakame seaweed
¼ cup plus 1 tablespoon rice vinegar
2 tablespoons low-sodium soy sauce
½ teaspoon turbinado or brown sugar

4 cups peeled and thinly sliced
    cucumber
1 tablespoon minced ginger

In a large bowl, soak the wakame in water for 8 minutes, or until rehydrated. Drain.

In the same bowl, combine the vinegar, soy sauce, and turbinado sugar. Stir until the sugar is dissolved.

Add the cucumber, ginger, and wakame and toss. Chill in the refrigerator for 15 minutes, stirring occasionally.

NUTRITION FACTS: 1 SERVING; Caloric Density 0.2; Calories (Kcal) 33; Protein (g) 1; Carbohydrate (g) 5; Total Fat (g) <1; Saturated Fat (g) 0.0; Monounsaturated Fat (g) 0.0; Polyunsaturated Fat (g) 0.0; Dietary Fiber (g) 1.4; Flavonoid and Other Phyto (mg) 0.0; Cholesterol (mg) 0; Sodium (mg) 386; Vitamin A (IU) 138; Vitamin C (mg) 3; Calcium (mg) 29; Iron (mg) 0.7; PERCENTAGE (%) Protein 19.4; Carbohydrate 74.2; Fat 6.4

Shiri-Shiri Carrot and Bitter Melon

SERVES 4

A simple family recipe in Okinawa, *shiri-shiri* consists of virtually any vegetable cut into thin matchstick shapes and cooked. It could be stir-fried, boiled, or used in salads with vinaigrette. The name comes from the "shiri-shiri" sound made when sticks were gathered and bound together.

1 teaspoon canola oil
2 free-range, omega-3 eggs or ½ cup
    egg substitute or egg white, beaten
    (optional)
Canola oil spray
2 cups julienned (matchstick-thin)
    carrot

1 cup cored and julienned (matchstick-
    thin) bitter melon
Pinch of sea salt
½ tablespoon low-sodium soy sauce
Freshly ground black pepper

Coat a large skillet with the canola oil. Heat on medium. Pour in the eggs and stir quickly, about 45 seconds to 1 minute. Transfer to a plate and set aside.

Increase the heat to medium-high and spray the skillet with canola oil. Add the carrot, bitter melon, and salt. Stirring continuously, cook for 7 minutes, or until the vegetables are crisp-tender. Stir in the egg. Season with the soy sauce and pepper.

NUTRITION FACTS: 1 SERVING, WITHOUT EGGS; Caloric Density 0.5; Calories (Kcal) 42; Protein (g) 1; Carbohydrate (g) 7; Total Fat (g) 1; Saturated Fat (g) 0.1; Monounsaturated Fat (g) 0.7; Polyunsaturated Fat (g) 0.4; Dietary Fiber (g) 2.5; Flavonoid and Other Phyto (mg) 0.0; Cholesterol (mg) 0; Sodium (mg) 165; Vitamin A (IU) 17,247; Vitamin C (mg) 25; Calcium (mg) 23; Iron (mg) 0.5; PERCENTAGE (%) Protein 8.8; Carbohydrate 65.2; Fat 26.0

Soy-Sake Shiitake Mushroom Steak

SERVES 4

As we've mentioned, shiitake mushrooms are a common food in Okinawan cuisine and make a good meat substitute due to their texture and flavor. They are often sautéed (as in this recipe) or added to simmered vegetable and seaweed dishes called *nitsuke*. Here we combine meaty shiitake mushrooms with a soy and sake sauce. Try serving this "steak" on top of rice or on a bun with lettuce, tomato, onion, or other veggies—like a shiitake burger.

Canola oil spray
1 tablespoon minced ginger
1 tablespoon minced garlic
20 fresh shiitake mushrooms, stems removed

2 tablespoons sake rice wine
1 tablespoon mirin sweet rice wine
1 tablespoon low-sodium soy sauce
3 tablespoons chopped green onion

Spray a large skillet with canola oil and cook the ginger and garlic over medium heat for 45 seconds to 1 minute, or until golden.

Increase the heat to medium-high. Add the shiitake mushrooms and cook, turning occasionally, for 2 minutes, or until crisp-tender.

Increase the heat to high and add the sake, mirin, and soy sauce. Toss to coat evenly. Cook for 2 to 4 minutes, or until the liquid is almost evaporated and the shiitake mushrooms are tender.

Garnish with green onion.

NUTRITION FACTS: 1 SERVING; Caloric Density 0.6; Calories (Kcal) 43; Protein (g) 1; Carbohydrate (g) 7; Total Fat (g) <1; Saturated Fat (g) 0.0; Monounsaturated Fat (g) 0.0; Polyunsaturated Fat (g) 0.0; Dietary Fiber (g) 2.2; Flavonoid and Other Phyto (mg) 1.2; Cholesterol (mg) 0; Sodium (mg) 156; Vitamin A (IU) 11; Vitamin C (mg) 1; Calcium (mg) 7; Iron (mg) 0.4; PERCENTAGE (%) Protein 12.7; Carbohydrate 63.9; Fat 4.8; Alcohol 18.6

Sautéed Shiitake and Konnyaku

SERVES 4

Konnyaku (also called *konjac*) is made from a combination of dried and powdered yam and water and has a unique elastic texture. Because of its high fiber content, it's long been considered a "stomach cleaner" in Japan, and is prominent in folklore. One legend has it that back around A.D. 930, a hardworking stonemason had a terrible pain in his stomach and was bedridden for days. His good wife prayed to the gods for his salvation, at which point she heard one say, "Your husband has stone dust stuck in his stomach, and since he is such a hardworking person, I will give you a powerful medicine to fix this problem." When she looked around, there was a ball of konnyaku lying on the table. She immediately cooked it up and fed it to her husband, who was instantaneously cured. These days you have to go to the store to get it—try an Asian market or Japanese food store. Konnyaku is a cake in a square shape, and it usually comes packed in a plastic bag with water. It also is sold as noodles, which are good for sukiyaki (see pages 274 and 293 for Nsunaba Sukiyaki and Nsunaba Sukiyaki Vegetarian).

8 ounces konnyaku yam cake
1 teaspoon canola oil
2 cloves garlic, minced
½ teaspoon red chili flakes (optional)
2 cups quartered fresh shiitake mushrooms

½ cup diced red bell pepper
1 tablespoon low-sodium soy sauce
1 tablespoon sake rice wine
Soy mayonnaise (optional)

Score the surfaces of the konnyaku lightly and dice into ½-inch pieces. Cook in a pot of boiling water for 2 minutes. Drain in a colander and run cold water over it to cool.

In a large skillet, heat the canola oil over high heat. Add the garlic and red chili flakes and cook for 20 seconds, or until the garlic is golden.

Add the diced konnyaku and cook for 3 minutes, or until the surface is lightly whitened. Shake and stir continuously, but be careful of spattering oil.

Stir in the shiitake mushrooms and red bell pepper. When the vegetables are coated evenly with oil, reduce the heat to low and add the soy sauce and sake. Cover and cook for 2 minutes, or until the red bell pepper is tender. Shake the skillet several times to season evenly.

Garnish with ½ tablespoon soy mayonnaise.

NUTRITION FACTS: 1 SERVING; Caloric Density 0.4; Calories (Kcal) 44; Protein (g) 1; Carbohydrate (g) 6; Total Fat (g) 1; Saturated Fat (g) 0.1; Monounsaturated Fat (g) 0.7; Polyunsaturated Fat (g) 0.3; Dietary Fiber (g) 3.3; Flavonoid and Other Phyto (mg) 0.0; Cholesterol (mg) 0; Sodium (mg) 158; Vitamin A (IU) 1086; Vitamin C (mg) 36; Calcium (mg) 32; Iron (mg) 0.6; PERCENTAGE (%) Protein 12.0; Carbohydrate 52.7; Fat 26.4; Alcohol 8.9

Cumin-Chili Cauliflower

SERVES 4

Cumin seeds are one of the most popular spices in the world. The "seeds" are actually the fruit of the cumin plant, which is related to parsley. In the United States, this spice is particularly common in Southwestern chili dishes; it is also used widely in Latin America, North Africa, and many Asian countries, especially India. Cumin contains high amounts of carotene and iron and has been used medicinally as a digestive aid and an anti-inflammatory. It has a strong, wonderful aroma that wafts through the air when the seeds are heated. This quick and easy vegetable side dish can also be served as an entrée when you don't feel like cooking a large meal but want to add low-CD veggies to the menu.

1 tablespoon canola oil	½ teaspoon chili powder
1 tablespoon dried cumin seeds	Pinch of sea salt
4 cups finely chopped cauliflower florets	

Over low heat, heat the canola oil in a large skillet. Add the cumin seeds and cook for 45 seconds to 1 minute, or until the aroma of cumin rises from the skillet.

Increase the heat to medium-high and add the cauliflower. Cook, stirring frequently, for 4 to 7 minutes, or until crisp-tender.

Stir in the chili powder and salt.

NUTRITION FACTS: 1 SERVING; Caloric Density 0.5; Calories (Kcal) 47; Protein (g) 2; Carbohydrate (g) 6; Total Fat (g) 2; Saturated Fat (g) 0.2; Monounsaturated Fat (g) 1.2; Polyunsaturated Fat (g) 0.7; Dietary Fiber (g) 2.8; Flavonoid and Other Phyto (mg) 0.0; Cholesterol (mg) 0; Sodium (mg) 104; Vitamin A (IU) 153; Vitamin C (mg) 47; Calcium (mg) 38; Iron (mg) 1.5; PERCENTAGE (%) Protein 16.9; Carbohydrate 44.7; Fat 38.3

Vinegar-Sautéed Shiitake Asparagus

SERVES 4

Shiitake mushrooms are popular in Okinawan and Asian cooking due to their distinctive fruity flavor and ease of preparation. Fresh shiitake are dark brown, with smooth velvety caps. They're best when the caps are thick, the flesh is firm and damp, and the cap edges are curled under. They also dry well and retain their excellent flavor. You'll love them in this *usachi*—vegetable dish with vinegar.

½ teaspoon sesame oil	1 teaspoon sake rice wine
½ teaspoon canola oil	1 tablespoon rice vinegar
1 tablespoon minced ginger	2 cups sliced fresh shiitake mushrooms
3 cups 1-inch-long asparagus pieces	⅓ cup dried fine bonito flakes
2 teaspoons low-sodium soy sauce	

Heat the sesame oil, canola oil, and ginger over medium heat for 45 seconds to 1 minute, or until the ginger is golden. Add the asparagus and cook, stirring frequently, for 4 to 6 minutes, or until crisp-tender.

In the meantime, whisk together the soy sauce, sake, and rice vinegar.

Stir the shiitake mushrooms into the skillet, then add ¼ cup water and cook for 1 minute. Add the soy sauce mixture to the vegetables and cook for 2 to 3 minutes, or until the shiitake mushrooms are coated with sauce and tender. Serve sprinkled with bonito flakes.

NUTRITION FACTS: 1 SERVING; Caloric Density 0.3; Calories (Kcal) 54; Protein (g) 4; Carbohydrate (g) 8; Total Fat (g) 2; Saturated Fat (g) 0.2; Monounsaturated Fat (g) 0.6; Polyunsaturated Fat (g) 0.5; Dietary Fiber (g) 3.7; Flavonoid and Other Phyto (mg) 0.0; Cholesterol (mg) 0; Sodium (mg) 105; Vitamin A (IU) 584; Vitamin C (mg) 13; Calcium (mg) 24; Iron (mg) 1.1; PERCENTAGE (%) Protein 24.1; Carbohydrate 50.8; Fat 22.8; Alcohol 2.3

Cumin-Flavored Fava Beans

SERVES 4

The fava bean, also called the *broad bean,* is a great summer treat. It is also one of the beans the Okinawan elders used to eat a lot when they were young. In those days, they grew all their own food, so beans were a relatively easy way of getting enough protein, iron, calcium, magnesium, copper, vitamins B_1, B_2, E, and dietary fiber. Fava beans were especially enjoyed in miso soup in those days.

2½ cups fava beans, outer skins removed, inner skins cut vertically to the black part	1 clove garlic, minced
	2 teaspoons dried cumin seeds
	Pinch of sea salt
Olive oil spray	

Bring a large pot of water to a boil. Cook the fava beans for 5 to 7 minutes, or until crisp-tender. Drain and remove the inner skins.

Spray a skillet with olive oil and cook the garlic and cumin seeds over medium heat for 45 seconds to 1 minute, or until the garlic is golden. Add the fava beans and cook for 2 minutes, or until the beans becomes slightly mashy. Season with salt.

NUTRITION FACTS: 1 SERVING; Caloric Density 0.8; Calories (Kcal) 55; Protein (g) 4; Carbohydrate (g) 9; Total Fat (g) 1; Saturated Fat (g) 0.1; Monounsaturated Fat (g) 0.2; Polyunsaturated Fat (g) 0.3; Dietary Fiber (g) 3.0; Flavonoid and Other Phyto (mg) 3.4; Cholesterol (mg) 0; Sodium (mg) 104; Vitamin A (IU) 254; Vitamin C (mg) 23; Calcium (mg) 27; Iron (mg) 2.0; PERCENTAGE (%) Protein 28.3; Carbohydrate 60.6; Fat 11.1

Genmai Tea, Shiitake, and Potato Medley

SERVES 4

Another folktale for your enjoyment: A young man was strolling down by the seaside of a northern Okinawan village when he happened upon a huge box. When he opened it, he discovered a monk inside, weak from lack of food and water. The young man carried the monk to his village spring for a bowl of water. The tasty water saved the monk's life, and he declared it good enough for tea making. Since that day, the spring's water has been widely used for tea. The spring tea is now called *sa-ga*, which means "tea spring."

8 dried shiitake mushrooms	2 cups ½-inch-thick zucchini slices
2 cups warm water	1 tablespoon sake rice wine
1 tea bag of Japanese *genmai* tea	2 tablespoons white miso
12 red-skinned new potatoes	

Rehydrate the shiitake mushrooms in the warm water for 15 minutes, or until tender. Reserve the soaking liquid. Cut the mushrooms in half or, if large, quarters.

In a large pot, bring the shiitake soaking liquid to a boil. Add the *genmai* tea bag, the potatoes, and 1 cup water; return to a boil. Remove the tea bag and reduce the heat to low. Cook for 10 minutes. Add the zucchini, sake, miso, and shiitake mushrooms. Bring to a boil over high heat. Reduce the heat to low and cook for 8 to 10 minutes, or until the zucchini is tender.

NUTRITION FACTS: 1 SERVING; Caloric Density 0.2; Calories (Kcal) 60; Protein (g) 3; Carbohydrate (g) 11; Total Fat (g) 1; Saturated Fat (g) 0.1; Monounsaturated Fat (g) 0.2; Polyunsaturated Fat (g) 0.4; Dietary Fiber (g) 2.5; Flavonoid and Other Phyto (mg) 20.6; Cholesterol (mg) 0; Sodium (mg) 332; Vitamin A (IU) 200; Vitamin C (mg) 9; Calcium (mg) 18; Iron (mg) 0.8; PERCENTAGE (%) Protein 16.9; Carbohydrate 67.7; Fat 9.3; Alcohol 6.1

Sprouts Stir-Fry (Maamina Chample)

SERVES 4

Maamina (Okinawan for "bean sprouts") are one of the healthiest and most esteemed vegetables in Okinawa, and they're used in most vegetable combination dishes. You'll always see *obaas* ("grandmas") in their eighties, nineties, and a few in their hundreds in the open market in the Okinawa capital of Naha, sitting on a mat and removing the beard (roots) of bean sprouts one by one. The corners where they sit are like havens of calm and quiet in the middle of the crowded, noisy market. The obaas treat the beautiful white plucked sprouts tenderly as they carefully pack them in plastic bags. You can buy the spouts for 100 yen a bag—and when you see those tiny obaas with their maamina, there's no way to resist making a purchase.

Canola oil spray	½ teaspoon chili powder
1 tablespoon minced ginger	Pinch of sea salt
1 cup julienned carrot	1 teaspoon low-sodium soy sauce
5 cups mung bean sprouts	1 tablespoon sake rice wine

Spray a skillet with canola oil. Cook the ginger over medium heat for 45 seconds to 1 minute, or until golden.

Increase the heat to medium-high. Add the carrot and cook for 3 to 4 minutes, or until tender.

Add the bean sprouts and cook, stirring continuously, for 5 minutes, or until the sprouts are tender. Add the chili powder, salt, soy sauce, and sake. Stir to season evenly and cook for an additional 1 to 2 minutes.

NUTRITION FACTS: 1 SERVING; Caloric Density 0.4; Calories (Kcal) 60; Protein (g) 4; Carbohydrate (g) 11; Total Fat (g) <1; Saturated Fat (g) 0.0; Monounsaturated Fat (g) 0.0; Polyunsaturated Fat (g) 0.1; Dietary Fiber (g) 3.4; Flavonoid and Other Phyto (mg) 0.0; Cholesterol (mg) 0; Sodium (mg) 140; Vitamin A (IU) 8720; Vitamin C (mg) 20; Calcium (mg) 27; Iron (mg) 1.4; PERCENTAGE (%) Protein 24.8; Carbohydrate 64.2; Fat 5.2; Alcohol 5.7

Goya Delight (Goya Nu Nimun)

SERVES 5

Recipe provided from: *Okinawan Mixed Plate: Generous Servings of Culture, Customs and Cuisine,* published by Hui O Laulima, August 2000. To order, call Bobbi Kuba at (808) 523-5858 or e-mail to: emkuba@yahoo.com / thelma@hawaii.rr.com

Goya (bitter melon) is the first vegetable that comes to mind when Japanese think about Okinawan cuisine. It's the chief ambassador of Okinawan vegetables. Goya grows easily in sunny Okinawan gardens. Locals rub its leaves on their skin to treat heat rash and drink its juice as a treatment for various ailments. This simmered goya recipe, though, is way beyond medicinal; it's a real traditional Okinawan favorite.

1 pound bitter melon
1 teaspoon sea salt
2 pieces aburage (a thin, deep-fried bean curd available in plastic bags at most Asian food stores)

2 cups bonito or kelp broth (see page 229)
3 teaspoons turbinado or brown sugar
½ teaspoon sake rice wine
1½ tablespoons white miso

Cut the bitter melon in half lengthwise and remove the seeds. Place in a colander, sprinkle with salt, and let stand for 20 minutes. Rinse under running water and drain well. Slice into pieces 1 to 1½ inches wide.

Blanch the aburage in hot water to remove its oil. Cut it into ¾-inch-wide pieces.

In a stockpot, place the bitter melon, aburage, broth, turbinado sugar, sake, and 1½ tablespoons miso and bring to a boil over high heat. Immediately reduce the heat to low and cook for 10 minutes.

NUTRITION FACTS: 1 SERVING; Caloric Density 0.7; Calories (Kcal) 65; Protein (g) 3; Carbohydrate (g) 8; Total Fat (g) 3; Saturated Fat (g) 0.4; Monounsaturated Fat (g) 0.6; Polyunsaturated Fat (g) 1.5; Dietary Fiber (g) 3.3; Flavonoid and Other Phyto (mg) 7.1; Cholesterol (mg) 0; Sodium (mg) 668; Vitamin A (IU) 349; Vitamin C (mg) 76; Calcium (mg) 70; Iron (mg) 1.1; PERCENTAGE (%) Protein 19.6; Carbohydrate 44.6; Fat 35; Alcohol 0.8

Baby Bok Choy Stir-Fry

SERVES 4

Stir-frying vegetables and tofu or small pieces of lean meat with just a hint of oil is called *chample* in Okinawa, and it's an extremely popular method of cooking all through the archipelago. But the reason Okinawa is often referred to as a "*chample* culture" is more for its role as a crossroads for China, Japan, and Southeast Asian cultures than for its cooking preferences. *Chample* literally means "mixture" or "combination," and Okinawa is indeed a wonderful mixture of Asian cultures.

Canola oil spray
1 tablespoon sesame oil
1 tablespoon thinly sliced ginger
2 tablespoons thinly sliced garlic

8 cups baby bok choy
¼ cup sake rice wine
3 tablespoons low-sodium soy sauce

Spray a large skillet with canola oil and add the sesame oil. Cook the ginger and garlic over medium heat for 45 seconds to 1 minute or until golden.

Increase the heat to medium-high. Add the bok choy, increase the heat to high, and cook for 1 minute, stirring. Add the sake and soy sauce and cook for 6 to 8 minutes, or until the bok choy is tender. Do not cook until the bok choy is brown and transparent.

Serve hot on a large plate.

NUTRITION FACTS: 1 SERVING; Caloric Density 0.4; Calories (Kcal) 63; Protein (g) 3; Carbohydrate (g) 6; Total Fat (g) 2; Saturated Fat (g) 0.3; Monounsaturated Fat (g) 0.7; Polyunsaturated Fat (g) 0.9; Dietary Fiber (g) 1.6; Flavonoid and Other Phyto (mg) 0.0; Cholesterol (mg) 0; Sodium (mg) 542; Vitamin A (IU) 4200; Vitamin C (mg) 64; Calcium (mg) 153; Iron (mg) 1.4; PERCENTAGE (%) Protein 17.2; Carbohydrate 32.5; Fat 26.8; Alcohol 23.3.

Okinawan Pumpkin Ragout (Nankwa Nbushi)

SERVES 6

Recipe provided from: *Okinawan Mixed Plate: Generous Servings of Culture, Customs and Cuisine,* published by Hui O Laulima, August 2000. To order, call Bobbi Kuba at (808) 523-5858 or e-mail to: emkuba@yahoo.com / thelma@hawaii.rr.com

This easy-to-make dish, cooked in the *nbushi* style, regularly appears on Okinawan dinner tables. Essentially, the veggies do all the work. You just put them in a pot, where they release their pleasing flavors into the mix. Pumpkins are an old Okinawan favorite because the climbing plant thrives in Okinawan soil, and one pumpkin is more than enough for several dinners. Okinawans also enjoy this carotene-rich vegetable in cakes, curry, and "pumpkin noodles," which are noodles stir-fried with thin pumpkin slices. *Kabocha* pumpkins have golden yellow flesh and dark-green skin.

2 pounds kabocha pumpkin, washed	**1 teaspoon canola oil**
2 tablespoons dried shrimp, chopped,	**1 tablespoon turbinado or brown sugar**
or ⅔ cup dried bonito flakes	**1 tablespoon low-sodium soy sauce**
(optional)	**Pinch of sea salt**

Microwave the pumpkin at high for 3 minutes. Cut it open and remove the seeds. Cut the pumpkin into 1-inch square pieces without removing the skin. Set aside.

In a large saucepan, place the dried shrimp, canola oil, and 2 cups water and bring to a boil. Reduce the heat and simmer for 5 minutes.

Add the pumpkin to the pan and cook for 8 to 10 minutes over low heat. Add the turbinado sugar, soy sauce, and salt. Toss the pumpkin pieces once without stirring, then cook for another 5 minutes, or until the pumpkin is tender.

NUTRITION FACTS: 1 SERVING; Caloric Density 0.3; Calories (Kcal) 69; Protein (g) 6; Carbohydrate (g) 12; Total Fat (g) 1; Saturated Fat (g) 0.1; Monounsaturated Fat (g) 0.5; Polyunsaturated Fat (g) 0.2; Dietary Fiber (g) 0.8; Flavonoid and Other Phyto (mg) 0.0; Cholesterol (mg) 0; Sodium (mg) 150; Vitamin A (IU) 2419; Vitamin C (mg) 14; Calcium (mg) 72; Iron (mg) 1.6; PERCENTAGE (%) Protein 29.9; Carbohydrate 58.7; Fat 11.4

Mediterranean Ratatouille

SERVES 4

Ratatouille is one of the tastiest and easiest ways to incorporate a large variety of vegetables in one dish. Eggplant, one of its main ingredients, is a terrific low-cal vegetable—a mere 20 calories per ½ cup. Cooked ratatouille is just as tasty after a day or two in the fridge, so make extra. It's perfect to have with a whole-wheat roll as a light but filling lunch.

1 tablespoon olive oil	**2 tablespoons tomato paste**
4 cloves garlic, minced	**½ tablespoon dried basil**
2 cups diced eggplant	**½ tablespoon dried oregano**
2 cups diced zucchini	**Pinch of sea salt**
3 medium ripe red tomatoes, chopped	**Freshly ground black pepper**
1 cup diced green bell pepper	

In a large pot, heat the olive oil and cook the garlic over medium heat for 45 seconds to 1 minute, or until golden.

Increase the heat to medium-high. Add the eggplant and zucchini; cook for 4 minutes, stirring continuously. Add the tomatoes and green pepper; cook 3 minutes.

Reduce the heat to low and add the tomato paste, basil, and oregano. Cook for 10 minutes. Add ¼ cup water if the ingredients are dry.

Season with salt and pepper. Cook another 5 minutes, or until vegetables are tender.

Serve warm or refrigerate overnight to set the flavor.

NUTRITION FACTS: 1 SERVING; Caloric Density 0.3; Calories (Kcal) 77; Protein (g) 3; Carbohydrate (g) 14; Total Fat (g) 2; Saturated Fat (g) 0.3; Monounsaturated Fat (g) 1.3; Polyunsaturated Fat (g) 0.4; Dietary Fiber (g) 4.2; Flavonoid and Other Phyto (mg) 0.8; Cholesterol (mg) 0; Sodium (mg) 88; Vitamin A (IU) 1310; Vitamin C (mg) 61; Calcium (mg) 46; Iron (mg) 1.6; PERCENTAGE (%) Protein 13.1; Carbohydrate 63.1; Fat 23.8

Kamato's Modern Herbal Marinade and Dressing

MAKES 1½ CUPS; 25 SERVINGS, 1 TABLESPOON EACH

1 cup olive oil
¼ cup lemon juice or red wine
   vinegar
⅓ cup fresh parsley leaves and
   tender stems
2 tablespoons finely chopped
   fresh marjoram

2 tablespoons finely chopped
   fresh basil
1 tablespoon finely chopped fresh
   thyme
½ teaspoon celery seed
1 clove garlic, chopped
Pinch of sea salt
½ teaspoon hot pepper sauce

In a blender, place the oil, lemon juice, parsley, marjoram, basil, thyme, celery seed, garlic, salt, hot pepper sauce, and ¼ cup water. On low speed, mix until nearly smooth. Switch to high speed for another 30 seconds.

Use the dressing for salad greens or to marinate cooked or raw vegetables.

Tip: Substitute 1 teaspoon dried herbs for 1 tablespoon fresh. Substitute ½ cup white wine vinegar for the lemon juice or the red wine vinegar and water.

Note: You can add zing to vegetables by marinating them overnight in a mixture of vinegar, lemon, or lime juice, and fresh chopped herbs and spices such as marjoram, basil, or thyme. This delightful marinade works as a dressing both for cold salads and for hot roasted or grilled vegetables.

NUTRITION FACTS: 1 SERVING; Caloric Density 5.2; Calories (Kcal) 78; Protein (g) <1; Carbohydrate (g) <1; Fat (g) 9

Special Herb Potato Gratin

SERVES 4

The key to this simple potato dish is the combination of herbs and the flavor of the vegetable broth. Remember when you choose the vegetable broth to look for a brand that has low or no salt and low or no fat. "Vegetarian" chicken broth is another option. If you can't find the prepared canned type, use a bouillon cube (approximately 1 cube per 2 cups warm water, or follow the instructions on the package).

¾ cup soymilk, plain
¾ cup low-sodium vegetable broth
1 dried bay leaf
Pinch of sea salt
Freshly ground black pepper
3 tablespoons soy Parmesan cheese
    alternative or real Parmesan cheese

3 tablespoons bread crumbs
2 tablespoons finely chopped fresh
    parsley or 1 tablespoon dried parsley
6 medium red new potatoes with skin,
    cut into ½-inch rounds
2 tablespoons dried rosemary
1 tablespoon dried thyme

Preheat the oven to 375°F.

In a saucepan, combine the soymilk and vegetable broth and cook over medium heat. When the liquid starts to bubble around the edge, reduce the heat to low. Add the bay leaf, salt, and pepper. Cook for another 3 minutes, then remove the pan from heat. Let stand.

In a small mixing bowl, combine the Parmesan cheese, bread crumbs, and parsley. Set aside.

Pour about half of the soymilk mixture into an 8 × 8-inch baking pan. Add the potato rounds. Sprinkle the rosemary and thyme over the potatoes. Pour the remaining soymilk over the potatoes. Bake for 40 minutes.

Top the potatoes with the Parmesan mixture. Raise the heat to 400°F. Bake another 10 to 15 minutes, until the bread crumbs are golden and the potatoes are thoroughly cooked.

NUTRITION FACTS: 1 SERVING; Caloric Density 0.6; Calories (Kcal) 82; Protein (g) 5; Carbohydrate (g) 10; Total Fat (g) 2; Saturated Fat (g) 0.3; Monounsaturated Fat (g) 0.3; Polyunsaturated Fat (g) 0.5; Dietary Fiber (g) 2.6; Flavonoid and Other Phyto (mg) 0.8; Cholesterol (mg) 0; Sodium (mg) 248; Vitamin A (IU) 1397; Vitamin C (mg) 8; Calcium (mg) 104; Iron (mg) 2.2; PERCENTAGE (%) Protein 25.5; Carbohydrate 51.2; Fat 23.3

Millet Brown Rice

SERVES 8

1 cup brown rice, uncooked   **½ cup hulled millet**

Rinse the brown rice in a colander.

Rinse the millet in a fine-mesh colander or strainer, dividing it into small batches.

Place the grains in a medium bowl with 2¾ cups water and let stand for 30 minutes.

Cook the grains in a rice cooker with the water. If you haven't got a rice cooker, place the grains and water in a medium pot and bring to a boil. Reduce the heat to very low and cook, covered, for 40 to 50 minutes, or until the grains are thoroughly cooked.

NUTRITION FACTS: ½ CUP; Caloric Density 1.1; Calories (Kcal) 133; Protein (g) 3; Carbohydrate (g) 27; Total Fat (g) 1; Saturated Fat (g) 0.2; Monounsaturated Fat (g) 0.3; Polyunsaturated Fat (g) 0.5; Dietary Fiber (g) 1.9; Flavonoid and Other Phyto (mg) 0; Cholesterol (mg) 0; Sodium (mg) 4; Vitamin A (IU) 0; Vitamin C (mg) 0; Calcium (mg) 10; Iron (mg) 0.8; PERCENTAGE (%) Protein 9.6; Carbohydrate 82.5; Fat 7.9

Soy Spinach Congee

SERVES 4

Congee is a rice porridge that is popular throughout Asia. It's often eaten for breakfast in China but usually comes at the end of a meal in Okinawa or Japan. Possible ingredients include fish, shrimp, chicken, eggs, sesame seeds, peanuts, and vegetables. Because it is easier to digest than regular cooked rice, congee is used as baby food and is often offered when someone has a cold in Okinawa—much like chicken soup in North America. Although congee is often made with white rice, we've made ours with brown and added spinach for extra vitamins and minerals. Try it as a light but filling breakfast—or lunch or dinner.

1½ cups cooked brown rice   **1 teaspoon low-sodium soy sauce**
3 cups chopped spinach

Bring 3 cups water to a boil and add the rice. Bring to a boil and cook for 3 minutes on high heat. Reduce heat to low and cook another 2 minutes. Stir in the spinach and cook for 1 minute, or until the spinach is tender. Add the soy sauce and stir.

NUTRITION FACTS: 1 SERVING; Caloric Density 0.3; Calories (Kcal) 87; Protein (g) 2; Carbohydrate (g) 18; Total Fat (g) <1; Saturated Fat (g) 0.1; Monounsaturated Fat (g) 0.2; Polyunsaturated Fat (g) 0.2; Dietary Fiber (g) 1.9; Flavonoid and Other Phyto (mg) 0.0; Cholesterol (mg) 0; Sodium (mg) 74; Vitamin A (IU) 1510; Vitamin C (mg) 6; Calcium (mg) 33; Iron (mg) 1.0; PERCENTAGE (%) Protein 10.8; Carbohydrate 82.1; Fat 7.0

Creamy Garlic Portobello

SERVES 4

The portobello mushroom is one of the most popular mushrooms around. It's the largest and hardiest of the cultivated mushrooms and is well known for its impressive 3- to 10-inch brown cap. Portobellos are more robust in texture and flavor than agaricus or crimini mushrooms, and their texture is very much like that of meat. In fact, portobellos make a great meat substitute; they taste a lot like steak when grilled. Although they're better known for their outstanding flavor than for their medicinal properties, portobello mushrooms have been used to treat diabetes in Asia and may, in fact, act as insulin sensitizers, helping the body process sugars better. Mushrooms are low in calories, virtually fat-free, and perfect for a low-CD meal. You'll often find this dish at Spanish tapas restaurants, but here, instead of using high-calorie heavy cream, we've brought out the flavor with low-CD soymilk and calorie-free spices.

1 teaspoon olive oil	**1 teaspoon low-sodium soy sauce**
2 cloves garlic, minced	**¼ teaspoon chili powder**
1½ pounds portobello mushrooms,	**Pinch of sea salt**
sliced	**Freshly ground black pepper**
1 cup soymilk, plain	

In a large skillet, heat the olive oil over medium heat and cook the garlic for 45 seconds to 1 minute, or until golden. Stir in the portobello mushrooms and sauté for 5 minutes.

Add the soymilk and soy sauce and bring to a boil. Immediately reduce the heat to low and gently simmer, stirring, for 7 minutes, or until the mushrooms are tender and the soymilk is reduced to ¼ cup.

Add the chili powder, salt, and pepper and cook another minute.

Evenly divide among 4 plates and serve.

NUTRITION FACTS: 1 SERVING; Caloric Density 0.4; Calories (Kcal) 94; Protein (g) 8; Carbohydrate (g) 10; Total Fat (g) 2; Saturated Fat (g) 0.3; Monounsaturated Fat (g) 1.0; Polyunsaturated Fat (g) 0.6; Dietary Fiber (g) 6.9; Flavonoid and Other Phyto (mg) 1.1; Cholesterol (mg) 0; Sodium (mg) 147; Vitamin A (IU) 76; Vitamin C (mg) 1; Calcium (mg) 87; Iron (mg) 1.2; PERCENTAGE (%) Protein 34.3; Carbohydrate 43.0; Fat 22.7

Zucchini and Mushroom Pancakes

SERVES 4 (MAKES 12)

This smooth pancake is perfect for breakfast or lunch. Zucchini, like other varieties of squash, were domesticated and cultivated by Native Americans long before the arrival of Europeans. A single plant can produce a lot of zucchini, which explains why those of us who grow it in our gardens always have lots to give away at harvest time. You can prepare this versatile recipe beforehand and reheat the pancakes later.

1 free-range, omega-3 egg or ¼ cup egg substitute or egg white	½ cup finely chopped onion
⅔ cup whole-wheat flour	½ clove minced garlic
1 teaspoon baking powder	3 tablespoons minced parsley
1 cup shredded zucchini	Pinch of sea salt
½ cup thinly sliced button mushrooms	Freshly ground black pepper
	Canola oil spray

In a large mixing bowl, combine the egg, flour, baking powder, and ½ cup water. Stir in the zucchini, mushrooms, onion, garlic, parsley, salt, and pepper. If the batter is too thick, add water, 1 tablespoon at a time, until correct consistency is achieved.

Spray a large skillet with canola oil. Set it over medium heat.

Add batter to the pan, using ¼ cup batter per pancake. Cook for 2 minutes or until golden on the bottom. Turn over the pancake and flatten with a spatula. Cook an additional 2 minutes or until set.

NUTRITION FACTS: 1 SERVING; Caloric Density 0.8; Calories (Kcal) 102; Protein (g) 5; Carbohydrate (g) 18; Total Fat (g) 2; Saturated Fat (g) 0.5; Monounsaturated Fat (g) 0.6; Polyunsaturated Fat (g) 0.4; Dietary Fiber (g) 3.4; Flavonoid and Other Phyto (mg) 9.0; Cholesterol (mg) 53; Sodium (mg) 180; Vitamin A (IU) 324; Vitamin C (mg) 8; Calcium (mg) 113; Iron (mg) 1.5; PERCENTAGE (%) Protein 19.0; Carbohydrate 66.0; Fat 14.9

Herbed Zucchini

SERVES 4

When you're thinking of reducing calories, using a small amount of vegetable broth is always an excellent low-CD alternative to cooking oil. Combined with zucchini, one of the great low-CD foods, you can't go wrong. Like other summer squash, zucchini is about 94 percent water, making its CD count only 0.1. One cup of raw sliced zucchini has less than 20 calories and is a good source of potassium, folate, and the antioxidants vitamin C and beta-carotene. Zucchini can be found year-round at almost any grocery store. Look for ones that feel firm and heavy. Although they can be refrigerated for a few days, zucchini spoils quickly, so use soon after buying to get the most out of this great vegetable.

⅓ cup low-sodium vegetable broth	Pinch of sea salt
⅓ cup minced white onion	1 dried bay leaf
⅓ cup minced celery	1 teaspoon dried oregano
1 can (14.5-ounce) low-sodium stewed tomatoes with liquid	1 teaspoon dried basil
	½ teaspoon ground turmeric
4 cups ½-inch zucchini rounds	⅓ cup fresh Italian parsley, chopped
1 cup diced yellow bell pepper	½ cup shredded soy mozzarella cheese

In a medium pot, bring the vegetable broth to a boil. Add the onion and celery and cook for 3 minutes, or until the onion is tender.

Add the tomatoes and their liquid and the zucchini, bell pepper, salt, bay leaf, oregano, and basil. Bring to a boil over medium-high heat, then reduce heat to low. Cover and simmer for 8 minutes, or until the zucchini is tender. Stir in the turmeric and parsley and turn off the heat. Remove the bay leaf.

Sprinkle the soy cheese over the vegetables and cover the pan. Let stand for 1 to 2 minutes, or until the cheese is melted.

NUTRITION FACTS: 1 SERVING; Caloric Density 0.3; Calories (Kcal) 104; Protein (g) 5; Carbohydrate (g) 19; Total Fat (g) 2; Saturated Fat (g) 0.6; Monounsaturated Fat (g) 0.9; Polyunsaturated Fat (g) 0.4; Dietary Fiber (g) 4.1; Flavonoid and Other Phyto (mg) 7.1; Cholesterol (mg) 0; Sodium (mg) 219; Vitamin A (IU) 1525; Vitamin C (mg) 111; Calcium (mg) 165; Iron (mg) 2.4; PERCENTAGE (%) Protein 17.4; Carbohydrate 64.4; Fat 18.2

Roasted Vegetables with Miso-Sesame Sauce

SERVES 4

A bowl of miso a day keeps the doctor away.

—FOURTEENTH-CENTURY JAPANESE SAYING

Miso, or fermented soybean paste, is consumed daily throughout Japan. Besides its healthy attributes and extraordinary flavor, another reason for miso's popularity is its role in unifying diverse ingredients into a whole greater than the sum of its parts. We promise you'll see what we mean when you try this delicious recipe, with its variety of heart-healthy roasted vegetables. And once again you'll see how easy it is to make a tasty low-calorie dish that contains your daily quota of vegetables.

8 thick slices pumpkin (preferably kabocha pumpkin) with skin, seeds removed

4 thin carrots, peeled, both ends removed, cut in half lengthwise

2 russet potatoes, cut lengthwise into 4 pieces each

2 medium zucchini, both ends removed and cut lengthwise into 4 strips each

Four ½-inch-thick horizontal slices of large eggplant, stem removed

Olive oil spray

2 tablespoons white miso

1 tablespoon white wine

½ teaspoon turbinado or brown sugar

2 tablespoons white sesame seeds

¼ teaspoon chili powder

Preheat the oven to 425°F.

Place parchment paper on 2 baking sheets. On one sheet put the pumpkin, carrots, and potatoes in a single layer. On the other sheet, put the zucchini and eggplant.

Spray olive oil over the vegetables. Place the pumpkin sheet on the oven's lower rack and the zucchini sheet on the higher rack. Roast for 20 minutes, or until all the vegetables are cooked through and tender.

In the meantime, in a small bowl whisk together the miso, wine, turbinado sugar, sesame seeds, chili powder, and ¼ cup water.

Evenly divide the vegetables among 4 dinner plates. Arrange them beautifully and top with the sauce.

NUTRITION FACTS: 1 SERVING; Caloric Density 0.3; Calories (Kcal) 134; Protein (g) 6; Carbohydrate (g) 29; Total Fat (g) 1; Saturated Fat (g) 0.2; Monounsaturated Fat (g) 0.2; Polyunsaturated Fat (g) 0.5; Dietary Fiber (g) 7.1; Flavonoid and Other Phyto (mg) 8.0; Cholesterol (mg) 0; Sodium (mg) 375; Vitamin A (IU) 32,850; Vitamin C (mg) 36; Calcium (mg) 88; Iron (mg) 2.7; PERCENTAGE (%) Protein 14.7; Carbohydrate 76.3; Fat 7.4; Alcohol 1.6

...bie's New-Style Oven-Roasted Vegetables with Herbs
SERVES 6

Roasted vegetables are simple to prepare and as satisfying as a visit to Grandma's house. This recipe shows how the sweet potato, a traditional Okinawan food, can be adapted for use with spices commonly used in the West. But truly, any vegetable will taste great prepared this way—try new potatoes or winter squash. Water-rich vegetables such as summer squash or mushrooms roast even more quickly and need only about 30 minutes to cook.

3 sweet potatoes, peeled and cut into 1-inch pieces
3 carrots, peeled, halved crosswise, then lengthwise
2 onions, cut into 8 wedges
1 garlic head, separated into cloves and peeled
¼ cup minced fresh rosemary leaves
¼ cup minced fresh thyme leaves
Olive oil spray
Sea salt and freshly ground black pepper

Preheat the oven to 400°F. In a large bowl, toss together the sweet potatoes, carrots, onions, garlic, rosemary, and thyme. Spray once with the olive oil and toss again. Spread the mixture on a large baking sheet and bake, stirring occasionally, for an hour, or until golden and tender. Add salt and pepper to taste, transfer to a platter, and serve.

NUTRITION FACTS: 1 SERVING; Caloric Density 0.6; Calories (Kcal) 138; Protein (g) 3; Carbohydrate (g) 31; Fat (g) <1

Brilliant Vegetarian Chili
SERVES 8

Eating healthily doesn't mean giving up all our favorite dishes. Vegetarian hamburger makes a great-tasting chili, high in protein and flavonoids but low in saturated fat and caloric density. In supermarkets, look for vegetarian hamburger patties in the frozen food or health food sections. Use it as you would regular hamburger, but reduce the cooking time and temperature, as vegetarian burgers cook more quickly.

Canola oil spray
2 cloves garlic, minced
2 cups chopped white onion
4 vegetarian hamburger patties, thawed if frozen and crumbled
½ to 1 teaspoon chili powder
1 teaspoon cumin seeds
1 can (15 ounces) black beans, drained
1 can (15 ounces) pinto beans, drained
1 can (14.5 ounces) low-sodium stewed tomatoes
Pinch of sea salt
Freshly ground black pepper

Spray a large pot with canola oil and heat over medium heat. Cook the garlic and onion for 5 minutes, or until the onion is tender and transparent. Add the hamburger crumbles, chili powder, and cumin seeds and cook for 3 minutes; stir well. Add the beans and tomatoes. Bring to a boil over medium-high heat. Reduce the heat to low and simmer, stirring occasionally, for 20 minutes, or until the mixture thickens. Adjust the seasoning with the salt, pepper, and chili powder.

NUTRITION FACTS: 1 SERVING; Caloric Density 0.7; Calories (Kcal) 168; Protein (g) 13; Carbohydrate (g) 26; Total Fat (g) 2; Saturated Fat (g) 0.1; Monounsaturated Fat (g) 0.4; Polyunsaturated Fat (g) 0.3; Dietary Fiber (g) 8.0; Flavonoid and Other Phyto (mg) 17.9; Cholesterol (mg) 0; Sodium (mg) 549; Vitamin A (IU) 230; Vitamin C (mg) 7; Calcium (mg) 108; Iron (mg) 3.0; PERCENTAGE (%) Protein 30.2; Carbohydrate 61.1; Fat 8.7

Dandelion Spring Rice

SERVES 4

Dandelion gets its name from the French *dent de lion,* meaning "lion's tooth," in reference to the jagged-edged leaves of this bright yellow-flowered "weed" that many of us dig out of our front lawns and discard. But, far from being useless, bright-green dandelion leaves are an excellent source of the antioxidants beta-carotene and vitamin C as well as the minerals iron and calcium. Called dandelion greens, the leaves have a slightly bitter, tangy flavor and add color and texture to salads. They can also be cooked and eaten much like spinach and have been used medicinally in Okinawa to treat stomach ailments.

1½ **cups soybean sprouts**
1½ **tablespoons rice vinegar**
½ **teaspoon chili powder**
½ **tablespoon low-sodium soy sauce**
Pinch of sea salt
Pinch of turbinado or brown sugar

2 **cups dandelion greens, available at large grocery stores and health food stores**
2 **cups cooked brown rice**
Sesame seeds

In a large pot of boiling water, cook the soybean sprouts for 2 minutes, or until crisp-tender. Drain. Squeeze out excess water.

In a large mixing bowl, whisk together the vinegar, chili powder, soy sauce, salt, and sugar.

Add the sprouts and the dandelion greens to the mixing bowl. Toss to coat evenly. Let stand for 5 to 10 minutes.

Toss in the rice. Garnish with sesame seeds.

NUTRITION FACTS: 1 SERVING; Caloric Density 1.0; Calories (Kcal) 159; Protein (g) 7; Carbohydrate (g) 29; Total Fat (g) 3; Saturated Fat (g) 0.5; Monounsaturated Fat (g) 0.7; Polyunsaturated Fat (g) 1.4; Dietary Fiber (g) 3.1; Flavonoid and Other Phyto (mg) 9.8; Cholesterol (mg) 0; Sodium (mg) 172; Vitamin A (IU) 3966; Vitamin C (mg) 14; Calcium (mg) 81; Iron (mg) 2.0; PERCENTAGE (%) Protein 15.9; Carbohydrate 68.9; Fat 15.2

Ogimi Village Sweet Potato Leaf Risotto

SERVES 4

Recipe provided from: "What I found in Grandma's Field [Japanese]," written by Emiko Kinjo, published by Kagawa Education Institute of Nutrition.

Ms. Emiko Kinjo is the owner-chef of a restaurant called Emi's Shop, which she started in 1990. As a dietitian, she worked mostly at hospitals and schools until she finally settled in one of the longevity villages of Okinawa called Ogimi, where her husband hails from. Just steps away from cheerful grandmas and grandpas, Emi-san uses vegetables freshly harvested from their fields. Emi-san says, "I never forget to tell our grandmas and grandpas that they are the village's treasures—and that learning and adopting their healing ways is my goal."

½ cup diced sweet potato
2 dried shiitake mushrooms
2⅔ cups bonito or kelp broth (see
    page 229)
⅓ cup julienned carrot
1¾ cups cooked brown rice
4 cups chopped sweet potato leaves or
    spinach

1 tablespoon white miso
1 tablespoon low-sodium soy sauce
2½ tablespoons kudzu powder or
    2 tablespoons arrowroot powder
1 teaspoon ground turmeric
3 tablespoons water

Steam the sweet potato for 5 to 8 minutes, until firmly cooked through.

In a small mixing bowl of water, soak the dried shiitake to rehydrate for 15 minutes or until tender. Drain and slice thinly.

In a medium pot, bring the bonito or kelp broth to a boil. Add the shiitake, carrot, and brown rice and bring to a boil, then immediately reduce the heat to low. Stir in the sweet potato leaves and sweet potato. Dissolve the miso using a ladle of liquid from the pot; stir the miso mixture into the pot along with the soy sauce. Cook for 2 to 4 minutes or until the sweet potato leaves are tender.

Dissolve the kudzu powder and turmeric with the 3 tablespoons of water in a small mixing bowl. Stir in the kudzu mixture and stir continuously until liquid is thick. Serve warm.

NUTRITION FACTS: 1 SERVING: Caloric Density 0.5; Calories (Kcal) 166; Protein (g) 5; Carbohydrate (g) 35; Total Fat (g) 1; Saturated Fat (g) 0.2; Monounsaturated Fat (g) 0.3; Polyunsaturated Fat (g) 0.5; Dietary Fiber (g) 3.8; Flavonoid and Other Phyto (mg) 14.4; Cholesterol (mg) 0; Sodium (mg) 329; Vitamin A (IU) 6556; Vitamin C (mg) 9; Calcium (mg) 38; Iron (mg) 1.5; PERCENTAGE (%) Protein 11.1; Carbohydrate 82.3; Fat 6.5

Hearty Bean Stroganoff

SERVES 4

Named after the nineteenth-century Russian diplomat Count Paul Stroganov, stroganoff usually consists of thin slices of beef, onions, and mushrooms, cooked with butter and combined with sour cream. If this sounds like a dish in the caloric density stratosphere, you're right—but using kidney beans, instead of beef, and soy sour cream gives us a much lower-CD meal with little of the cholesterol and saturated fat found in the usual stroganoff. Okra, one of the great low-cal vegetables, is high in folate, calcium, and potassium and also is a rich source of the antioxidant vitamins A and C.

Canola oil spray
2 cloves garlic, minced
1 cup sliced yellow onion
2 cups low-sodium vegetable broth
¼ cup red wine
1 can (15 ounces) drained red kidney
   beans, half whole, half mashed
2 teaspoons dried thyme
1 teaspoon dried rosemary

1 teaspoon dried tarragon
2 dried bay leaves
Freshly ground black pepper
1 tablespoon low-sodium soy sauce
2 tablespoons kudzu powder or
   1½ tablespoons arrowroot powder
2 cups sliced okra
½ cup soy sour cream or nonfat sour
   cream

Spray a large pot with canola oil. Cook the garlic and onion over medium heat for 5 minutes, or until the onion is tender and half transparent.

Add the broth and wine; increase the heat to medium-high and slowly bring to a boil.

Add the beans, thyme, rosemary, tarragon, bay leaves, black pepper, and soy sauce. Bring to a boil. Immediately reduce the heat to low and simmer for 10 to 15 minutes, or until the liquid is reduced by one-quarter.

Combine the kudzu powder and 2 tablespoons water. Mix well to dissolve. Stir in the kudzu mixture, okra, and sour cream and cook for 2 more minutes, stirring continuously, until the liquid is thickened. Serve over brown rice, combined with cooked whole-wheat macaroni and baked in the oven, or over whole-grain noodles.

NUTRITION FACTS: 1 SERVING; Caloric Density 0.5; Calories (Kcal) 184; Protein (g) 8; Carbohydrate (g) 34; Total Fat (g) <1; Saturated Fat (g) 0.1; Monounsaturated Fat (g) 0.1; Polyunsaturated Fat (g) 0.3; Dietary Fiber (g) 7.2; Flavonoid and Other Phyto (mg) 26.2; Cholesterol (mg) 1; Sodium (mg) 640; Vitamin A (IU) 1744; Vitamin C (mg) 18; Calcium (mg) 131; Iron (mg) 3.0; PERCENTAGE (%) Protein 18.3; Carbohydrate 73.6; Fat 2.9; Alcohol 5.2

Goya Sushi Roll

SERVES 4

Sushi, of course, is one of most popular Japanese foods. Now you can make your own. Simple sushi rolls are the easiest kind to make—just place whatever you want on top of a sheet of seaweed and roll it up with rice. This Okinawan sushi roll uses the wonderfully healthy Okinawan vegetable bitter melon. To make this or other rolled sushi, you'll need a special rolling tool called a *makisu*, which is a thin, square-shaped bamboo rolling mat about 4 × 4 inches. It makes rolling up the sushi easier than you'd ever imagine and is available at most Asian food stores and kitchenware stores. Have fun!

1 cup peeled, seeded, thinly sliced bitter melon	**12 baby carrots, cooked in the microwave on high for 3 minutes**
½ teaspoon sea salt	**½ avocado, peeled and pitted, sliced**
4 sheets of nori laver seaweed	**1 tablespoon white sesame seed**
2 cups cooked short-grain brown rice	**4 teaspoons low-sodium soy sauce**
	Wasabi (Japanese horseradish paste)

In a bowl, sprinkle the bitter melon with the salt. Rub and press with your hands to soften. When the bitter melon is tender, transfer it to a colander and rinse off the salt under running water. Squeeze off excess water.

Place a *makisu* bamboo rolling mat on the counter. Place 1 nori sheet on the mat. Evenly spread ½ cup rice on the sheet, leaving a 1½-inch-wide space on the edge away from you. Over the rice, lay out a quarter of the bitter melon, 3 carrots, and a quarter of the avocado in lines from left to right.

Roll the mat and the ingredients, holding the ingredients in place; do not roll in the mat. Repeat steps with the remaining sheets and fillings.

Cut each roll into 8 portions and arrange on serving plates. Serve with 1 teaspoon soy sauce per serving and wasabi on the side.

NUTRITION FACTS: 1 SERVING; Caloric Density 0.9; Calories (Kcal) 195; Protein (g) 5; Carbohydrate (g) 33; Total Fat (g) 5; Saturated Fat (g) 1.0; Monounsaturated Fat (g) 2.6; Polyunsaturated Fat (g) 1.4; Dietary Fiber (g) 6.5; Flavonoid and Other Phyto (mg) 0.0; Cholesterol (mg) 1; Sodium (mg) 218; Vitamin A (IU) 9180; Vitamin C (mg) 28; Calcium (mg) 61; Iron (mg) 1.7; PERCENTAGE (%) Protein 10.4; Carbohydrate 65.1; Fat 24.5

Fresh Garden Quiche

SERVES 4

Quiche is ideal for lunch, and our healthier version, made with heart-healthy omega-3 eggs, flavonoid-rich tofu, and a veritable storehouse of healing herbs and spices, will easily see you through until dinnertime. Soy cheese is a great substitute for regular cheese because it's similar in texture but cholesterol-free and lower in fat than cheese from dairy sources. For those who wish to avoid all milk products, check the label on soy cheeses carefully, as most contain some milk protein. Vegan varieties, though, are available at health food stores, and in the health food sections of most regular supermarkets.

7 ounces water-packed silken light tofu
1 free-range, omega-3 egg (optional; if using egg, reduce tofu to 3 ounces)
¼ cup low-sodium vegetable broth
⅓ teaspoon dried basil
⅓ teaspoon dried oregano
⅓ teaspoon dried rosemary
½ teaspoon low-sodium soy sauce
Freshly ground black pepper
Canola oil spray
1 clove garlic, minced
1½ cups quartered white mushrooms

2 cups cooked brown rice
4 cups chopped spinach
1 cup diced tomato
Pinch of sea salt
½ cup shredded soy mozzarella cheese

TOPPING (OPTIONAL)
⅓ cup bread crumbs
2 tablespoons finely chopped fresh parsley
2 tablespoons grated soy Parmesan cheese or dairy Parmesan cheese

Preheat the oven to 375°F.

In a blender, process the tofu, egg, broth, basil, oregano, rosemary, soy sauce, and pepper until smooth.

Spray a large skillet with canola oil and cook the garlic over medium heat for 45 seconds to 1 minute, or until golden. Increase the heat to medium-high. Add the mushrooms and brown rice to the skillet and cook for 2 minutes. Add the spinach, tomato, salt, and pepper to taste and cook for 2 minutes, or until the spinach is tender.

Transfer the rice mixture to a 9-inch pie plate and pour the tofu mixture over the rice. Bake for 15 minutes. Top with soy mozzarella cheese and optional bread crumb mixture and bake for 2 more minutes, or until the cheese is melted and the bread crumbs are golden brown.

Allow to cool for 10 minutes and serve.

NUTRITION FACTS: 1 SERVING; Caloric Density 0.7; Calories (Kcal) 199; Protein (g) 11; Carbohydrate (g) 30; Total Fat (g) 4; Saturated Fat (g) 0.9; Monounsaturated Fat (g) 1.3; Polyunsaturated Fat (g) 1.3; Dietary Fiber (g) 3.6; Flavonoid and Other Phyto (mg) 10.2; Cholesterol (mg) 53; Sodium (mg) 173; Vitamin A (IU) 2636; Vitamin C (mg) 18; Calcium (mg) 276; Iron (mg) 2.7; PERCENTAGE (%) Protein 22.0; Carbohydrate 60.1; Fat 17.9

Painted Bean Casserole

SERVES 8

Pinto means "painted" in Spanish, and pinto beans are so called because of the streaks of reddish brown that appear brushed on the beige bean. Grown in the southwestern United States, they're a popular item in many Spanish dishes, and because they're such a good source of protein, calcium, and iron, they're a staple in many parts of the world where animal protein is scarce. Here they make for a healthy, tasty, and filling casserole.

Canola oil spray
2 cloves garlic, minced
1½ cups sliced white onion
9 ounces low-fat meat substitute or
   crumbled veggie burger
2 15-ounce cans pinto beans, drained
1 can (14.5 ounces) low-sodium stewed
   tomatoes with liquid

½ cup finely chopped green bell pepper
½ teaspoon dried oregano
1 dried bay leaf
Pinch of sea salt
Freshly ground black pepper
1 cup cooked whole-wheat macaroni
½ cup shredded soy cheese

Preheat the oven to 350°F.

Spray a large pot with canola oil. Cook the garlic and onion over medium heat for 5 minutes, or until the onion is tender and transparent. Stir frequently.

Add the meat substitute and cook for 4 minutes. Add the pinto beans, the tomatoes with their liquid, and the bell pepper, oregano, bay leaf, salt, and pepper. Bring to a boil over medium-high heat. Stir in the macaroni.

Transfer the mixture to a large baking pan, top with soy cheese, and bake for 10 minutes. Remove the bay leaf before serving.

NUTRITION FACTS: 1 SERVING; Caloric Density 0.8; Calories (Kcal) 203; Protein (g) 14; Carbohydrate (g) 32; Total Fat (g) 3; Saturated Fat (g) 0.5; Monounsaturated Fat (g) 0.7; Polyunsaturated Fat (g) 0.5; Dietary Fiber (g) 9.0; Flavonoid and Other Phyto (mg) 14.0; Cholesterol (mg) 0; Sodium (mg) 567; Vitamin A (IU) 352; Vitamin C (mg) 15; Calcium (mg) 153; Iron (mg) 3.2; PERCENTAGE (%) Protein 26.7; Carbohydrate 62.4; Fat 10.9

Hijiki Brown Rice

SERVES 4

Hijiki is a mineral-rich, high-fiber seaweed that looks like thin, black, needle-shaped short noodles. It contains about 20 percent protein and is very high in calcium (approximately 1400 mg /100 g dry weight). In Japan, hijiki is mostly rehydrated and added to rice, simmered with soybeans and konnyaku, or mixed with tofu to make tofu balls. You'll find it in all health food stores, Asian groceries, and Japanese food stores.

12 medium dried shiitake mushrooms
¼ cup plus 2 tablespoons dried hijiki
**   seaweed**
1 teaspoon canola oil
Several drops of sesame oil
1 tablespoon minced ginger
½ teaspoon red chili flakes (optional)

3 tablespoons low-sodium soy sauce
¼ cup sake rice wine
1 tablespoon mirin sweet rice wine
½ cup frozen edamame green soybeans
2 cups cooked medium-grain brown rice
2 cups arugula, torn

In a large mixing bowl, soak the shiitake mushrooms in plenty of water to rehydrate. Let stand for 15 to 30 minutes, or until tender. Save 1 cup of the soaking water. Slice the shiitake thinly.

In a small mixing bowl, soak the hijiki in plenty of water to rehydrate. Let stand for 10 minutes. Drain and lightly wash.

In a large skillet, heat the canola oil and sesame oil over medium heat. Add the ginger and red chili flakes and cook for 45 seconds to 1 minute, or until the ginger is golden. Add the shiitake and hijiki and cook for 2 minutes, stirring continuously. Add the soy sauce, sake, and mirin and bring to a boil. Reduce the heat to low and cook for 10 minutes. Add the edamame and cook, stirring occasionally, another 8 to 10 minutes, or until the liquid is almost gone.

Place the brown rice in a large mixing bowl and stir in the shiitake mixture and arugula. Toss to mix evenly.

NUTRITION FACTS: 1 SERVING; Caloric Density 1.3; Calories (Kcal) 223; Protein (g) 7; Carbohydrate (g) 39; Total Fat (g) 4; Saturated Fat (g) 0.4; Monounsaturated Fat (g) 1.3; Polyunsaturated Fat (g) 1.3; Dietary Fiber (g) 4.3; Flavonoid and Other Phyto (mg) 9.6; Cholesterol (mg) 0; Sodium (mg) 462; Vitamin A (IU) 296; Vitamin C (mg) 6; Calcium (mg) 62; Iron (mg) 1.7; PERCENTAGE (%) Protein 12.2; Carbohydrate 66.7; Fat 14.1; Alcohol 7.1

Creamed Spinach and Broccoli on Soba

SERVES 4

This interesting blend of East and West combines traditional Japanese noodles and creamed vegetables—worthy contributions from both cultures. Soba, or buckwheat noodles, provide the fiber, and the soymilk and broccoli provide healthy flavonoids. Spinach is also rich in carotenoids and iron. And the combination of colors—the dark brown of the noodles, the white of the soymilk, the green of the spinach and broccoli, and the red of the paprika—turns this dish into a visual delight as well as an incredibly healthy meal.

8 ounces Japanese soba (buckwheat) noodles, dry	1 cup soymilk, plain
	1 tablespoon whole-wheat flour
Canola oil spray	Pinch of sea salt
2 cloves garlic, minced	Freshly ground black pepper
1 shallot, minced	2 cups chopped spinach
3 cups finely chopped broccoli	1 teaspoon ground paprika

Cook the soba noodles as instructed on the package.

Spray a large skillet with canola oil and cook the garlic and shallot over medium heat for 1 minute, or until the shallot is half transparent. Add the broccoli and cook, stirring frequently, for 5 minutes or until thoroughly cooked.

Increase the heat to medium-high and add the soymilk. Cook for 2 minutes, or until just before the liquid boils. Immediately reduce the heat to low. Do not allow the liquid to boil. Stir in the flour, salt, and pepper. Cook for 1 minute, or until the liquid is thickened. Stir in the spinach and cook for 1 minute or until spinach is soft.

Evenly divide the soba noodles among 4 plates. Ladle sauce over the noodles and garnish with paprika.

NUTRITION FACTS: 1 SERVING; Caloric Density 1.2; Calories (Kcal) 248; Protein (g) 13; Carbohydrate (g) 50; Total Fat (g) 2; Saturated Fat (g) 0.3; Monounsaturated Fat (g) 0.4; Polyunsaturated Fat (g) 0.8; Dietary Fiber (g) 6.1; Flavonoid and Other Phyto (mg) 6.2; Cholesterol (mg) 0; Sodium (mg) 556; Vitamin A (IU) 2337; Vitamin C (mg) 67; Calcium (mg) 76; Iron (mg) 3.2; PERCENTAGE (%) Protein 18.9; Carbohydrate 74.4; Fat 6.8

Tomato Broth Soba Noodles

SERVES 4

Buckwheat has played such an important part in Japanese culture that there is no end to the folktales surrounding it. Here's one of our favorites: One chilly winter morning, in the days when plants could still talk, an old man approached a deep river and needed help getting across. He asked a stalk of wheat to carry him over to the other side, but the wheat refused. The old man then asked a stalk of buckwheat, who happily obliged. Because the river was freezing cold and flowing rapidly, the buckwheat's legs became red. When they got to the other side, the old man revealed that he was no ordinary mortal but actually the god of grain! "Buckwheat," he said, "you have done a very kind deed for someone you didn't even know. From now on, I will let you grow under brilliant sunshine in the summertime." Thus, from that day forward, buckwheat grows in the summertime and is harvested by autumn, while ordinary wheat has to endure the winter cold before spring harvest. Enjoy this benevolent noodle.

3 tablespoons dried wakame seaweed	½ cup fresh diced tomato
2½ cups bonito or kelp broth (see page 229)	3 tablespoons low-sodium soy sauce
	2 tablespoons sake rice wine
1-inch-long dried kelp strip (kombu)	1 tablespoon mirin sweet rice wine
3 cups chopped fresh spinach	8 ounces dried soba buckwheat noodles
1 cup canned diced no-salt-added tomato	½ cup chopped green onion

In a large bowl, soak the wakame in water for 10 minutes. Drain.

Warm the broth. Turn off the heat, add the kelp, and let stand for 10 minutes. Bring to a boil. Immediately remove the kelp and cut it into thin strips. Set it aside.

Steam the spinach, tightly covered, and set it aside.

Add the canned tomato and fresh tomato to the broth and bring to a boil. Stir in the soy sauce, sake, and mirin.

Cook the soba noodles as directed on the package. Evenly divide the noodles among 4 deep bowls. Divide the kelp strips, wakame, and green onion among the noodle bowls and pour the broth over all. Serve.

NUTRITION FACTS: 1 SERVING; Caloric Density 0.7; Calories (Kcal) 257; Protein (g) 12; Carbohydrate (g) 54; Total Fat (g) 1; Saturated Fat (g) 0.1; Monounsaturated Fat (g) 0.1; Polyunsaturated Fat (g) 0.3; Dietary Fiber (g) 5.1; Flavonoid and Other Phyto (mg) 2.8; Cholesterol (mg) 0; Sodium (mg) 1076; Vitamin A (IU) 2151; Vitamin C (mg) 18; Calcium (mg) 83; Iron (mg) 3.7; PERCENTAGE (%) Protein 17.5; Carbohydrate 76.7; Fat 2.9; Alcohol 2.9

Baked Sweet Potatoes

SERVES 4

...in Okinawa is as loved and revered as the sweet potato. Hot baked potatoes are sold from roaming trucks outfitted with a flaming oven in the back, and from autumn through spring, the cry of the sweet-potato man is as familiar to Okinawan neighborhoods as the ice cream truck bell is in America. In the old days, this Okinawan lifesaver was eaten root, stems, leaves, and all—especially in the countryside, where people were poor and couldn't afford rice. Even when consuming several pounds of sweet potatoes a day, people remained fit and lean. Indulge yourself with this healthy lightweight.

2 pounds sweet potatoes, peeled and cut into ½-inch slices	**1½ cups soymilk, plain**
Canola oil spray	**½ teaspoon garlic powder**
3 tablespoons tomato paste	**½ teaspoon dried oregano**
	Freshly ground black pepper

Preheat the oven to 375°F.

Layer the sweet potatoes in a canola-sprayed 1-quart baking dish.

In a small bowl, whisk together the tomato paste, soymilk, garlic powder, oregano, and pepper. Pour over the sweet potatoes. Bake for 40 minutes or until thoroughly cooked.

NUTRITION FACTS: 1 SERVING; Caloric Density 0.8; Calories (Kcal) 256; Protein (g) 6; Carbohydrate (g) 54; Total Fat (g) 2; Saturated Fat (g) 0.3; Monounsaturated Fat (g) 0.4; Polyunsaturated Fat (g) 1.1; Dietary Fiber (g) 7.9; Flavonoid and Other Phyto (mg) 1.6; Cholesterol (mg) 0; Sodium (mg) 48; Vitamin A (IU) 41295; Vitamin C (mg) 48; Calcium (mg) 56; Iron (mg) 2.1; PERCENTAGE (%) Protein 9.7; Carbohydrate 81.9; Fat 9.5

Bean and Rice Burritos

SERVES 4

Burritos, standard Mexican fare, are also popular among immigrant Okinawan populations throughout the Spanish-speaking Americas. A burrito is a folded flour tortilla that contains pinto beans that are mashed, then fried in melted lard. Our refried pinto beans and soybeans contain little fat and are loaded with other essential nutrients, including calcium, iron, phosphorus, potassium, and B vitamins—which will keep you in much better shape for dancing the tango.

1 cup cooked brown rice	**1⅓ cups Okinawa-Style Refried Beans (see page 288) or low-fat, low-sodium refried beans**
1 cup low-fat tomato soup	
8 small or 4 large soft whole-grain flour tortillas, fat-free or low-fat, warmed	**2 cups shredded romaine lettuce**
	½ cup chopped yellow onion

In a microwavable container, combine the brown rice and tomato soup. Cook in the microwave at high for 3 to 5 minutes, or until the rice absorbs the tomato soup. Let cool.

Place a tortilla on a flat board. Spread one-eighth of the refried beans on the tortilla, then top with ¼ cup brown rice mixture, ¼ cup lettuce, and 1 tablespoon onion. (Double these amounts if you are using large tortillas.)

Roll up the tortilla, tucking in both sides. With the remaining ingredients, make 7 more burritos.

NUTRITION FACTS: 1 SERVING; 2 SMALL OR 1 LARGE BURRITO(S).; Caloric Density 1.0; Calories (Kcal) 289; Protein (g) 13; Carbohydrate (g) 53; Total Fat (g) 3; Saturated Fat (g) 0.4; Monounsaturated Fat (g) 0.6; Polyunsaturated Fat (g) 1.3; Dietary Fiber (g) 24.9; Flavonoid and Other Phyto (mg) 24.9; Cholesterol (mg) 0; Sodium (mg) 449; Vitamin A (IU) 3269; Vitamin C (mg) 12; Calcium (mg) 113; Iron (mg) 4.2; PERCENTAGE (%) Protein 18.5; Carbohydrate 73.5; Fat 8.0

Edamame Basil Spaghetti

SERVES 4

The soybean first made its way to America in the early 1800s aboard clipper ships from China, which used soybeans as inexpensive ballast. Upon arrival, the beans were thrown overboard. American farmers took the discarded beans and planted them in tillable soil. By 1900, hundreds of farmers in the United States were utilizing the almost effortlessly grown and easily harvested soybeans as a feed crop for cattle. Since that time the soybean has found many new niches, particularly in the vegetable oil industry. In this interesting combination of East and West—edamame and pasta—the fresh green (immature) soybeans take the place of chopped vegetables, and each bite provides a dose of antioxidants and whole-grain fiber at the same time.

1 cup frozen green soybeans (not the ones in pods)
8 ounces dry whole-wheat spaghetti
4 cloves garlic

1 cup fresh basil leaves
1 tablespoon olive oil
Pinch of sea salt

Defrost the soybeans in the microwave. Place them in a large bowl.

Cook the spaghetti according to the directions on the package.

In a food processor, process the garlic, basil, olive oil, salt, and ⅓ cup water until smooth.

Add the spaghetti and basil sauce to the bowl with the soybeans and toss until evenly coated.

NUTRITION FACTS: 1 SERVING; Caloric Density 1.2; Calories (Kcal) 290; Protein (g) 14; Carbohydrate (g) 47; Total Fat (g) 7; Saturated Fat (g) 0.9; Monounsaturated Fat (g) 3.1; Polyunsaturated Fat (g) 2.0; Dietary Fiber (g) 9.3; Flavonoid and Other Phyto (mg) 19.1; Cholesterol (mg) 0; Sodium (mg) 80; Vitamin A (IU) 477; Vitamin C (mg) 10; Calcium (mg) 109; Iron (mg) 3.0; PERCENTAGE (%) Protein 18.2; Carbohydrate 61.3; Fat 20.5

Roasted Tomato Pasta

SERVES 4

Spaghetti was first taken to Japan in 1895 by a Japanese chef who'd studied cooking in Italy, but it didn't become common until more than half a century later and even then was eaten as an afternoon snack more than as a meal. Roasted tomato has a special, dense summer sunshine flavor that can't be beat. By cooking tomatoes with oil, you can absorb the maximum amount of their lycopene, a carotenoid antioxidant associated with lower risk for prostate and breast cancer. This recipe also works as an appetizer when served with thin garlic toast instead of spaghetti.

3 cloves garlic, minced	Freshly ground black pepper
¼ cup finely chopped Italian parsley	1½ pounds ripe red tomatoes, stems
½ teaspoon dried basil	removed, halved horizontally
½ teaspoon dried oregano	8 ounces whole-wheat spaghetti
2 tablespoons olive oil	1 tablespoon balsamic vinegar
Pinch of sea salt	¼ cup finely chopped Italian parsley

Preheat the oven to 375°F.

In a small bowl, combine the garlic, parsley, basil, oregano, olive oil, salt, and pepper; set aside.

Place the tomatoes on a baking sheet, cut side facing up. Pour the olive oil mixture over the tomatoes and bake for 35 minutes, or until starting to brown on top.

Beginning 20 minutes after the tomatoes go in the oven, cook the spaghetti according to the directions on the package.

When the tomatoes are cooked, transfer them to a large bowl and crush. Toss in the balsamic vinegar.

Drain the spaghetti and toss it with the tomato mixture.

Garnish each serving with chopped parsley.

NUTRITION FACTS: 1 SERVING; Caloric Density 0.9; Calories (Kcal) 297; Protein (g) 10; Carbohydrate (g) 51; Total Fat (g) 8; Saturated Fat (g) 1.2; Monounsaturated Fat (g) 5.2; Polyunsaturated Fat (g) 1.2; Dietary Fiber (g) 9.3; Flavonoid and Other Phyto (mg) 0.0; Cholesterol (mg) 0; Sodium (mg) 92; Vitamin A (IU) 1479; Vitamin C (mg) 43; Calcium (mg) 53; Iron (mg) 3.1; PERCENTAGE (%) Protein 12.7; Carbohydrate 64.0; Fat 23.3

Desserts

People everywhere love sweets, and the world's longest-lived people are no exception. Older Okinawans often balance sips of tart jasmine tea with small bites of raw brown cane sugar. As youths, they had little else to satisfy a sweet tooth—there certainly was nowhere near the broad array of sweets available to us today. Treating yourself to a sweet every now and then is an enjoyable part of a healthy lifestyle, particularly if you choose carefully and select a sweet that's not packed with calories. Here are our simple guiding principles for enjoying healthy desserts:

1. **Fruit, fruit, and more fruit!** Fruit is a great low-CD dessert in and of itself and when added to other more traditional desserts, such as puddings and cakes. The more fruit added, the lower the CD of the dessert becomes.

2. **Feel the natural sweet.** In the majority of store-bought desserts, the sugar content is so high that you can't even get a feel for the real taste of the ingredients. Why ruin the delicate natural taste of sweet potatoes or strawberries with too much sugar? Gradually cut back on your sugar use until you retrain your taste buds to be sensitive to subtle sweets.

3. **Bag the butter!** Butter and shortening are loaded with artery-clogging saturated fat. Most margarines are even worse because they are full of trans fatty acids—the nastiest kind of fat around. Substituting canola or olive oil for butter, shortening, or margarine will not only add to your intake of heart-healthy oils, but you may even be surprised at the added flavor.

4. **Go for the soy.** Nowadays, soy substitutes for cream, cheese, yogurt, and milk have progressed to the point that we can use them in the same ways we use dairy. It's a win-win situation: Lower caloric density and cholesterol and saturated fat levels at the same time you increase cancer-fighting flavonoids and heart-healthy omega-3 and monounsaturated fat levels.

Watermelon Fizz

Roasted Summer Peach

Cantaloupe and Grapefruit Sorbet

Darjeeling Pudding

Mugwort Rice Cake (Fuchiba Nantu)

Green Tea Panna Cotta

Okinawan Steamed Bean Cake (Mushi Manju)

Tropical Mango Pudding

Mochi on a Leaf

October Pumpkin Soufflé

Chocolate Chip Cookies

Sweet Potato Mousse with Green Tea Sauce

Fruitful Frozen Yogurt

Tapioca Sweet Potato Dessert

Can't-Be-Easier Chocolate Fruit Pudding

Tofu Key Lime Pie

Sweet Amagashi Beans

Watermelon Fizz

SERVES 6

Instead of serving plain slices of watermelon (which we also love), we highly recommend this refreshing alternative. Watermelon is a very low-CD food (only 0.3), and it also contains lycopene, a carotenoid thought to lower the risk of certain diseases. Enjoy this low-cal, cancer-fighting, cooling dessert on a sultry summer evening.

2 tablespoons turbinado or brown sugar
5 cups watermelon balls, chilled

3 cups lemon-flavored unsweetened carbonated water, chilled
Sprigs of fresh mint leaves

Combine 2 tablespoons water and the turbinado sugar in a small cup and cover it with plastic wrap. Microwave at low for 1 minute and stir to dissolve.

In a large glass bowl or in 6 individual dessert glasses, mix the watermelon balls, carbonated water, and sugar syrup. Float mint leaves on the liquid.

NUTRITION FACTS: 1 SERVING; Caloric Density 0.2; Calories (Kcal) 53; Protein (g) 1; Carbohydrate (g) 12; Total Fat (g) 1; Saturated Fat (g) 0.1; Monounsaturated Fat (g) 0.1; Polyunsaturated Fat (g) 0.2; Dietary Fiber (g) 0.7; Flavonoid and Other Phyto (mg) 0.0; Cholesterol (mg) 0; Sodium (mg) 5; Vitamin A (IU) 482; Vitamin C (mg) 12; Calcium (mg) 31; Iron (mg) 0.3; PERCENTAGE (%) Protein 5.6; Carbohydrate 85.8; Fat 8.6

Roasted Summer Peach

SERVES 4

A peach makes a tasty and versatile dessert ingredient. With its low CD count of 0.4, it's a wonderful base for pies, cobblers, and fruit salads and terrific served fresh, chilled, and sliced. Peaches are a good source of the antioxidant vitamins A and C, and they are high in fiber—particularly pectin, a soluble fiber that helps lower blood cholesterol. This dessert is simple, takes little time to prepare, and is especially yummy when topped with a small scoop of vanilla soy ice cream.

1 tablespoon turbinado or brown sugar
1 teaspoon ground cinnamon

5 medium peaches, peeled and sliced
1 egg white

Preheat the oven to 400°F.

In a small mixing bowl, combine the turbinado sugar and cinnamon.

Place the peach slices on a baking sheet. Brush them with the egg white and sprinkle the sugar mixture on top. Bake for 6 to 8 minutes, or until soft.

NUTRITION FACTS: 1 SERVING; Caloric Density 0.5; Calories (Kcal) 67; Protein (g) 2; Carbohydrate (g) 17; Total Fat (g) <1; Saturated Fat (g) 0.0; Monounsaturated Fat (g) 0.0; Polyunsaturated Fat (g) 0.1; Dietary Fiber (g) 0.0; Flavonoid and Other Phyto (mg) 0.0; Cholesterol (mg) 0; Sodium (mg) 15; Vitamin A (IU) 657; Vitamin C (mg) 8; Calcium (mg) 16; Iron (mg) 0.4; PERCENTAGE (%) Protein 9.5; Carbohydrate 88.9; Fat 1.6

Cantaloupe and Grapefruit Sorbet

SERVES 8

Finish a warm meal with this light, cool dessert. Cantaloupes are high in the antioxidant beta-carotene. Four ounces of cantaloupe also provide about 45 milligrams of vitamin C and 320 milligrams of potassium. When buying cantaloupe, check the stem area for a smooth, slightly sunken scar; this indicates the melon was ripe when picked and will yield its best flavor. Grapefruits are also high in vitamin C, potassium, and several carotenoids, including beta-carotene. Their white pith contains pectin and bioflavonoids, which makes them an excellent antioxidant food as well. Cantaloupe and grapefruit together make for an unbeatable antioxidant sorbet.

1 tablespoon agar-agar powder or 1 envelope gelatin powder, unflavored	4 cups cubed cantaloupe
	1 cup white grapefruit juice with pulp
3 tablespoons turbinado or brown sugar	2 tablespoons honey

Warm ½ cup water in the microwave on low for 1 minute. Stir in the agar-agar powder and turbinado sugar to dissolve.

In a blender, process the cantaloupe, grapefruit juice, and honey until smooth. Add the agar-agar mixture and process again to mix evenly.

Transfer to a baking pan, cover with plastic wrap, and freeze for 1 to 1½ hours, or until solid.

Using a wooden spatula, break the frozen mixture into pieces. Process them in the blender until soft but not melted. Return the mixture to the container and freeze for 1 hour. Repeat this step 2 to 3 times.

NUTRITION FACTS: 1 SERVING, ABOUT ½ cup; Caloric Density 0.5; Calories (Kcal) 72; Protein (g) 2; Carbohydrate (g) 17; Total Fat (g) <1; Saturated Fat (g) 0.1; Monounsaturated Fat (g) 0.0; Polyunsaturated Fat (g) 0.1; Dietary Fiber (g) 0.8; Flavonoid and Other Phyto (mg) 0.0; Cholesterol (mg) 0; Sodium (mg) 11; Vitamin A (IU) 2581; Vitamin C (mg) 43; Calcium (mg) 15; Iron (mg) 0.3; PERCENTAGE (%) Protein 8.4; Carbohydrate 88.7; Fat 3.0

Darjeeling Pudding
8 RAMEKINS OR 1 9-INCH PIE PAN

Agar-agar, called *kanten* in Japanese, is made of agar-agar seaweed (*Gracilaria*) and comes flaked, powdered, and in solid bars. Available in health food stores, powdered agar-agar is the easiest to prepare—use it just like gelatin. Gelatin is made of animal bones, cartilage, tendons, and skin, so agar-agar is a great solution for vegetarian jelly desserts. In Japan, agar-agar is also used to make a traditional summer snack food called *tokoro-ten*.

2 tablespoons black tea leaves, such as Darjeeling, Ceylon, or Earl Grey	2½ cups soymilk, plain
1½ tablespoons agar-agar powder or 1½ envelopes gelatin powder, unflavored	¼ cup turbinado or brown sugar
	1 vanilla bean, split vertically in half, or 1 teaspoon vanilla extract
	2 tablespoons amaretto liqueur

Place the tea leaves and ½ cup water in a microwavable cup and microwave at high for 3 minutes. Let stand for 5 minutes. Strain and place the infusion in a medium pot.

Add the agar-agar and 1 cup water. Cook over low heat, stirring frequently, for 5 minutes, or until thickened.

Stir in the soymilk and turbinado sugar. Scoop out the seeds from the vanilla bean and add together with the pod. Cook over medium heat for 6 to 8 minutes, or until the liquid starts bubbling. Stir continuously to avoid burning. Turn off the heat.

Add the amaretto to the thickened tea mixture and stir well to dissolve. Strain with a fine strainer into a medium mixing bowl. Let cool.

Transfer the cooled mixture into 8 ramekins (about ⅓ cup each), cover, and refrigerate for 1 to 2 hours or until set.

Optional: Spoon 1 teaspoon caramel sauce on top and serve.

CARAMEL SAUCE
½ cup turbinado or brown sugar   4 tablespoons bubble-boiling water

In a small saucepan, combine the turbinado sugar and 3 tablespoons water and cook over low heat.

When the liquid starts bubbling, shake the saucepan continuously for 1 minute, or until the liquid is golden brown. Do not stir. Immediately remove from the heat and add the bubble-boiling water. Shake the pan to distribute the water evenly.

NUTRITION FACTS: 1 SERVING, 1 RAMEKIN OR ⅛ pie pan; Caloric Density 0.6; Calories (Kcal) 90; Protein (g) 3; Carbohydrate (g) 15; Total Fat (g) 1; Saturated Fat (g) 0.2; Monounsaturated Fat (g) 0.2; Polyunsaturated Fat (g) 0.6; Dietary Fiber (g) 1.0; Flavonoid and Other Phyto (mg) 2.0; Cholesterol (mg) 0; Sodium (mg) 17; Vitamin A (IU) 24; Vitamin C (mg) 0; Calcium (mg) 17; Iron (mg) 0.7; PERCENTAGE (%) Protein 12.0; Carbohydrate 65.6; Fat 13.7; Alcohol 8.6

Mugwort Rice Cake (Fuchiba Nantu)

SERVES 12

Recipe from *Okinawan Mixed Plate: Generous Servings of Culture, Customs and Cuisine,* published by Hui O. Laulima, August 2000. To order, call Bobbi Kuba at (808) 523-5858 or e-mail to: emkuba@yahoo.com / thelma@hawaii.rr.com

This traditional mugwort cake is an Okinawan New Year favorite, said to bring health and good fortune. *Nantu* is an Okinawan version of *mochi* (Japanese sticky rice cake) and tastes almost the same. The real difference is that Japanese mochi is made by pounding cooked rice with a huge wooden mallet, while Okinawan nantu is made by combining rice flour with water, then steaming—a much easier technique that results in lower caloric density.

⅓ cup fresh mugwort leaf, chrysanthemum leaf, or dandelion greens, or similar leaves

1⅓ cups glutinous rice flour (available at many Asian food stores, also called mochi-ko)

½ cup turbinado or brown sugar

Pinch of sea salt

2 tablespoons potato starch or all-purpose unbleached flour

Place the mugwort and 1 cup water in a blender and process until blended.

In a large mixing bowl, place the rice flour, turbinado sugar, and salt and mix well. Add the mugwort mixture and stir with a wooden spoon.

Line a steamer with a wet cloth or cheesecloth (folded over twice). The cloth should drape over the steamer's edge. Pour the mugwort mixture onto the cloth, smooth it out, and fold the cloth over to cover the mixture.

Steam, tightly covered, for 45 to 50 minutes, or until set.

Sprinkle the work surface with the potato starch. Turn out the mugwort mixture onto the potato starch. Let cool. Slice into 1 × 2 × ½-inch pieces. Dredge each slice in the starch. Serve with jasmine or green tea.

NUTRITION FACTS: 1 SERVING; Caloric Density 1.9; Calories (Kcal) 91; Protein (g) 1; Carbohydrate (g) 22; Total Fat (g) <1; Saturated Fat (g) 0.0; Monounsaturated Fat (g) 0.0; Polyunsaturated Fat (g) 0.0; Dietary Fiber (g) <1; Flavonoid and Other Phyto (mg) 30; Cholesterol (mg) 0; Sodium (mg) 30; Vitamin A (IU) 43; Vitamin C (mg) <1; Calcium (mg) 11; Iron (mg) 0.4; PERCENTAGE (%) Protein 5.3; Carbohydrate 93.0; Fat 1.7

Green Tea Panna Cotta

8 RAMEKINS OR 1 9-INCH PIE PAN

Panna cotta is an Italian dessert; the name means "cooked cream." It resembles a cream pudding but is thicker, smoother, and richer than most other puddings. Panna cotta has recently become trendy in Japan, and many restaurant chefs have been competing to make their own original panna cottas the best. We think we've come up with the winner. Our unique recipe uses green tea powder, and its deep emerald color is beautiful when the panna cotta is served in glass or white ceramic dessert bowls—and, of course, the taste is superb, too.

1½ cups half-and-half or cream substitute
1 cup soymilk, plain
⅓ cup turbinado or brown sugar
1 vanilla bean, split vertically in half, or 1 teaspoon vanilla extract
¼ cup boiling water

2 tablespoons green tea powder (matcha), unsweetened
1 cup cold water
1 tablespoon agar-agar powder or 1 envelope gelatin powder, unflavored
2 tablespoons white rum

In a large pot, combine the half-and-half, soymilk, and turbinado sugar. Scoop out the seeds from the vanilla bean and add both seeds and pod to the milk mixture. Cook over medium heat, continuously stirring to avoid burning, for 8 minutes, or until the milk starts steaming. Do not allow to boil.

In the meantime, whisk together the boiling water and green tea powder in a medium mixing bowl.

In a separate, small mixing bowl, whisk together the cold water and the agar-agar powder.

Transfer the milk mixture to the bowl containing the green tea. Whisk together. Whisk in the agar-agar mixture and the rum.

Fill a large bowl with cold water and plenty of ice. Place the bowl containing the green tea mixture on top. Be careful not to let the water flow into the green tea mixture. Allow to cool for about 10 minutes, then refrigerate for 30 to 45 minutes, or until the mixture becomes thick. Stir to make sure the green tea powder is distributed evenly.

Transfer the mixture to 8 ramekins, cover with plastic wrap, and refrigerate again for 1 to 1½ hours, or until it has the desired consistency.

NUTRITION FACTS: 1 SERVING, 1 RAMEKIN OR ⅛ pie pan; Caloric Density 0.8; Calories (Kcal) 97; Protein (g) 3; Carbohydrate (g) 9; Total Fat (g) 5; Saturated Fat (g) 2.8; Monounsaturated Fat (g) 1.4; Polyunsaturated Fat (g) 0.4; Dietary Fiber (g) 1.9; Flavonoid and Other Phyto (mg) 0.7; Cholesterol (mg) 14; Sodium (mg) 27; Vitamin A (IU) 778; Vitamin C (mg) 3; Calcium (mg) 71; Iron (mg) 1.0, PERCENTAGE (%) Protein 11.6; Carbohydrate 35.0; Fat 45.2; Alcohol 8.1

Okinawan Steamed Bean Cake (Mushi Manju)

MAKES 16

Recipe provided from: *Okinawan Mixed Plate: Generous Servings of Culture, Customs and Cuisine*, published by Hui O. Laulima, August 2000. To order, call Bobbi Kuba at (808) 523-5858 or e-mail to: emkuba@yahoo.com / thelma@hawaii.rr.com

Fiber-rich adzuki beans have long been enjoyed in Japan and Okinawa. Because their bright red color symbolizes good fortune in the Okinawan culture, "adzuki rice" (white rice tinged pink by the beans) is served at weddings, baby showers, birthdays, and other celebratory occasions. Adzuki beans slow-cooked with sugar make one of the oldest and most revered sweets of Okinawa. The dish is very low in calories because it is steamed rather than baked with oil, which makes it water-rich rather than fat-rich—a real plus.

1 cup whole-wheat flour	**2 egg whites**
1 cup all-purpose unbleached flour	**⅓ cup soymilk, plain**
½ cup turbinado or brown sugar	**½ cup adzuki bean paste (also called**
1 tablespoon baking powder	**tsubushi-an or koshi-an) or**
1 tablespoon canola oil	**low-sodium smooth peanut butter**

In a large mixing bowl, combine both flours, the sugar, and the baking powder.

In a medium mixing bowl, beat together the canola oil, egg whites, and soymilk. Pour this mixture over the dry ingredients and mix well with a wooden spoon. Divide into 16 portions, each the size of a golf ball.

Line a steamer with wet cheesecloth. Make 16 wax paper pieces, each 2 inches square. Divide the adzuki bean paste into 16 portions.

In the palm of your hand, flatten the dough into a 3-inch round. Place a portion of adzuki bean paste in the center and pinch the edges together to seal. Place on a wax paper square. Repeat this step to make 15 more balls.

Steam the balls, tightly covered, for 12 minutes, or until the dough is set.

NUTRITION FACTS: 1 SERVING, 1 PIECE; Caloric Density 2.6; Calories (Kcal) 105; Protein (g) 2.7; Carbohydrate (g) 21; Total Fat (g) 1; Saturated Fat (g) 0.1; Monounsaturated Fat (g) 0.5; Polyunsaturated Fat (g) 0.4; Dietary Fiber (g) 1.2; Flavonoid and Other Phyto (mg) 0.1; Cholesterol (mg) 0; Sodium (mg) 98; Vitamin A (IU) 2; Vitamin C (mg) 0; Calcium (mg) 73; Iron (mg) 1.0; PERCENTAGE (%) Protein 10.3; Carbohydrate 80.0; Fat 9.8

Tropical Mango Pudding

SERVES 4

The tropical scent and deep orange-red color of mangos always reminds us of the hot Okinawan summer sun. Like other orange or deep yellow fruits, mangos are exceptionally high in beta-carotene. They are also a good source of vitamin C, vitamin E, iron, and potassium. Ripe mangos work best for this recipe. You can tell when a mango is ripe when the skin is orange or red and the flesh gives a little when pressed. For maximum sweetness put the mango in a paper bag and leave it in a cool spot for a couple of days. If a mango is very ripe, use it right away or refrigerate, as mangos turn sour when overripe. This tropical dessert is perfect after a spicy dinner.

3 large mangos, peeled and diced
3 tablespoons half-and-half or cream substitute
1 tablespoon agar-agar powder or 1 envelope gelatin powder, unflavored

2 tablespoons turbinado or brown sugar

Place 2 tablespoons diced mango in each of 4 dessert bowls or ramekins.

Purée the remaining mango and the half-and-half until smooth. Transfer to a mixing bowl.

Warm ½ cup water in a saucepan and add the agar-agar powder and turbinado sugar. Mix well, add to the mango mixture, and mix well again.

Pour the mixture evenly into the mango-lined dessert bowls, about ¾ cup each. Cover with plastic wrap and refrigerate for 45 minutes, or until set.

NUTRITION FACTS: 1 SERVING; Caloric Density 0.7; Calories (Kcal) 134; Protein (g) 1; Carbohydrate (g) 32; Total Fat (g) 2; Saturated Fat (g) 0.3; Monounsaturated Fat (g) 1.0; Polyunsaturated Fat (g) 0.1; Dietary Fiber (g) 2.8; Flavonoid and Other Phyto (mg) 0.0; Cholesterol (mg) 0; Sodium (mg) 15; Vitamin A (IU) 6055; Vitamin C (mg) 43; Calcium (mg) 21; Iron (mg) 0.3; PERCENTAGE (%) Protein 2.5; Carbohydrate 88.1; Fat 9.4

Mochi on a Leaf

SERVES 8

Mochi is a Japanese word for "cake," but this cake is very different from the kind we know in North America. Mochi is a small, round sticky rice cake made from steamed and pounded glutinous rice. It's eaten with condiments, such as *kinako* (roasted soybean flour) or *anko* (sweet red bean paste). Okinawans serve this dessert on a getto leaf (*sannin* in Okinawan), which comes from a plant in the ginger family and has a mild, sweet aroma similar to ginger. They say the leaf is coated with natural bactericidal oil and helps preserve any food wrapped in it. You could try presenting this unusual dessert on a beautiful dark green bamboo leaf, or any other wide, pretty edible leaf that's readily available in your area.

1¼ cups kudzu powder or tapioca starch
⅔ cup turbinado or brown sugar
⅓ cup soy flour

Bamboo leaves or other beautiful edible leaves for decoration, such as leaves from ginger-family plants

Sift the kudzu powder. In a medium pot, place the kudzu powder and turbinado sugar. Slowly add 2½ cups water, stirring continuously. Cook over medium heat until small bubbles rise at the edge. Reduce heat to low and simmer for 15 to 20 minutes, or until the mixture becomes transparent. Keep stirring with a wooden spatula to avoid burning. Remove from the heat.

Sprinkle a 9-inch pie dish (preferably glass) with half the amount of soy flour. Immediately pour in the kudzu mixture. Let cool. Sprinkle with the remaining soy flour and cover with plastic wrap. Refrigerate for 40 minutes to 1 hour.

Slice into 8 wedges. Serve on a plate lined with bamboo leaf.

NUTRITION FACTS: 1 SERVING; Caloric Density 1.2; Calories (Kcal) 138; Protein (g) 2; Carbohydrate (g) 32; Total Fat (g) 1; Saturated Fat (g) 0.1; Monounsaturated Fat (g) 0.2; Polyunsaturated Fat (g) 0.5; Dietary Fiber (g) 1.1; Flavonoid and Other Phyto (mg) 48.4; Cholesterol (mg) 0; Sodium (mg) 8; Vitamin A (IU) 5; Vitamin C (mg) 0; Calcium (mg) 29; Iron (mg) 0.6; PERCENTAGE (%) Protein 4.3; Carbohydrate 90.1; Fat 5.7

October Pumpkin Soufflé

SERVES 8

Free-range, omega-3 eggs are ideal for health-conscious egg lovers. They come from uncaged chickens that are given heart-healthy omega-3 fatty acids in their feed. They pass those healthy eating habits along to you in the form of a great-tasting and healthier egg. Healthy, fit chickens produce a bright orange yolk with a deep taste, in contrast to broiler chickens' eggs, with their lifeless, pale yellow yolk. The pumpkin is packed with nutrition too—its bright orange color tells us it's loaded with the antioxidant beta-carotene. Colorful and healthy—a winning combination!

12 ounces pumpkin, peeled, cored and diced into 1 × 1-inch squares, or 2 cups canned unsweetened pumpkin
3 tablespoons canola oil
2 tablespoons honey
1 teaspoon ground nutmeg
1 cup soymilk, plain
2 free-range, omega-3 eggs, separated, or ½ cup egg substitute
⅓ cup chopped or sliced almonds
⅓ cup raisins

Preheat the oven to 350°F.

Steam the pumpkin, tightly covered, in a steamer for 15 to 18 minutes, or until tender. Mash or process the pumpkin in a food processor. Make 2 cups mashed pumpkin. (Skip this step if using canned pumpkin.)

In a large mixing bowl, whisk together the canola oil, honey, and nutmeg and whisk vigorously until the mixture becomes cloudy. Add the pumpkin, soymilk, and egg yolks (if using whole eggs) and mix.

Beat the egg white (or the egg substitute, if using) until stiff. Fold into the pumpkin mixture along with the almonds and raisins.

Spray a 2-quart baking dish with canola oil and transfer the pumpkin mixture to the dish. Bake for 45 to 60 minutes, or until firm. Serve warm.

NUTRITION FACTS: 1 SERVING; Caloric Density 1.4; Calories (Kcal) 144; Protein (g) 4; Carbohydrate (g) 12; Total Fat (g) 10; Saturated Fat (g) 1.1; Monounsaturated Fat (g) 5.3; Polyunsaturated Fat (g) 2.6; Dietary Fiber (g) 1.5; Flavonoid and Other Phyto (mg) 0.5; Cholesterol (mg) 53; Sodium (mg) 22; Vitamin A (IU) 771; Vitamin C (mg) 4; Calcium (mg) 35; Iron (mg) 1.1; PERCENTAGE (%) Protein 11.0; Carbohydrate 30.9; Fat 58.1

Chocolate Chip Cookies

MAKES 24; SERVES 12

This is an emergency treat for those who *really* need chocolate chip cookies. With heaps of almond butter, tofu, turbinado sugar, and carrot, we've transformed traditional chocolate chip cookies into low-cal healthy ones. Conventional store-bought chocolate chip cookies are about 4.7 to 5.0 on the Caloric Density Index, with some of the healthier ones at 4.0 to 4.3; our chocolate chip cookies are only 2.7. But just because we've halved the usual caloric density of chocolate chip cookies doesn't mean you can eat twice as many. Enjoy— in moderation.

⅓ cup almond butter, crunchy or smooth
4½ ounces water-packed silken light tofu
3 tablespoons soymilk, plain
1 cup turbinado or brown sugar
1 teaspoon vanilla extract
⅔ cup whole-wheat flour

½ teaspoon sea salt
1 teaspoon baking powder
⅔ cup rolled oats
⅓ cup shredded carrot
⅓ cup chocolate chips, preferably dairy-free
Canola oil spray

Preheat the oven to 375°F.

In a blender, process the almond butter, tofu, soymilk, turbinado sugar, and vanilla until smooth.

In a large bowl, mix together the flour, salt, baking powder, and rolled oats.

Transfer the tofu mixture to a large mixing bowl. Add the flour mixture, the carrots, and the chocolate chips. Combine with a wooden spoon. Do not overmix.

Spray a baking sheet with canola oil. Drop the dough onto the baking sheet by large spoonfuls. Bake for 5 minutes, rotate the sheet front to back, and then bake for another 4 minutes.

Keep the cookies on the baking sheet for 5 minutes before transferring them to a wire rack.

NUTRITION FACTS: 1 SERVING, 2 COOKIES; Caloric Density 2.7; Calories (Kcal) 148; Protein (g) 4; Carbohydrate (g) 29; Total Fat (g) 6; Saturated Fat (g) 1.3; Monounsaturated Fat (g) 3.3; Polyunsaturated Fat (g) 1.2; Dietary Fiber (g) 2.0; Flavonoid and Other Phyto (mg) 2.2; Cholesterol (mg) 0; Sodium (mg) 114; Vitamin A (IU) 114; Vitamin C (mg) 0; Calcium (mg) 92; Iron (mg) 1.0; PERCENTAGE (%) Protein 8.3; Carbohydrate 61.7; Fat 30.0

Sweet Potato Mousse with Green Tea Sauce

SERVES 4

The Okinawan dish called *umunii* is essentially a mashed sweet potato dessert. Made with taro, it's an important ceremonial food appearing in the life-passage celebrations that occur every twelve years, according to the old Chinese zodiac. Plain umunii is served at the forty-ninth and sixty-first birth year celebrations, and rice flour is added for the seventy-third and eighty-fifth birth year celebrations. Umunii is usually garnished with getto leaves (a plant of the ginger family). Our recipe is a Western version of umunii, with a flavonoid-rich green tea sauce.

8½ ounces peeled sweet potato (approximately 1½ cups), cut into 1-inch-thick rounds
1 cup soymilk, plain
2 tablespoons turbinado or brown sugar
1 tablespoon agar-agar powder or 1 envelope gelatin powder, unflavored
1 teaspoon white rum (optional)

SAUCE
5 ounces water-packed silken light tofu
1½ tablespoons tahini paste
½ teaspoon green tea powder
1 tablespoon honey or desired substitute
¼ teaspoon vanilla extract

Steam the sweet potatoes, tightly covered, for 15 to 18 minutes, or until tender, or cook in the microwave on high for 6 minutes.

In the meantime, warm the soymilk. Do not allow it to boil. Stir in the sugar, agar-agar, and rum.

In a food processor, process the sweet potatoes and soymilk mixture until smooth. Transfer to 4 ramekins or other desired container. Refrigerate for 1 hour, or until set.

In a food processor, process the tofu, tahini, green tea powder, honey, and vanilla until smooth.

Serve the mousse chilled and garnished with the sauce.

NUTRITION FACTS: 1 SERVING; Caloric Density 0.9; Calories (Kcal) 162; Protein (g) 7; Carbohydrate (g) 24; Total Fat (g) 4; Saturated Fat (g) 0.5; Monounsaturated Fat (g) 1.2; Polyunsaturated Fat (g) 1.8; Dietary Fiber (g) 3.4; Flavonoid and Other Phyto (mg) 8.4; Cholesterol (mg) 0; Sodium (mg) 50; Vitamin A (IU) 12,793; Vitamin C (mg) 14; Calcium (mg) 165; Iron (mg) 1.4; PERCENTAGE (%) Protein 16.9; Carbohydrate 57.7; Fat 23.7; Alcohol 1.6

Fruitful Frozen Yogurt

SERVES 4

The combination of strawberries and bananas with yogurt is a natural. You can give it an interesting twist by adding tiny baby bananas, monkey bananas, or apple bananas. The skin is usually a little darker in these bananas than the regular kind, and they smell of island mornings when peeled. This type of banana is called *shima banana* in Okinawa, which means "island banana"; in Indonesia, they're called *pisang susu*—"milky banana"—which nicely describes their taste.

⅔ cup strawberries or a combination of several berries, frozen overnight
1½ cups soy yogurt, plain
2 teaspoons turbinado or brown sugar

⅔ cup chopped banana, frozen overnight
½ cup low-fat granola
Fresh mint leaves (optional)

In a blender, process the berries, ⅔ cup soy yogurt, and 1 teaspoon of the turbinado sugar until smooth. Set aside in the refrigerator.

Rinse the blender container with water and process the banana and the remaining soy yogurt and turbinado sugar until smooth.

Place 2 tablespoons of granola in the bottom of 4 dessert glasses. Top with 3 tablespoons banana yogurt. Layer with 3 tablespoons berry yogurt. Repeat with 2 tablespoons berry and banana yogurt each and garnish with small mint leaves.

NUTRITION FACTS: 1 SERVING; Caloric Density 0.9; Calories (Kcal) 150; Protein (g) 4; Carbohydrate (g) 30; Total Fat (g) 2; Saturated Fat (g) 0.2; Monounsaturated Fat (g) 0.2; Polyunsaturated Fat (g) 0.6; Dietary Fiber (g) 2.5; Flavonoid and Other Phyto (mg) 2.6; Cholesterol (mg) 0; Sodium (mg) 47; Vitamin A (IU) 225; Vitamin C (mg) 19; Calcium (mg) 295; Iron (mg) 1.2; PERCENTAGE (%) Protein 9.0; Carbohydrate 77.0; Fat 14.0

Tapioca Sweet Potato Dessert

SERVES 4

Almost any sweet potato will work in this recipe, although the ones with firmer flesh are best. As always, we recommend the purple sweet potatoes with white skin, if you can find them. You could also substitute the same amount of fresh pumpkin or 5 ounces unsweetened canned pumpkin. Not surprisingly, this dessert is hugely popular in Hawaii, where there's a large population of Okinawan immigrants.

⅓ cup dry small tapioca pearls
1 pound sweet potatoes
1 cup water

1 cup light soymilk, vanilla-flavored
1 tablespoon turbinado or brown sugar
Fresh mint leaves

In a large saucepan, bring plenty of water to a boil and add the tapioca pearls. Boil, stirring occasionally, for 7 to 10 minutes, or until the pearls are transparent.

In the meantime, wrap the sweet potatoes with paper towel, then with plastic wrap. Microwave at high for 5 to 7 minutes, or until cooked. Peel and dice.

In a blender, process two-thirds of the sweet potato, the water, soymilk, and turbinado sugar until smooth.

In a large mixing bowl, combine the remaining diced sweet potato, tapioca pearls, and sweet potato mixture. Chill for 30 minutes, or until the liquid is thickened a little. Garnish with mint leaves.

NUTRITION FACTS: 1 SERVING; Caloric Density 1.0; Calories (Kcal) 193; Protein (g) 4; Carbohydrate (g) 42; Total Fat (g) 2; Saturated Fat (g) 0.2; Monounsaturated Fat (g) 0.2; Polyunsaturated Fat (g) 0.7; Dietary Fiber (g) 4.3; Flavonoid and Other Phyto (mg) 1.0; Cholesterol (mg) 0; Sodium (mg) 23; Vitamin A (IU) 22,770; Vitamin C (mg) 26; Calcium (mg) 32; Iron (mg) 1.3; PERCENTAGE (%) Protein 7.2; Carbohydrate 85.9; Fat 6.8

Can't-Be-Easier Chocolate Fruit Pudding

SERVES 4

This elegant chocolate dessert is wonderful when served with bananas and raspberries. The addition of fruit lowers the caloric density and ups the flavor and nutrients. Chocolate aficionados will find this low-fat chocolate fruit pudding rich and satisfying, and the lovely sheen on the pudding provides a nice bonus for the visual sense—especially when garnished with a sprig of mint. This dessert works equally well with Grand Marnier, Kahlúa, or rum. Teetotalers, just skip all three.

1 packet (1 ounce) instant fat-free, sugar-free, reduced-calorie chocolate pudding mix	2 cups cold soymilk, plain
	1 tablespoon white rum (optional)
	2 ripe bananas, diced
3 tablespoons unsweetened cocoa powder	1 cup raspberries

Combine the pudding mix and cocoa powder. Prepare the pudding, following directions on the package, substituting the soymilk for dairy milk. Stir in the rum.

In each of 4 dessert cups, spoon in ¼ cup pudding. Evenly divide the banana over the pudding. Cover the banana with the remaining pudding, about ¼ cup per serving. Top with ¼ cup raspberries per serving. Chill and serve.

NUTRITION FACTS: 1 SERVING; Caloric Density 0.7; Calories (Kcal) 158; Protein (g) 4; Carbohydrate (g) 34; Total Fat (g) 2; Saturated Fat (g) 0.7; Monounsaturated Fat (g) 0.5; Polyunsaturated Fat (g) 0.7; Dietary Fiber (g) 5.0; Flavonoid and Other Phyto (mg) 5.2; Cholesterol (mg) 0; Sodium (mg) 226; Vitamin A (IU) 89; Vitamin C (mg) 13; Calcium (mg) 25; Iron (mg) 1.4; PERCENTAGE (%) Protein 8.1; Carbohydrate 76.1; Fat 11.2; Alcohol 4.6

Tofu Key Lime Pie

SERVES 8

Key lime pie is the quintessential American dessert—wickedly delicious but loaded with calories. Try our healthier version, made with phytoestrogen-rich tofu and heart-healthy omega-3 eggs instead of heavy cream laden with saturated fat and high-cholesterol conventional eggs. Your taste buds will never know the difference, but the rest of your body will surely appreciate it!

8 ounces soy cream cheese or low-fat cream cheese

8 ounces water-packed silken light tofu

⅓ cup Key lime juice

1 tablespoon grated lime zest

¼ cup turbinado or brown sugar

1 free-range, omega-3 egg or ¼ cup egg substitute or egg white

½ teaspoon vanilla extract

2 tablespoons cornstarch

1 9-inch graham cracker pie crust

8 thin lime slices

Preheat the oven to 350°F.

In a blender, process the cream cheese, tofu, lime juice, lime zest, turbinado sugar, egg, vanilla, and cornstarch until smooth. Pour the mixture into the pie crust.

Bake for 40 minutes, or until a toothpick inserted in the center comes out clean. Refrigerate. Serve chilled, garnished with the lime slices.

NUTRITION FACTS: 1 SERVING; Caloric Density 2.5; Calories (Kcal) 197; Protein (g) 3; Carbohydrate (g) 17; Total Fat (g) 13; Saturated Fat (g) 2.8; Monounsaturated Fat (g) 2.4; Polyunsaturated Fat (g) 7.7; Dietary Fiber (g) 0.5; Flavonoid and Other Phyto (mg) 5.0; Cholesterol (mg) 27; Sodium (mg) 240; Vitamin A (IU) 42; Vitamin C (mg) 6; Calcium (mg) 14; Iron (mg) 0.6; PERCENTAGE (%) Protein 5.1; Carbohydrate 34.6; Fat 60.4

Sweet Amagashi Beans

SERVES 4

On a hot and sleepy afternoon in the Okinawan islands, people seek shade in a corner café to enjoy an *ammaa's* (mother's) recipe of chilled *amagashi* with crushed ice. It's a true island treat that goes hand in hand with *hari* (dragon-boat racing season) at the beginning of hot weather in May. On the hari festival day, Okinawans eat amagashi with chopsticks made of fresh calamus stalks (a kind of climbing palm) because it is believed that calamus protects people from disease. This treat can also be eaten hot, a nice way to warm up on a cold winter's day.

½ cup dried mung beans
½ cup pearled barley
½ cup turbinado or brown sugar

1 teaspoon ginger juice, squeezed from grated ginger
¼ cup small tapioca pearls

Soak the mung beans and barley in separate bowls with at least 1½ cups water each for 5 to 6 hours or overnight. Drain.

In a large pot, bring 4½ cups water to a boil. Add the beans and barley and cook over medium heat. When the water reaches a slow boil, reduce the heat to low and cook covered for 40 to 60 minutes, or until the beans are tender. Do not allow to boil rapidly. This is to avoid broken beans.

Stir in the turbinado sugar and the ginger juice. Cover, remove from heat, and let stand for 10 minutes.

Cook the tapioca pearls in at least 2 cups boiling water over low heat. When the pearls become clear, drain them in a fine strainer and rinse under cold water.

Serve the beans and tapioca pearls together, chilled or warm, in individual dessert bowls.

NUTRITION FACTS: 1 SERVING; Caloric Density 0.6; Calories (Kcal) 197; Protein (g) 7; Carbohydrate (g) 41; Total Fat (g) 1; Saturated Fat (g) 0.1; Monounsaturated Fat (g) 0.1; Polyunsaturated Fat (g) 0.3; Dietary Fiber (g) 5.0; Flavonoid and Other Phyto (mg) 0.0; Cholesterol (mg) 0; Sodium (mg) 18; Vitamin A (IU) 57; Vitamin C (mg) 0; Calcium (mg) 42; Iron (mg) 2.4; PERCENTAGE (%) Protein 13.8; Carbohydrate 82.9; Fat 3.3

Teas and Snacks

These low-cal snacks and teas are for those times when you feel like having a little something but aren't quite ready for a full meal. They're perfect for grazing between meals, nibbling while preparing dinner, munching while watching TV, or sipping when curled up with a good book.

BEST STEEPING TEAS AND MATCHA

For simple, everyday healthy teas we turn to Okinawa and Japan. The importance of tea in Japanese culture is illustrated by its place in folklore. According to one story, when Okinawan delegates to China returned home they would thank the Ocean God for the safe trip by offering tea. There were so many successful trips and so many tea offerings, that there is now a huge rock on the north shore of Zamami, a small island just off the coast of the main island of Okinawa, which is said to be made entirely of discarded tea leaves from these offerings. The rock is called Ucha-Kashi, literally, "discarded tea leaf."

Jasmine Tea

Green Tea

Matcha

Soy Masala Chai

Tomato Juice Frappé

Apricot-Yogurt Soy Smoothie

Spiced Cranberry Cider

Miso and Dill Dip

Tofu Hummus

Cucumber and Avocado
Hors d'Oeuvre

Snacking Pita Pizza

Spinach Wedges

Orange-Glazed Sesame Carrots

Caramel Sweet Potato Chips

Cajun Hot Popcorn

Hearty Granola

Jasmine Tea

SERVES 4

There are two main kinds of tea: fermented (black tea), and unfermented (green tea). Jasmine tea, the most popular tea in Okinawa, is slightly fermented. It has the freshness of green tea but the wonderful aroma that comes from fermentation. The intoxicating scent of jasmine flowers contributes to this tea's unique aroma and refreshing taste.

1 heaping tablespoon jasmine tea leaves

In a kettle bring at least 2 quarts water to a boil. Fill a teapot and 4 mugs with about 1 cup of the boiling water each to warm. Wait 1 minute and discard the water from the teapot. In the meantime, return the kettle to the stove and maintain a boil over high heat. Place the jasmine tea leaves in the teapot and pour in approximately 4 cups of the boiling water. Steep for 2 minutes. Discard the water from the mugs and pour the tea into each cup, little by little, alternating mugs to make sure each gets the same strength tea.

Approximate flavonoid content: 16.8 milligrams in 1 mug

Green Tea

SERVES 4

In Japan, green tea is usually referred to as *ryoku-cha*—"general green tea"—but several grades are available. *Gyokuro,* literally, "a drop of jewelry," which comes from Shizuoka Prefecture, the major source of good tea, is considered to be the best. Steeped green tea is a beautiful earthy green color and is considered very relaxing. Tea bags are frowned upon (it's thought to compromise the taste of tea), so every household has a special decorative tea can or two for loose-leaf green tea.

4 teaspoons green tea leaves of the best quality available, preferably gyokuro

In a kettle bring 1 quart water (soft water is recommended) to a boil. Fill a teapot and four 6-ounce teacups with boiling water to warm. Wait 30 seconds and discard the water from the teapot. Place the green tea leaves in the teapot. Transfer the water from the teacups to the teapot. Steep for 1 minute. Pour the tea into each teacup, little by little, alternating teacups to make sure each gets the same strength tea.

Approximate flavonoid content: 1 milligram per 1 teacup

Matcha

SERVES 4

Matcha is ground green tea leaf in powder form. While *ryoku-cha* is steeped and its leaves discarded, matcha is combined with hot water and drunk in its entirety. The world-famous Japanese tea ceremony has been practiced with matcha since the fifteenth century. Because of its powdery form, modern Japanese love to use it in various desserts, including puddings, cakes, and cookies. Matcha can be found in some regular supermarkets and most Asian food stores.

KOI-CHA (STRONG GREEN TEA)
3 teaspoons green tea powder (matcha)

In a kettle, bring at least 2 quarts water (soft water recommended) to a boil.

Fill 4 tea bowls, café au lait cups, or teacups and a medium mixing bowl with boiling water to warm. When the mixing bowl is hot, discard the water from it.

Place green tea powder in the bowl with ¼ cup water from the kettle and whisk together. Add 2¾ cups water and whisk vigorously, making small white bubbles on the surface.

Discard the water from the tea bowls and pour the tea.

Approximate flavonoid content: 1 milligram per tea bowl

USU-CHA (WEAK GREEN TEA)
1½ teaspoons green tea powder (matcha)

In a kettle, bring at least 2 quarts water (soft water recommended) to a boil.

Fill 4 tea bowls, café au lait cups, or teacups and a medium mixing bowl with boiling water to warm. When the mixing bowl is hot, discard the water from it.

Place the green tea powder in the bowl, add 3 cups water from the kettle, and whisk vigorously, making bubbles on the surface.

Discard the water from the tea bowls and pour the tea.

Approximate flavonoid content: 0.5 milligram per tea bowl

Soy Masala Chai

SERVES 4

Chai, though sometimes thought of as a complicated mysterious mixture of exotic ingredients, is essentially tea. But different cultures add their own touch to the globally popular beverage. This recipe most closely resembles the chai of India and incorporates some of the amazing spices that were brought to Japan by enterprising Okinawan merchants in the ancient days of the Ryukyu Kingdom. Its primary spice is cardamom, one of the most common and delightful Indian spices. Cardamom has been used in India for over a millennium as a digestive aid, and the folkloric claims run the gamut from headache and nausea cures to heart stimulant. The incredible flavor and aroma of the spice is hard to describe—all we can say is that it whispers of India in the most wonderful way possible. Once you try this tea, we guarantee you'll be hooked.

2 tablespoons unflavored, fine-cut black tea (note: Earl Grey is flavored)
3 cups soymilk, plain
½ teaspoon ground cardamom
¼ teaspoon ground cloves
¼ teaspoon ground cinnamon
Pinch of ground ginger
1 tablespoon turbinado or brown sugar

In a small saucepan bring ½ cup water to a boil. Add the black tea leaves and reduce the heat to low. Continue to boil for 1 minute.

Add the soymilk and spices and simmer over medium-low heat for 3 minutes, or until bubbles rise around the edge. Do not allow to boil. Turn off the heat, stir in the sugar, strain, and serve.

1 SERVING: Caloric Density 0.2; Calories 72; Protein 5g; Carbohydrate 7g; Fat 3g

Tomato Juice Frappé

SERVES 4

This tomato juice is best if you use fresh, organic, very ripe tomatoes. In Okinawa, there is an expression: "The redder a tomato becomes, the paler a doctor becomes"; a pale doctor, of course, being one whose potential clients are so healthy he's out of a job. There's no doubt some truth to the adage. Tomatoes are loaded with vitamins A, B_1, B_2, C, and lycopene, among other nutrients. If you can, use vine-ripened tomatoes from your own garden or the farmers' market for the best flavor and aroma.

4 large red tomatoes, peeled and sliced in half	1 tablespoon turbinado or brown sugar
2 cups ice cubes	Pinch of sea salt
	4 celery sticks

In a blender, process the tomatoes, ice cubes, turbinado sugar, and salt. Serve with a celery stick in each glass

1 SERVING: Caloric Density 0.2; Calories 38; Protein 1g; Carbohydrate 9g; Fat <1g

Apricot-Yogurt Soy Smoothie

SERVES 4

This flavonoid-laden snack is a refreshing treat for a sleepy summer afternoon. Soy yogurt, like dairy yogurt, is made by adding live bacteria cultures to milk—in this case, soymilk. One cup of soy yogurt contains 12 grams of lactose-free and cholesterol-free protein. Soy yogurt can be eaten plain or flavored with your favorite fruit. Apricots are a rich source of vitamin C and are high in iron and potassium, a mineral essential for proper nerve and muscle function, blood pressure control, and balance of body fluids. If apricots are not in season, 1 cup of fresh peach slices will do the trick.

6 ounces water-packed silken light tofu	1 tablespoon turbinado or brown sugar
6 ounces soy yogurt, plain	1 tablespoon lemon juice
4 apricots, peeled and sliced	½ cup crushed ice

In a blender, process the tofu, yogurt, apricots, turbinado sugar, lemon juice, and crushed ice until smooth. Serve immediately, or freeze for later use.

1 SERVING: Caloric Density 0.4; Calories 69; Protein 4g; Carbohydrate 11g; Fat 1g

Spiced Cranberry Cider

SERVES 4

There is nothing like a mug of warm cranberry cider to warm up your bones on a cold winter afternoon. High in flavonoids and other antioxidants, cranberry juice has long been used as a home remedy for cystitis (bladder infections) and may also help prevent kidney and bladder stones. Highly recommended!

2 cups apple cider
2 cups vitamin C–fortified cranberry
   juice
2 dried whole cloves, crushed

1 dried whole allspice, crushed
1 cinnamon stick
½ teaspoon vanilla extract

Place everything in a stockpot and bring to a boil over medium-high heat. Turn off the heat and let stand for 10 minutes. Strain and serve warm.

Variation: Use 1 quart apple cider and 1 quart cranberry juice. Add 2 more cloves, 1 more allspice, and ½ teaspoon more vanilla. Serve with cinnamon sticks.

1 SERVING, 1 CUP: Caloric Density 0.5; Calories 116; Protein <1g; Carbohydrate 19g; Fat <1g

Miso and Dill Dip

MAKES 16 SERVINGS, 1 TABLESPOON EACH

Dill gets its name from the old Norse word *dilla,* "to lull" because of its reputed sedative effects. In the Middle Ages, the herb was a popular ingredient in potions and magic spells and was also employed as a charm against sorcery. Today it works magic in pickles, salad dressings, soups, and fish dishes. Dill also contains a pinch of cancer-fighting flavonoids, which makes this already healthy dip even a little more magical.

5 ounces water-packed silken light tofu
2 tablespoons white miso or your
   favorite kind
¼ cup soymilk, plain

⅓ cup finely chopped dill weed
Pinch of sea salt
Pinch of chili powder

In a blender, process the tofu, miso, soymilk, dill weed, salt, and chili powder until smooth. Serve with vegetable sticks or spread over bread.

1 serving: Caloric Density 0.7; Calories 11; Protein 1g; Carbohydrate 1g; Fat <1g

Tofu Hummus

MAKES 16 SERVINGS, 1 TABLESPOON EACH

The nutty-flavored garbanzo bean, also called *chickpea,* is a staple of Middle Eastern, Mediterranean, and Indian cuisine. Hummus, made of pureed garbanzo beans, garlic, olive oil, and sesame paste, is one of the most popular Middle Eastern foods in North America. It is great as a veggie dip or bread spread (especially on pita). We make it with tofu for a flavonoid boost and smoother texture.

1 can (15 ounces) garbanzo beans,
   drained and rinsed
3 ounces water-packed firm light tofu
1 clove garlic, minced
⅓ cup canned black olives, pitted

½ teaspoon ground cumin
1 tablespoon tahini paste
2 tablespoons olive oil
¼ cup lemon juice
Pinch of sea salt

In a blender, process the beans, tofu, garlic, olives, cumin, tahini, olive oil, lemon juice, and salt until smooth. Add water little by little if the mixture is too thick. Serve with vegetables, pita breads, or crackers.

1 SERVING: Caloric Density 1.4; Calories 58; Protein 2g; Carbohydrate 7g; Fat 3g

Cucumber and Avocado Hors d'Oeuvre

SERVES 4

The calorie-busting cucumber helps balance the fatty avocado to lower the caloric density of this recipe, so you can still enjoy this healthy fruit (packed with essential monounsaturated fatty acids) for its rich flavor and smooth texture. When possible, choose Florida avocados, which contain half the fat of California avocados. This dip can also be used on vegetable sticks, toast, sandwiches, or as a side dish.

⅓ cup finely chopped cucumber	12 low-sodium, low-fat crackers
⅓ cup finely chopped avocado	⅓ teaspoon ground paprika
1 tablespoon lime juice	Fresh dill weed, chopped

In a small mixing bowl, combine the cucumber, avocado, and lime juice. Top each cracker with approximately ⅔ tablespoon of the cucumber mixture. Garnish with a pinch of paprika and a tiny bit of dill weed.

1 SERVING: Caloric Density 1.7; Calories 90; Protein 2g; Carbohydrate 15g; Fat 3g

Snacking Pita Pizza

SERVES 4

You can use practically any vegetable for this versatile recipe. Fresh veggies, of course, are best. Chop, dice, slice, and add as a last-minute pizza topping. More vegetables mean more taste and fewer calories. What's even better is that you can place all the ingredients on plates and just let people prepare their own afternoon snack when they want it. A healthy treat for busy people.

¼ cup tomato paste	½ cup chopped tomatoes
¼ cup salsa	¼ cup sliced olives (optional)
4 small whole-grain pita breads	½ cup shredded soy mozzarella cheese
½ cup sliced white onion	Olive oil spray
½ cup chopped green bell pepper	Tabasco sauce (optional)

Preheat the oven to 350°F.

Combine the tomato paste and salsa and spread the mixture over the pita breads.

Arrange the onion, green pepper, tomatoes, and olives on the pita breads and cover with soy cheese. Spray each pizza with olive oil.

Bake for approximately 10 minutes, or until the vegetables are done to your preference. Sprinkle with Tabasco when serving.

1 SERVING, 1 PIZZA: Caloric Density 1.0; Calories 116; Protein 6g; Carbohydrate 23g; Fat 2g

Spinach Wedges

SERVES 4

This is a kind of pancake, ideal for a light snack. Instead of spinach, you can use almost any green veggie—for example, watercress, dandelion, leek, green onion, or finely chopped celery. You can also serve this snack with hummus, soy mayonnaise, or mustard instead of the lime-soy sauce. A good opportunity for creativity.

4 cups chopped spinach
7 ounces water-packed silken light tofu
1 free-range, omega-3 egg
2 tablespoons whole-wheat flour
Pinch of sea salt

Freshly ground black pepper
Canola oil spray
¼ cup lime juice
1 tablespoon low-sodium soy sauce

Cook the spinach in boiling water for 30 seconds. Rinse under running water immediately. Squeeze out extra water.

In a blender, process the tofu, egg, flour, salt, and pepper. Combine with the spinach in a medium bowl.

Spray a large skillet with canola oil and heat it over medium heat. Pour the spinach batter into the skillet, making a round shape with a wooden spatula. Cook for 2 minutes, or until the bottom is golden. Turn over and cook for another 2 minutes.

Cut the pancake into wedges. Combine the lime juice and soy sauce; serve with the pancake.

1 SERVING: Caloric Density 0.5; Calories 61; Protein 6g; Carbohydrate 6g; Fat 2g

Orange-Glazed Sesame Carrots

SERVES 4

Sesame seeds are popular in Japan as a longevity food. They're a good source of fiber and are high in iron, protein, and calcium: 1 ounce of sesame seeds contains as much calcium as 1 cup of milk. They're also high in caloric density and fat, but it's mostly the good, heart-healthy mono- or polyunsaturated fat, so when they are used in moderation, sesame seeds make a healthy addition to your diet.

3 cups baby carrots
2 tablespoons white sesame seeds
Juice of 2 oranges

1 tablespoon turbinado or brown sugar
Pinch of cinnamon
Canola oil spray

Steam the carrots, tightly covered, for 6 minutes, or until crisp-tender. Do not overcook.

Place the sesame seeds in a flat plate or a baking dish.

In a medium skillet, bring the orange juice and turbinado sugar to a boil over medium-high heat. Reduce the heat to low and simmer for 2 minutes, or until the liquid is thickened and darkened in color a bit. Stir by shaking the skillet, without using a spoon or spatula.

Add the carrots, cinnamon, and a few sprays of canola oil. Toss to coat with the orange glaze. Transfer to the plate of sesame seeds and roll to coat. Separate the carrots and let cool.

1 SERVING: Caloric Density 0.7; Calories 95; Protein 2g; Carbohydrate 16g; Fat 3g

Caramel Sweet Potato Chips

SERVES 8

This recipe is a great low-cal snack and could even be served at your next Thanksgiving dinner. It would be a welcome change from standard holiday candied sweet potato recipes that often include a lot of unnecessary sugar and fat. Sweet potatoes are highly nutritious, and their natural sweet flavor belies their overall healthy constituents and low G.I. They do spoil quickly, though, and any that have moldy spots or are shriveled should be thrown away. To prevent spoiling, store sweet potatoes in a cool place, but never in the refrigerator —temperatures below 50°F will make them hard and tasteless.

Canola oil spray
1 pound sweet potatoes, peeled and
   thinly sliced

3 tablespoons turbinado or brown sugar

Preheat the oven to 350°F.

Spray two baking sheets with canola oil and set the sweet potato slices on them in a single layer. Bake for 10 to 15 minutes.

In the meantime, combine the turbinado sugar and ½ cup water in a small saucepan and bring to a boil. Reduce the heat to low and simmer for 1 to 2 minutes, or until the liquid is thickened and darkened in color a bit. Stir by shaking the skillet, without using a spoon or spatula.

Once the sweet potatoes are done, turn the slices over and brush the tops with the caramel. Switch the baking sheets from top to bottom and bake for 10 to 15 minutes more.

1 SERVING: Caloric Density 0.9; Calories 73; Protein 1g; Carbohydrate 17g; Fat <1g

Cajun Hot Popcorn

SERVES 4

Popcorn, everyone's favorite movie-time snack food, is a special variety of corn that grows on a cob smaller than the usual sweet corn. Using air-popped popcorn is *very* important when thinking low-CD. Check this math: 2 cups of air-popped popcorn is 61 calories (CD 3.8), while the same amount of oil-popped popcorn is 110 calories (CD 5.0)—and oil-popped buttered popcorn is a whopping 146 calories (CD 5.2)! Once you try this low-cal popcorn with our special seasoning, you will never go back to the ordinary fattening kind. Try it at your next movie party!

2 teaspoons paprika	**½ teaspoon ground allspice**
1 teaspoon chili powder	**Pinch of sea salt**
1 teaspoon onion powder	**8 cups air-popped popcorn**
½ teaspoon garlic powder	**Canola oil spray**

In a small mixing bowl, combine the paprika, chili powder, onion powder, garlic powder, allspice, and salt.

Place the popcorn in a large bowl. Spray it evenly with canola oil. Sprinkle with the spices little by little, tossing to coat evenly.

1 SERVING, 2 cups: Caloric Density 3.7; Calories 72; Protein 2g; Carbohydrate 14g; Fat 1g

Hearty Granola

SERVES 16

Say the words *health food,* and what's the first thing you think of? For many, it's granola. Although granola has an image as the ultimate health food, and is, in fact, high in fiber, many granolas are loaded with fat and sugar. Whip up a batch of this tasty granola and avoid the problem. It's got lots of oat bran, the soluble fiber that helps lower blood cholesterol levels and helps the body utilize insulin more efficiently. This granola is terrific on yogurt, with fruit and chilled soymilk, and even with soy ice cream, and it is great as a party dessert, snack, or breakfast cereal. That's versatility!

2 cups rolled oats	**⅓ cup raisins**
1 cup oat bran	**⅓ cup chopped dried apple or prune**
1 cup wheat flakes	**⅓ cup honey**
½ cup wheat germ	**⅓ cup boiling water**
½ cup sliced or chopped almonds	**1 teaspoon vanilla extract**

Preheat the oven to 300°F.

In a large mixing bowl, combine the oats, oat bran, wheat flakes, wheat germ, almonds, raisins, and dried apple.

In a smaller bowl, stir together the honey, boiling water, and vanilla.

Add the liquid ingredients to the dry and mix well. Spread in a 13 × 9-inch baking dish. Bake for 40 to 50 minutes, or until golden brown, stirring occasionally.

1 SERVING, ⅓ CUP: Caloric Density 3.1; Calories 137; Protein 5g; Carbohydrate 26g; Fat 4g

Appendix A

The Eight-Week Phase-In Plan: A Mini Guide

We recognize that the Okinawa diet probably represents a fairly significant change from the way you're used to eating and thinking about food. By phasing in to this new approach over eight weeks, you can monitor the results of your regimen and also incorporate the other elements of a healthier lifestyle, like a good exercise program. After eight weeks, take stock of your progress. If the weight loss isn't enough to make you a convert for life, the improved energy level and long-term health benefits will. Begin by reviewing the following core concepts of the Okinawa diet.

Hot Reading Topics	*Where to Find the Info*
Causes of obesity	Chapter 2, pages 18–39
Obesity and health risks	Chapter 2, pages 18–19
Caloric density	Chapter 1, pages 13–14; chapter 4, pages 57–64, 100–107
Energy balance	Chapter 2, pages 25–30; chapter 6, pages 171–172

Getting Yourself Ready	*Where to Find the Info*
Assess your motivation and plan ways to overcome your barriers.	Chapter 6, pages 166–168
Calculate your BMI (and body fat percent) and estimate how much fat weight you need to lose to reach a healthy goal. Plan on roughly 10 to 25 pounds. The more weight you lose above these limits, the more likely it is to be water and muscle, not fat.	Chapter 1, page 6. See also Body Mass Index Calculator website on page 406.
Calculate your energy balance: Output (baseline calorie burn plus exercise burn) minus input.	Chapter 6, pages 171–175
Consider having a basic biomarker profile done by your physician.	Chapter 2, pages 39–46

Important Activities	*Where to Find the Info*
Clean up the kitchen: Eliminate all cooking oils except cold-pressed, extra-virgin olive oil and canola oil. Toss out all butter, margarines, and vegetable shortenings, except margarines that are *extremely* low in trans fatty acids, such as Benecol® and Take Control®. (Low levels of trans are 0.5 grams per serving or less.)	Chapter 4, pages 81, 84, 87–89
Empty the house of CD heavyweights, except a few in mini-size packs for emergency cravings. Also select some low-calorie snacks from the Okinawa Diet Pantry list and buy enough for one week.	Chapter 7, pages 186–193
Copy the Caloric Density pyramid and paste it on the fridge.	Chapter 3, page 58
Add some bowls of healthy fruit around the house.	Chapter 5, pages 137–139
Check to see if your local grocery has a good Asian section. Also try to locate a good health or Asian food store in your area. Refer to the Yellow Pages, ask friends or the managers of your local Asian restaurants. (Also see "Recommended Readings" on page 405 for a list of websites and potential stores in your area.)	Okinawan Restaurants, page 407
Check to see if you have a wok or a deep skillet. If not, buy a stainless-steel wok. Look for nonstick types,which allow for less oil use, and try to avoid aluminum, since there are still some questions about its health implications.	Find out about woks at www.i-clipse.com/woks.asp and www.fantes.com/coolware.htm.
Buy or borrow a blender (food processor) and an electric rice cooker, which makes hassle-free, perfectly cooked rice. Just put in the rice and water, close the lid, and press COOK. Electric cookers have auto-sensors that detect when the rice is ready and switch the temperature to warm mode automatically. Look for styles with a simple COOK/WARM switch and avoid the fancy computerized timers. Good brands include National/Panasonic and Zojirushi. Microwave rice cookers are also good.	Visit the National/Panasonic website at www.panasonic.com and Zojirushi at www.zojirushi.com
Make sure you have exercise gear and a good pair of walking shoes.	Learn about athletic shoes at www.mayoclinic.com/invoke.cfm?id=HQ00885 and about gear at www.mayoclinic.com/invoke.cfm?id=SM00027

Important Activities	*Where to Find the Info*
Buy a weight scale that also calculates body fat. (The Tanita body fat scale is excellent and is available in most sporting goods stores or over the Web.) Remember to weigh yourself naked (or in the same clothes) at the same time of day. Measurements on these scales can vary as much as 10 percent during the day and depend on many factors. Don't get hung up on too frequent weigh-ins or taking too many body fat measurements. Body fat drops more slowly than pounds. Look for long-term trends and be consistent.	Visit Tanita at www.tanita.com/ indexUS.shtml.
Buy a notebook for a fitness/wellness diary to record your weight, body fat percent, thoughts, feelings, and accomplishments daily. Also use the page we provide to calculate your calories burned.	Chapter 6, page 181
Write down your goals in your journal. If your goal is healthy weight loss, follow the calorie guide for your activity level and aim for 500–1,000 calories a day less than you need. Over seven days you will drop one to two pounds of fat (not water). If you lose more than three pounds per week, it's likely to be water and muscle loss, both of which your body needs.	Chapter 6, page 172
Go over the Okinawa Diet Pantry list and start stocking up on the basic foods, herbs, spices, and condiments.	Chapter 7, pages 186–189

WEEKS 1 AND 2: LET'S GET MOVING!

Here we go. Now you're prepared and it's time to get moving toward a lifelong healthy weight.

Hot Reading Topics	*Where to Find the Info*
Good carbs, bad carbs, and how to tell the difference	Chapter 2, pages 33–37; chapter 4, pages 89–95
Glycemic index	Chapter 2, page 34; chapter 4, pages 91–94
Insulin index	Chapter 2, page 35
Minimum protein requirements: how to calculate	Chapter 4, pages 64–65
Differences between plant and animal protein foods	Chapter 4, pages 67, 69–70, 70–80
Good fats, bad fats	Chapter 4, pages 80–89

Important Activities	*Where to Find the Info*
Choose two weeks from the eating tracks or plan your own meals.	Chapter 7, pages 194–205
Prepare your diet journal by entering your daily calorie goal, energy balance calculations, and exercise plan.	Chapter 6, pages 180–181 183–184
Start your exercise program.	Chapter 6, pages 176–182

WEEKS 3 AND 4: WORKING OUT THE KINKS

Congrats! You're still here and have diligently stuck to the plan (well, mostly) for two weeks. By now you should have lost a few pounds and be well into the groove. These are the weeks where we really get down to the business of healthy weight and where flexibility counts. This week you'll also be able to make some decisions about what has worked for you and what hasn't, what changes you'd like to incorporate into your life, and what more you can do to enhance your healthy weight loss and further sculpt your body and hone your mind.

Hot Reading Topics	*Where to Find the Info*
Motivation and self-belief	Chapter 6, page 170
Calorie busters	Chapter 4, pages 115–117
Reading food labels	Chapter 3, pages 50–51
Dining out	Learn tips at the American Heart Association website, www.american heart.org/presenter.jhtml? identifier=4538.

Important Activities	*Where to Find the Info*
Choose two different weeks from the eating tracks or plan your own meals.	Chapter 7, pages 194–205
Continue to write down daily totals (food consumed, exercise accomplished, energy balance, thoughts and feelings).	Chapter 6, pages 180–181, 183–184
Shop for some new clothes that you will be wearing in a couple of weeks.	

WEEKS 5 AND 6: GETTING OVER THE HUMP

You've made it halfway and have done well! But this is the time when it's easy to slip, so watch yourself closely. The initial pounds came off fairly easily in weeks one and two, then a bit more slowly in weeks three and four—but now it can get tricky. The weight you're losing now consists of more fat and less water, so stick to it. There are big rewards just ahead.

Hot Reading Topics	**Where to Find the Info**
Cravings, food triggers, compulsive overeating, stress and emotions	Chapter 6, pages 168–169
Effective ways for dealing with stress	Chapter 6, pages 166–167
Dietary ways to cut cravings	Chapter 3, pages 49–50, 52, 54–55

Important Activities	**Where to Find the Info**
Deal with your sweet tooth.	Chapter 4, pages 121–122
Practice meditation.	Chapter 6, page 171

WEEKS 7 AND 8: THE HOME STRETCH

Fantastic—you made it to week 7. You have now entered a phase in which you can build on what you have learned. You should be feeling great about yourself. You're healthier, closer to an optimum weight, and feeling a renewed inner strength. These weeks allow you to consolidate the gains you've made over the previous six weeks. If you started out on the Western eating track, experiment with some of the East–West Fusion foods or try a week on the Okinawan/ Eastern track. Make up a few of your own recipes. Now is the time to expand your wellness efforts. Let's take the next step.

Hot Reading Topics	**Where to Find the Info**
Fad diets (e.g., low-carb diets)	Chapter 2, pages 36–37, 38–39, 55–56
Group weight-loss programs	See websites, page 406
Herbal and nonprescription remedies	Chapter 4, pages 107–113; chapter 5, page 163
Finding dependable resources	See websites, page 406
Weight-loss winners	Chapter 6, page 178

Important Activities	**Where to Find the Info**
Modify a recipe.	Chapter 7
Overcoming setbacks.	Chapter 6, pages 169–170
Find a source of support.	See websites, page 406
Re-evaluate goals.	Chapter 6, pages 167–169

You did it! Eight weeks have passed and you've gained invaluable knowledge, lost unwanted pounds, and should be fitting yourself for some new clothes about now. You have several powerful new tools at your disposal to help prepare you for a lifetime of healthy weight. Use them wisely, and if you start to regain some of that weight, go back to week 1!

Appendix B

Recipe Index by Calories

200 calories and up

Creamy Split Pea and Sweet Potato Soup	218
Fragrant Soy Go Vegetable Soup	230

Chicken

100 to 200 calories

Poached Chicken with Herb Dressing	103
Chilled Chicken Wontons	139
Okinawan Coq au Vin	140
Winter Soy Chicken with Vegetables	143
Chicken and Peanut Stir-Fry in Oyster Sauce	152
Spicy Stewed Chicken	185

200 calories and up

Nasi Goreng Ayam (Chicken Rice) (with rice)	206
Walnut-Dressed Chicken	229
Simple and Easy Tandoori Chicken	235
Chicken Asparagus Cordon Bleu	281
Chicken and Mushroom Linguine (with pasta)	308
Chicken Edamame Curry (with rice)	367

Fish and Seafood

Under 100 calories

Sea Bream Carpaccio with Turmeric Sauce	66
Garlic Mussels with White Wine Sauce	99

100 to 200 calories

Poached White Fish with Honey-Lime Sauce	121
Cod Wa no Ichi	122
Ryukyu Fish Curry	123
Hawaiian Lemon-Ahi Poke	135
Baked Salmon Mousse	142
Cheesy Scallops and Potatoes	147
Spicy Garlic Shrimp	179
Papaya and Shrimp Spring Roll	184
Miso Salmon with Vegetables	188
Grilled Fish with Grated Radish	190

200 calories and up

Teriyaki Yellowtail with Rice (with rice)	260
Shrimp and Broccoli Penne (with pasta)	335
Salmon with Nuts and Rice (with rice)	418

Lean Meats

100 to 200 calories

Beef in Oyster Sauce	140
Balsamic Pork with Mushrooms	155
Pork Daikon	156
Nsunaba Sukiyaki	160
Shabu Shabu Pork with Herb Sauce	165
Sloppy Tofu with Beef	170
Veggieful Beef Stew	185
Veggie Pork Pita (with bread)	190

200 calories and up

Beef à la Crème	215
Bambou Short Ribs	298

Tofu

Under 100 calories

Turmeric-Marinated Tofu with Chard	48
Ginkgo-Tofu Supreme	77
Ryukyu Scrambled Eggs II	81
Spicy Tofu and Summer Vegetables	82

Desserts

Under 100 calories

Watermelon Fizz	53
Roasted Summer Peach	67
Cantaloupe and Grapefruit Sorbet	72
Darjeeling Pudding	90
Mugwort Rice Cake (Fuchiba Nantu)	91
Green Tea Panna Cotta	97

100 to 200 calories

Okinawan Steamed Bean Cake (Mushi Manju)	105
Tropical Mango Pudding	116
Mochi on a Leaf	138
October Pumpkin Soufflé	144
Chocolate Chip Cookies	148
Fruitful Frozen Yogurt	150
Can't-Be-Easier Chocolate Fruit Pudding	158
Sweet Potato Mousse with Green Tea Sauce	162
Tapioca Sweet Potato Dessert	193
Tofu Key Lime Pie	197
Sweet Amagashi Beans	197

Teas and Snacks

Under 100 calories

Best Steeping Teas and Matcha	0
Miso and Dill Dip	11
Tomato Juice Frappé	38
Tofu Hummus	58
Spinach Wedges	61
Apricot-Yogurt Soy Smoothie	69
Cajun Hot Popcorn	72
Soy Masala Chai	72
Caramel Sweet Potato Chips	73
Cucumber and Avocado Hors d'Oeuvre	90
Orange-Glazed Sesame Carrots	95

100 to 200 calories

Snacking Pita Pizza	116
Spiced Cranberry Cider	116
Hearty Granola	137

Notes

CHAPTER 1. OKINAWA: LEAN PEOPLE, LONG, HEALTHY LIVES

1. Shangri-la metaphor: We chose James Hilton's "Shangri-la," as portrayed in his book *Lost Horizon,* as a metaphor for the Okinawan successful aging phenomenon. Like Hilton's mythical valley where the robust inhabitants lived unknown to the outside world and counted their ages in centuries, not decades, Okinawa has been an isolated island nation, first mentioned in Chinese records in A.D. 605, and, until recently, largely unknown to U.S. gerontologists. This is beginning to change as we publish more of our Okinawan studies in English-language scientific journals. Unlike Hilton's version of Shangri-la, or the version of Okinawa seen in some popular television infomercials that portray Okinawans as disease-free and routinely living to their hundreds, Okinawans certainly can fall prey to modern diseases. But they do have markedly lower risk for the chronic diseases of aging such as cardiovascular disease and cancer, and they do have the longest healthy life expectancy in Japan, which has the longest healthy life expectancy in the world. See Mathers, C., Ritu, S., Salomon, J., et al. Healthy life expectancy in 191 countries, 1999. *Lancet* 2001; 357:1685-91. Willcox, B.J., Willcox, D.C., and Suzuki, M. Built to last? Past medical history of Okinawan-Japanese centenarians. *J Am Geriatr Soc* 2002; 50(4):394. And unlike in Shangri-la, there are good data to back up age claims in Okinawa. See Willcox, B.J., Willcox, D.C., and Suzuki, M. Evidence-based extreme longevity. The case of Okinawa, Japan. *J Am. Geriatr Soc* 2001; 49(4):397. Thus, if a case can be made for a real Shangri-la, Okinawa appears to be it. See www.okicent.org for more information.

2. World's Longest-Lived People Claim: The world's longest-lived population is a much-coveted title, and many lay claim to it. If we are to take an evidence-based gerontological approach, it is clear that Japan is the world's longest-lived country, according to the World Health Organization. In fact, Japan is currently the only country to have achieved a life expectancy of over eighty years for men and women combined (see World Health Statistics Annual 2000. World Health Organization, Geneva). It is also clear from life expectancy data calculated from life table data from the Japan Ministry of Health, Labor, and Welfare that Okinawa has been the longest-lived prefecture (state) in Japan since life expectancy data were routinely calculated in the 1920s. While the pre–World War II data have been criticized for underreporting infant mortality in Okinawa, adding some artifactual increase to Okinawa's life expectancy at birth, the modern data set has no such problems. Mortality statistics are standardized throughout Japan. They are currently among the world's most reliable sources of information for research on demographic trends in longevity. See Kannisto, V. On the survival of centenarians and the span of life. *Population Studies* 1988; 42(3):389–406. Wilmoth, J.R. Is the pace of Japanese mortality decline converging toward international trends? *Pop Development Rev* 1998; 24(3):593–600. Unfortunately, the mortality trends for younger Okinawans, which are higher than the national (Japan) average, are resulting in slower life expectancy gains for Okinawa. It is the outstanding health of the elders (ages seventy-plus) that has given men and women in Okinawa their mortality advantage versus other Japanese and Americans, but future generations are in peril due to vastly different lifestyles.

3. "Concentrations" of centenarians are usually measured in terms of prevalence (numbers per 100,000), often simply referred to as *centenarian ratio*. Centenarian ratios are open to multiple sources of bias. These include in-migration and out-migration, size of particular birth cohorts, and lower reliability of the age database at exceptionally old ages. Okinawa's high centenarian ratio persists despite out-migration of the older age cohort and large numbers of youth due to the highest birth rate in Japan, and all centenarians are age-validated. Even 116-year-old Kamato Hongo, born in 1887 on Tokuno Island, part of the Ryukyu (Okinawa) archipelago annexed by Japan in the seventeenth century, has a valid birth certificate. Japan began recording these data in 1872 and Okinawa in 1879 in a national family registry (*koseki*) system. Other problems with many centenarian studies include illiteracy, cognitive impairment, and age exaggeration. As far back as 1939, Bowerman noted the spurious but strong correlation of centenarian prevalence with illiteracy rates by state in the United States (Bowerman, W.G. Centenarians. *Transactions of the Actuarial Society of America*. 1939; XL:360–78). Cognitive disability also limits the ability of some centenarians to report their ages accurately. Even in 1909, Clark reported that cultural factors affected an individual's knowledge of his or her true age (Clark, F.C. The problem of centenarianism. *The Providence Medical Journal* 1909; 10:143–58). In the U.S. census data, there is undoubtedly some tendency of extremely aged persons (and their relatives and friends) to overstate their ages out of a sense of pride in long living. Alter reported in the 1990 U.S. census that 83% of centenarians reported ages 100–104, 9% ages 105–109, and 7% ages 110 and over. Of 1505 whites who reported ages 110 and over in the 1990 census, 68% reported no mobility or personal care limitations; 30% lived alone; and 41% were married (Alter, G. Old age mortality and age misreporting in the United States, 1900–1940. *Working Paper* #24. Population Institute for Research and Training, Indiana University,1990)—all of which cast severe doubt on the validity of most of the supercentenarian age reports in the 1990 U.S. census.

4. Supercentenarians: *Semi-supercentenarian* and *supercentenarian* are terms that are now in use by gerontologists that study exceptional longevity, also called *exceptional survival*, and refer to centenarians who are at least 105 years old and 110 years old respectively. Once exceedingly rare, they are becoming more common as the number of centenarians grows. Currently, in most Western countries the centenarian population is growing at a rate that averages 8% per year (Vaupel, J.W., and Jeune, B. 1995, "The emergence and proliferation of centenarians," in Jeune, B., and Vaupel, J.W. eds. *Validation of Exceptional Longevity*, Odense University Press, Odense, Denmark). For a good review, see Robine, J.M., and Vaupel, J.W. Supercentenarians: slower aging individuals or senile elderly? *Exp Gerontol* 2001; 36:915–30. There is some debate in the gerontological community as to what constitutes a reliable age database for estimating numbers of exceptionally aged individuals, such as centenarians or supercentenarians. Various factors contribute to an upward bias in ages, but men appear particularly prone to age-exaggeration, since a certain pride seems to be attached to attaining a very old age. Age verification via a birth certificate is vitally important. When a birth registration database has been in existence for over 110 years, then it becomes much easier to validate the reliability of exceptional survivors. Registration of births became compulsory in Japan in 1872, England and Wales in 1874, Germany in 1876. These countries possess reliable databases for estimating numbers of exceptional survivors. The U.S. did not have national birth registration until 1940, making the database reliability at very old ages suspect to many gerontologists. Currently, up to twenty-five countries, including Japan, qualify as having reliable data, depending on the researchers queried. After the 1970s, when Japan's birth database (which includes Okinawa) approached 110 years in existence, the data on exceptional longevity and centenarian prevalence became highly reliable, leaving little doubt about Okinawa's longevity claims. For review, see Kannisto, V. *Population Studies* 1988; 42:389–406, and Coale, A., and Kisker, E. Mortality cross-overs: reality or bad data? *Population Studies* 1986; 40:389–401. Kannisto, V. Development of oldest-old mortality, Monographs on Population Aging, 1. 1994, Odense University Press.

5. Okinawa's most recently validated centenarian prevalence was 39.5 per hundred thousand (Japan

Ministry of Health, Labor, and Welfare. Statistics and Information Division, 2002), based on annual review of birth certificates from city and village offices. Our last review of centenarian prevalence in Okinawa was in 2001 and found prevalence rates of 33.6 per hundred thousand (Willcox, B.J., Willcox, D.C., and Suzuki, M. Evidence-based extreme longevity. The case of Okinawa, Japan. *J Am Geriatr Soc* 2001; 49(4):397). Centenarian prevalence rates in the U.S. are not known with precision. Estimates vary from a high of 26 per hundred thousand (U.S. Department of Health and Human Services, National Institutes of Health, National Institute on Aging. Centenarians in the United States. 1990. U.S. Census Bureau.) to a more likely figure of 10 per hundred thousand. The latter figure is based on validation of birth certificates from a population-based study in New England in 1999 (Perls, T.T., Bochen, K., Freeman, M., et al. Validity of reported age and centenarian prevalence in New England. *Age and Aging* 1999; 28:193–7 and is likely closer to the actual figure for the U.S. because it consists of age-validated centenarians similar to the Okinawan data. For further review of this topic, see Jeune, B., and Vaupel, J.W., eds. *Validation of Exceptional Longevity.* Odense, Denmark: Odense University Press.

6. We found links between high levels of prostate-specific antigen and saturated fat intake as well as other dietary factors. See Willcox, B.J., Jenkins, D.J.A., Fuchigami, K., et al. Serum fatty acid profiles and PSA in Japanese and Canadian men. *FASEB J* 1996; 10:A550(3170). Willcox, B.J., Fuchigami, K., Willcox, D.C., et al. Isoflavone intake in Japanese and Japanese-Canadians. *Am J Clin Nutr* 1995; 61(4):901. Willcox, B.J., Jenkins, D.J.A., Fuchigami, K., et al. Dietary Westernization and chronic disease in Japan. *FASEB J* 1995; 9(3):A445. Mr. Oyakawa was touted as the oldest man in Ontario, the largest province of Canada, and was likely the oldest man alive at that time. While Mr. Oyakawa had birth documentation in Japan and a Canadian passport that verified his age, the lack of a national database of age-validated centenarians in Canada makes it difficult to verify that he was actually the oldest man alive in Canada at that time.

7. Disability-free life expectancy: As mentioned in Note 1, Okinawans have the longest disability-free life expectancy in Japan (Japan Ministry of Health, Labor, and Welfare. Statistics and Information Division, 2000), and the Japanese have the world's longest disability-free life expectancy for a country. See Mathers, C., Ritu, S., Salomon, J., et al. Healthy life expectancy in 191 countries, 1999. *The Lancet* 2001; 357:1685–91. Willcox, B.J., Willcox, D.C., Suzuki, M. Built to last? Past medical history of Okinawan-Japanese centenarians. *J Am Geriatr Soc* 2002; 50(4):394. This allows Okinawans a strong population-based claim to having the world's longest healthy life expectancy. Cross-national data are open to some bias depending on how the country itself measures disability, and there may be very healthy groups of people within countries or states that could make such a claim as well (see note 8). Of interest, our research collaborators at the Pacific Health Research Institute have also found that Japanese-American men (including Okinawan-Americans), many of them hardworking plantation laborers, much like Okinawan farmers, are also highly functional at older ages. They ate an East-West dietary blend similar in many ways to the Okinawan diet, were physically active for most of their lives, and have reported much lower disability rates at older ages compared to the average American. See Rantanen, T., Guralnik, J.M., Foley, D., et al. Midlife hand grip strength as a predictor of old age disability. *JAMA* 1999; 10:281:558–60. Rodriguez, B.L., D'Agostino, R., Abbott, R.D., et al. Risk of hospitalized stroke in men enrolled in the Honolulu Heart Program and the Framingham Study: A comparison of incidence and risk factor effects. *Stroke* Jan 2002; 33(1):230–6. And see note 8.

8. Claims of longevity regions in the old Soviet Union, the Hunza Valley in Pakistan, and the village of Vilcabamba in Ecuador have been thoroughly discredited (see Leaf, A. Long-lived populations: Extreme old age. *J Am Geriatr Soc* 1982; 30:485–87). However, certain U.S. sub-populations such as Japanese-Americans, Seventh-day Adventists, and Mormons also have very long lives, mostly due to their healthy lifestyles. For further reading, see Curb, J.D., Reed, D.M., Miller, F.D., and Yano, K. Health status and life style in elderly Japanese men with a long life expectancy. *J Gerontol.* 1990; 45(5): S206–11. Grundmann, E. Cancer morbidity and mortality in USA Mormons, and Seventh-day Adventists. *Arch Anat Cytol Pathol* 1992; 40(2–3):73–8.

Fraser, G.E., and Shavlik, D.J. Ten years of life: Is it a matter of choice? *Arch Intern Med* 2001; 9:161(13):1645–52.

9. Most of these publications have been in Japanese. For recent English publications, see Akisaka, M., Asato, L., Chan, Y.C., et al. Energy and nutrient intakes of Okinawan centenarians. *J Nutr Sci Vitaminol* 1996; 42:241–48. Akisaka, M., Suzuki, M., and Inoko, H. Molecular genetic studies on DNA polymorphism of the HLA class II genes associated with human longevity. *Tissue Antigens* 1997; 50:489–93. Chan, Y.C., Suzuki, M., and Yamamoto, S. Nutritional status of centenarians assessed by activity and anthropometric, hematological and biochemical characteristics. *J Nutr Sci Vitaminol* 1997;43:73–81. Itokazu, D., Willcox, B.J., Willcox, D.C., et al., eds. Okinawa International Conference on Longevity Abstracts. *Journal of Okinawa Chubu Hospital.* 2001; 27(suppl.2). Naka, K., Willcox, D.C., Todoriki, H., and Kageyama, T. Suicide in Okinawa from an international perspective: A consideration of socio-cultural factors. *Ryukyu Med J* 1998; 18:1–10. Suzuki, M., Willcox, B.J., Willcox, and D.C. Implications from and for food cultures for cardiovascular disease: longevity. *Asia Pacific J Clin Nutr* 2001; 10(2):165–171. Willcox, B.J., Willcox, D.C., and Suzuki, M. Evidence-based extreme longevity. The case of Okinawa, Japan. *J Am Geriatr Soc* 2001; 49(4):397. Willcox, B.J., Willcox, D.C., and Suzuki, M. Built to last? Past medical history of Okinawan-Japanese centenarians. *J Am Geriatr Soc* 2002; 50(4):394. Willcox, B.J., Willcox, D.C., and Suzuki, M. Defining cardiovascular health in a large population-based study of exceptional survivors. *Circulation* 2003. In press. See our website at www.okicent.org for our latest publications.

10. See *The Okinawa Program: How the World's Longest-Lived People Achieve Everlasting Health—and How You Can Too.* New York: Clarkson Potter, 2001.

11. Weight gain with age has been cited by a recent expert panel on caloric restriction as potentially the most reliable method of gauging whether a human population was actually calorically restricted (CR) over an extended period. More precisely, it represents energy balance—that is, how many calories we ate versus how many we burned off in physical activity. But it's probably one of the best estimates we have for gauging long-term calorie intake in large populations. Nutrition questionnaires for measuring caloric intake are often of suspect reliability because people tend to underreport their true calorie (energy) intake by 20 percent or more. Even dieticians underreport by an average of 10 percent. See Hoidrup, S., Andreasen, A.H., Osler, M., et al. Assessment of habitual energy and macronutrient intake in adults: Comparison of a seven-day food record with a dietary history interview. *EJCN* 2002; 56(2):105–113. For a review of weight gain with age and CR, see Lee, I.M., Blair, S.N., Allison, D.B., et al. Epidemiologic data on the relationships of caloric intake, energy balance, and weight gain over the life span with longevity and morbidity. *J Gerontol A Biol Sci Med Sci* 2001; 56:7–19. The fact that the Okinawan centenarians were part of a birth cohort who did not gain significant weight with age demonstrates that they kept in energy balance, largely through low caloric intake but also through physical activity. Therefore, the Okinawans are frequently mentioned as the best example of a human population that has been calorically restricted but not to the point of malnutrition or constant hunger. We believe this had a substantial contribution to their healthy long lives. See Akisaka, M., Asato, L., Chan, Y.C., et al. Energy and nutrient intakes of Okinawan centenarians. *J Nutr Sci Vitaminol* 1996; 42:241-48. Kagawa, Y. Impact of Westernization on the nutrition of Japanese: Changes in physique, cancer, longevity and centenarians. *Prev Med* 1978; 7(2):205-17. Suzuki, M., Willcox, B.J., and Willcox, D.C. Implications from and for food cultures for cardiovascular disease: longevity. *Asia Pacific J Clin Nutr* 2001; 10(2):165–171. Weindruch, R., and Sohal, R. Caloric intake and aging. *N Engl J Med* 1997; 337:986–94. Willcox, B.J., Willcox, D.C., and Suzuki, M. Nutrition and aging in Okinawa: Is there a diet that extends health span? *Am Diet Assoc Pulse* 2001; 20(2):5–8.

12. While many countries, such as India or China, have large populations that did not gain weight with age due to caloric restriction, this is usually associated with malnutrition. In Okinawa, due to a healthy nutrient-rich diet low in caloric density, there was large-scale "undernutrition" (low calorie intake or "caloric restriction") without large-scale malnutrition. This persisted until the

1970s when significant westernization took hold, and only in the elders (ages 70-plus) does some semblance of the traditional diet exist. Data sources for the traditional diet, East-West fusion diet, modern Okinawa diet, and modern American diet, respectively, are: U.S. National Archives, 1949; Japan National Nutrition Survey, 1972; Japan Ministry of Health and Welfare; Okinawa Prefectural Nutrition Survey, 1992, Department of Health and Welfare, Okinawa Prefecture; U.S. 1994–96 Continuing Survey of Food Intakes by Individuals, USDA. Per capita food supply trends: progress toward dietary guidelines. *Food Review* 2001; 23:2–14. U.S. food supply providing more food and calories. *Food Review* 1999; 22:2–12.

13. Lee, I.M., Blair, S.N., Allison, D.B., et al. Epidemiological data on the relationships of caloric intake, energy balance, and weight gain over the life span with longevity and morbidity. *J Gerontol A Biol Sci Med Sci* 2001; 56:7–19.

14. For an excellent online review of this topic, see Masoro, E.J. Subfield history: caloric restriction, slowing aging, and extending life. *Science* 2003; (SAGE KE) 299(8). For other recent reviews, see Koubova, J., and Guarente, L. How does energy restriction work? *Genes and Dev* 2003; 17:313–21. A classic book for both general reader and scientist alike is from Roy Walford, one of the true legends in the CR field; see Walford, R. *Beyond the 120-year diet.* New York–London: Four Walls Eight Windows, 2000. Although now getting somewhat dated a classic scientific text is Weindruch, R., and Walford, R.L. *The Retardation of Aging and Disease by Dietary Restriction.* Springfield, IL.: CC Thomas, 1988. Further evidence for the efficacy of a CR diet in humans has been published by Walford in a series of papers resulting from his Biosphere 2 experience: see Walford, R.L., Mock, D., Verdery, R., and MacCallum, T. Energy restriction in Biosphere 2. Alterations in physiologic, hematologic, hormonal, and biochemical parameters in humans restricted for a 2-year period. *J Gerontol Biol Sci* 2002; 57(6):B211–24.

15. McCay, C.M., Cromwell, M.F., and Maynard, L.A. The effects of retarded growth upon the length of life and upon ultimately body size. *J Nutr* 1935; 10:63–79.

16. Mattison, J.A., Lane, M.A., Roth, G.S., and Ingram, D.K. Calorie restriction in rhesus monkeys. *Experimental Gerontology* 2003; 38:35–46; Poehlman, E.T., Turturro, A., Bodkin, N., et al. Caloric restriction mimetics. Physical activity and body composition changes. *J Gerontol Series A* 2001; 56:45–54. Roth, G.S., Ingram, D.K., and Lane, M.A. Energy restriction in primates and relevance to humans. *Ann NY Acad Sci* 2001; 928:305–15.

17. Johannes, L. "Lean times: The surprising rise of radical, calorie-cutting diet." *Wall Street Journal,* June 4, 2002.

18. Kagawa, Y. Impact of Westernization on the nutrition of Japanese: Changes in physique, cancer, longevity and centenarians. *Prev Med* 1978; 7(2):205–17; Willcox, B.J., Willcox, D.C., and Suzuki, M. Built to last? Past medical history of Okinawan-Japanese centenarians. *J Am Geriatr Soc* 2002; 50(4):394. Willcox, B.J., Willcox, D.C., and Suzuki, M. Defining cardiovascular health in a large population-based study of exceptional survivors. *Circulation Online* June 2003. For more information on biomarkers of longevity in humans, see Roth, G.S., Lane, M.A., Ingram, D.K., et al. Biomarkers of caloric restriction may predict longevity in humans. *Science* 2002; 297(5582):811. Butler, R., ed. *Biomarkers of Aging: From Primitive Organisms to Man.* New York: International Longevity Center-USA, 2001

19. For a good review, see: Mitteldorf, J. Can experiments on caloric restriction be reconciled with the disposable soma theory of evolution of senescence? *Evolution* 2001; 55:1902–05.

20. Putnam, J. U.S. food supply providing more food and calories. *Food Review* 1999; 22(3):2–12; Okinawa Centenarian Study Nutrition Database. For Okinawa data, see note 12.

21. U.S. Department of Health and Human Services. The Surgeon General's call to action to prevent and decrease overweight and obesity. Rockville, MD: U.S. Department of Health and Human Services, Public Health Service, Office of the Surgeon General, 2001. Available from: US GPO, Washington. Available by order from the Superintendent of Documents, U.S. Government Printing Office, http://bookstore.GPO.gov, (866) 512-1800; (202) 512-1800; Stop SSOP, Washington, D.C., 20402-0001.

22. Kenchaiah, S., Evans, J.C., Levy, D., et al. Obesity and the risk of heart failure. *N Engl J Med* Aug 2002; 347(5):305–13.

23. Fraser, G.E., and Shavlik, D.J. Ten years of life: Is it a matter of choice? *Arch Intern Med* July 9 2001; 161(13):1645–52.

24. See the *Action Plan for Aging Research, Strategic Plan for Fiscal Years 2001–2005.* National Institutes of Health, National Institute on Aging, NIH Publication N. 01-4951. May 2001; 161:1645–52.

25. Bell, E.A., and Rolls, B.J. Energy density of foods affects energy intake across multiple levels of fat content in lean and obese women. *Am J Clin Nutr* Jun 2001; 73(6):1010–8.

26. The 236-calories/day increase in U.S. calorie intake reported in the text comes from the Continuing Survey of Food Intakes by Individuals (CSFII), a national nutrition survey conducted by the U.S. Department of Agriculture (USDA). CSFII uses a two-day food record where individuals are asked to record their food intake for two nonconsecutive days. See Lin, B.H., Frazao, E., and Guthrie J. Away-from-home foods increasingly important to quality of American diet. Agricultural Information Bulletin No. 749. USDA and US Department of Health and Human Services. Research Summary in: *Family Economics and Nutrition Review* 1999; 12:85–89. We don't place much stock in the precise numbers of calories reported in most population nutrition surveys, as people tend to underreport their actual intake. Obese people tend to underreport more than non-obese people. Heitmann, B.L., Lissner, I., Osler, M. Do we eat less fat, or just report so? *Int J Obes Relat Metab Disord* April 2000; 24(4):435–42. So how do we actually know how many calories Americans are eating? The answer is that nobody knows precisely, but we can make an educated guess. For example, in 1995 the CSFII estimated Americans ate 2,043 calories per day. The National Health and Nutrition Examination Survey (NHANES), conducted by the National Center for Health Statistics (NCHS), Centers for Disease Control and Prevention, using a single 24-hour recall estimate of food intake, estimated that Americans ate 2,200 calories per day in 1990. Food supply (or "food disappearance") data are also used by the USDA to estimate population caloric intake and usually has the opposite problem—overestimation of caloric intake. This is because calorie intake is reported as total food produced in the US minus food exported divided by the total population. Obviously there is some waste (e.g., restaurant scraps), spoilage, etc., and restaurants don't only serve U.S. residents (i.e., tourists and visitors consume food in the U.S. as well). The best anyone can say with certainty is that Americans eat somewhere between what the USDA reports in its CSFII surveys (2,043 calories), the CDC reports in its NHANES surveys (2,200 calories), and the USDA reports in its food supply data (2,700 calories when adjusted for waste/spoilage). USDA, Economic Research Service. Putnam, J. U.S. food supply providing more food and calories. *Food Review* Sept–Dec 1999; 22(3):2–12. Since 24-hour recall and food records underestimate by up to 20 percent the real figure is likely around 2,500 calories per day for the average American adult (men/women combined).

27. Jequier, E., and Tappy, L. Regulation of body weight in humans. *Physiol Rev* 1999; 79:451–80.

28. Nielsen, S.J., and Popkin, B.M. Patterns and trends in food portion sizes, 1977–1998. *JAMA* 2003; 289(4):450–3.

29. Jacobson, M., Hurley, J. *Restaurant Confidential.* New York: Workman, 2002.

30. Rolls, B.J., Morris, E.L., and Roe, L.S. Portion size of food affects energy intake in normal-weight and overweight men and women. *Am J Clin Nutr* Dec 2002; 76(6):1207–13.

31. "New survey shows Americans ignore importance of portion size in managing weight." American Institute for Cancer Research press release; March 31, 2000.

32. Lee, T., Oliver, J.E. "Obesity not seen as serious health problem in U.S." Kennedy School of Government Working Paper Number: RWP02-017.

33. A recent paper from the Framingham Study showed that large decreases in life expectancy were associated with being overweight (BMI 25–29.9 kg/m^2) or obese (BMI 30 or more kg/m^2) during adulthood. Overweight 40-year-old men and women lost 3.1 and 3.3 years of life, respectively. Those men and women who smoked lost 5.8 and 7.1 years of life. Being obese

approximately doubled that risk again where obese male and female nonsmokers lost 6.7 and 7.2 years respectively and obese smokers lost 13.7 and 13.3 years respectively. These data show the powerful independent effect body fat has on our health but do not address the further potential gains in life expectancy with caloric restriction (CR). CR's mechanism of action is not precisely known but may be related to both low body-fat levels and to a more efficient metabolism, which lowers blood glucose levels, insulin signaling, and free radical production and affects a multitude of other processes. See Peeters, A., Barendregt, J.J., and Willekens, F., et al. *Annals of Internal Medicine* 2003; 138:24–32 for further reading on this study; and Bluher, M., Kahn, B.B., and Kahn, C.R. Extended longevity in mice lacking the insulin receptor in adipose tissue. *Science* 2003; 299:572–4 for a recent study on caloric restriction, body fat, and mortality.

34. Willcox, B.J., Willcox, D.C., and Suzuki, M. Nutrition and aging in Okinawa: Is there a diet that extends health span? *Am Diet Assoc Pulse* 2001; 20(2):5–8.

35. USDA and DHHS, 2000. *Nutrition and Your Health: Dietary Guidelines for Americans.* Fifth Edition. Home and Garden Bulletin No. 23.

CHAPTER 2. NEW FINDINGS FOR HEALTHY WEIGHT

1. For a general review of how obesity affects health and life expectancy, see Fontaine, K.R., Redden, D.T., Wang, C., et all. Years of life lost due to obesity. *JAMA* 2003; 289:187–93. Willcox, B.J., Willcox, D.C., and Suzuki, M. Nutrition and aging in Okinawa: is there a diet that extends health span? *Am Diet Assoc Pulse* 2001; 20(2):5–8. For a review of how obesity contributes to diabetes see Marx, J. Unraveling the causes of diabetes. *Science* 2000; 296:686–9.

2. Sturm, R. The effects of obesity, smoking, and drinking on medical problems and costs. Obesity outranks both smoking and drinking in its deleterious effects on health and health costs. *Health Aff* (Millwood) 2002; 21:245–53.

3. For further information see Lyon, C.J., Law, R.E., and Hsueh, W.A. Minireview: adiposity, inflammation, and atherogenesis. *Endocrinology* Jun 2003; 144(6):2195–200. Guerre-Millo, M. Adipose tissue hormones. *J Endocrinol Invest.* Nov 2002; 25(10):855–61. Abel, E.D., Peroni, O., Kim, J.K., et al. Adipose-selective targeting of the *GLUT4* gene impairs insulin action in muscle and liver. *Nature* 2001; 409:729–33.

4. For reviews see Bray, G.A. The underlying basis for obesity: relationship to cancer. *J Nutr* Nov 2002; 132(11 Suppl):3451S–3455S. Kaaks, R., Lukanova, A., and Kurzer, M.S. Obesity, endogenous hormones, and endometrial cancer risk: a systematic review. *Cancer Epidemiol Biomarkers Prev.* Dec 2002; 11(12):1531–43.

5. The American Federation for Aging Research, one of the leading nonprofit funding organizations for aging research maintains an excellent website information center on biomarkers of aging at www.infoaging.org/b-biomark-home.html. For an outstanding review of research on aging-related biomarkers, see the International Longevity Center (ILC) report at www.ilcusa.org. The ILC is a nonprofit research institute headed by former National Institute on Aging director Dr. Robert Butler. Recently the ILC published the proceedings of a comprehensive workshop on biomarkers of aging. Butler, R., ed. Biomarkers of aging: from primitive organisms to man. International Longevity Center, New York, 2001. See also Ingram, D., Nakamura, E., Smucny, D., et al. Strategy for identifying biomarkers of aging in long-lived species. *Exp Gerontol* 2001; 36(7):1025–34.

6. Willcox, B.J., Willcox, D.C., and Suzuki, M. Defining cardiovascular health in a large population-based study of exceptional survivors. *Circulation* 2003. In press.

7. Akisaka, M., Suzuki, M., and Inoko, H. Molecular genetic studies on DNA polymorphism of the HLA class II genes associated with human longevity. *Tissue Antigens* 1997; 50:489–93. Takata, H., Suzuki, M., Ishii, T., et al. Influence of major histocompatibility complex region genes on human longevity among Okinawan-Japanese centenarians and nonagenarians. *Lancet* Oct 1987; 2(8563):824–6.

8. For an excellent review, see Rankinen, T., Perusse, L., Weisnagel, S., et al. The human obesity gene map: the 2001 update. *Obes Res* 2002; 10:196–243. Also see Pi-Sunyer, X. A clinical view of the obesity problem. *Science* Feb 2003; 299(5608):859–60. Niswender, K.D., and Schwartz, M.W. Insulin and leptin revisited: adiposity signals with overlapping physiological and intracellular signaling capabilities. *Front Neuroendocrinol* Jan 2003; 24(1):1–10. Schrauwen, P., Walder, K., and Ravussin, E. Human uncoupling proteins and obesity. *Obes Res.* Jan 1999; 7(1):97–105.

9. Tschop, M., and Heiman, M.L. Rodent obesity models: an overview. *Exp Clin Endocrinol Diabetes.* 2001; 109(6):307–19.

10. Mokdad, A.H., Serdula, M.K., Dietz, W.H., et al. The spread of the obesity epidemic in the United States, 1991–1998. *JAMA* 1999; 282:1519–22.

11. Rankinen, T., Perusse, L., Weisnagel, S.J., et al. The human obesity gene map: the 2001 update. *Obes Res.* March 2002; 10(3):196–243.

12. Atwood, L., Heard-Costa, N., Cupples, A., et al. Genome-wide linkage analysis of body mass index across 28 years of the Framingham Heart Study. *Am J Hum Genet* 2002; 71:1044–50. Fabsitz, R.R., Nam, J.M., Gart, J., et al. Invited anniversary review: HLA associated diseases. *Hum Immunol* 1997; 53:1–11. HLA associations with obesity. Fabsitz, R.R., Nam, J.M., Gart, J., et al. *Hum Hered* 1989; 39(3):156–64.

13. Mizushima, S., Moriguchi, E.H., Nakada, Y., et al. The relationship of dietary factors to cardiovascular diseases among Japanese in Okinawa and Japanese immigrants, originally from Okinawa, in Brazil. *Hypertens Res* 1992; 15:45–55. Moriguchi, Y. Japanese centenarians living outside Japan. In Tauchi, H., Sato, T., and Watanabe, T., eds. *Japanese Centenarians: Medical Research for the Final Stages of Human Aging.* Aichi, Japan: Institute for Medical Science of Aging, 1999, 85–94.

14. *Okinawa Centenarian Study,* Anthropometric Database, 2003; Japan Ministry of Health, Labor and Welfare 2000. Statistics and Information Division.

15. Arakaki, H., and Sho, H. Nutritional survey on Kumejima. *The Science Bulletin of the Division of Agriculture, Home Economics & Engineering* 1962; 9:327–34. Okinawa, Japan: University of the Ryukyus.

16. Todoriki, H., Willcox, D.C., Kinjo, Y., et al. The nutrition transition in postwar Okinawa: changes in body weight and fat intake. The IEA XVI World Congress of Epidemiology, Montreal, Canada, August, 2002. *Okinawa Centenarian Study,* Anthropometric Database, 2003. Japan Ministry of Health, Labor and Welfare 2000. *Okinawa Prefectural Health and Nutrition Survey,* 1998. Statistics and Information Division, Okinawa, Japan: Prefecture of Okinawa, 2000.

17. *Okinawa Centenarian Study,* Nutrition Database; U.S. National Archives. 1949. *Prefectural Health and Nutrition Survey for Year 1998.* Department of Health and Welfare, Okinawa, Japan: Prefecture of Okinawa, 2000.

18. Chopra, M., Galbraith, S., and Darnton-Hill, I. A global response to a global problem: the epidemic of overnutrition. *Bull World Health Organ* 2002; 80:952–8.

19. For one of the most comprehensive reviews on diet and obesity, particularly energy efficiency and macronutrient balance, see Jequier, E., and Tappy, L. Regulation of body weight in humans. *Physiological Rev* 1999; 79:451–80. For an excellent recent review of the life-shortening health risks of obesity see Fontaine, K.R., Redden, D.T., Wang, C., et al. Years of life lost due to obesity. *JAMA* 2003; 289:187–93.

20. Fermi, E. Thermodynamics. In *Lectures at Columbia University,* 1937. New York: Dover Publications; 1956, ix.

21. For an excellent review of set point theory, see Weinsier, R.L. Etiology of obesity: methodological examination of the set-point theory. *J Parenter Enteral Nutr* 2001; 25:103–10. Weinsier, R.L., Nagy, T.R., Hunter, G.R., et al. Do adaptive changes in metabolic rate favor weight regain in weight-reduced individuals? An examination of the set-point theory. *Am J Clin Nutr* 2001; 73:655–8.

22. Hill, J.M., Wyatt, H.R., Reed, G.W., and Peters, J.C. Obesity and the environment: where do we go from here? *Science* 2003; 299:853–5.

23. Yanovski, S.Z., and Yanovski, J.A. Obesity. *N Engl J Med.* Feb 2002; 346(8):591–602.

24. Merry, B.J. Molecular mechanisms linking calorie restriction and longevity. *Int J Biochem Cell Biol* 2002; 34:1340–54. Schrauwen, P., Walder, K., and Ravussin, E. Human uncoupling proteins and obesity. *Obes Res.* Jan 1999; 7(1):97–105.

25. Kim, J.D., McCarter, R.J., and Yu, B.P. Influence of age, exercise, and dietary restriction on oxidative stress in rats. *Aging* (Milano) Apr 1996; 8(2):123–9.

26. CDC/NCHS Press Office. HHS issues new report on American's overall physical activity levels: one in five (17%) adults engage in high level of activity, but one in four are generally inactive. News Release, United States Department of Health and Human Services, May 14, 2003.

27. Trichopoulou, A., and Lagiou, P. Healthy traditional Mediterranean diet: an expression of culture, history, and lifestyle. *Nutr Rev* 1997; 55:383–9.

28. Dietary fat consensus statements [Consensus Development Conference review]. *Am J Med* 2002; 113 Suppl 9B:5S–8S.

29. Dr. Atkins had a long and colorful history in the fad diet world. He had somewhat of a metamorphosis himself when he finally accepted that there are healthy forms of fat and carbohydrate. He reinvented his nefarious original diet (*Dr. Atkins' Diet Revolution: The High Calorie Way to Stay Thin Forever,* Bantam Books, New York, 1972) which proclaimed carbohydrates as the root cause of obesity and encouraged readers to eat all the fat and protein they wished. The new diet limits the amount of bacon and other foods high in saturated fat followers can eat. He encourages more consumption of healthy fats, such as monounsaturated and omega–3 fat and also incorporates low glycemic index carbs based on Dr. Jenkins' work and called them Atkins' carbs. The new Atkins Diet is still far too high in protein and saturated fat but it's a vast improvement on the original Atkins Diet and there are certainly healthier ways to lose weight, eating healthy foods and preserving your muscle tissue at the same time. See Atkins, R.C. *Dr. Atkins' New Diet Revolution,* New York: Avon Books, 2001. Atkins' new diet was gaining popularity because it induces an early weight loss (about half of it fat and the rest water and lean muscle) so the early "success" helps motivate people to stick to the diet. But the diet really began to take off when popular health writer Gary Taubes wrote a *New York Times Magazine* article entitled "What If It's All Been a Big Fat Lie." (July 7, 2002, p. 8). In the article Taubes does a serious job of misquoting a number of key researchers in the obesity field and generates a lot of controversy as he tries to support the diet based on rather flimsy evidence. A critical review of his article appears in Liebman, B. Big fat lies: the truth about the Atkins Diet. *Nutrition Action Health Letter* Nov 2002. For the view of the American Heart Association see Jeor, S.T., Howard, B.V., Prewitt, T.E., et al. Dietary protein and weight reduction: a statement for healthcare professionals from the Nutrition Committee of the Council on Nutrition, Physical Activity, and Metabolism of the American Heart Association. *Circulation* 2001; 104:1869–74.

30. Lin, L., Martin, R., Schaffhauser, A.O., and York, D.A. Acute changes in the response to peripheral leptin with alteration in the diet composition. *Am J Physiol Regul Integr Comp Physiol* Feb 2001; 280(2):R504–9. Madiehe, A.M., Schaffhauser, A.O., Braymer, D.H., et al. Differential expression of leptin receptor in high- and low-fat-fed Osborne-Mendel and S5B/Pl rats. *Obes Res* Sep 2000; 8(6):467–74. Lin, L., Martin, R., Schaffhauser, O, and York, D.A. Acute changes in the response to peripheral leptin with alteration in the diet composition. *Am J Physiol* 2001; 280:R504–R509.

31. Recently two important research studies on low-carb diets were published in the *New England Journal of Medicine* which the media pounced upon as evidence that the diet "works" (Samaha, F.F., Iqbal, N., Seshadri, P., et al. A low-carbohydrate as compared with a low-fat diet in severe obesity. *N Engl J Med* 2003; 348(21):2074–81. Foster, G.D., Wyatt, H.R., Hill, J.O., et al. A randomized trial of a low-carbohydrate diet for obesity. *N Engl J Med* 2003; 348(21):2082–90). The diets showed that people who were given copies of the new Atkins Diet rather than simply told to

eat a low-fat diet lost more weight on the Atkins Diet in the first six months but were no better off at the end of a year on either diet. The studies did not record caloric intake or tell us what kind of weight was lost. The media took this as support for the Atkins Diet. What this demonstrates is that some people find it easier to cut out carbs than to cut out fat. Considering the dietary advice on the low-carb diet was to cut out almost all carbs, which drops caloric intake by about 50 percent (carbs form about half our diet) versus the low-fat advice to keep fat below 30 percent of calories (it is about 33 percent at present) which drops caloric intake by less than 10 percent its no wonder more weight was lost initially on the new Atkins Diet. The low-carb advice results in a much lower intake of calories than low-fat advice and extra water/lean muscle loss so it's not surprising that the low-carb dieters initially lost more weight. Any diet that lowers calories will cause you to lose weight. Keeping the weight off is the challenge.

32. Peters, J.C. Dietary fat and body weight control. *Lipids* Feb 2003; 38(2):123–7. Jequier, E., and Tappy, L. Regulation of body weight in humans. *Physiological Rev* 1999; 79:451–80.

33. Flatt, J.P. Importance of nutrient balance in body weight regulation. *Diabetes Metab Rev* 1988; 4:571–81.

34. Flatt, J.P. The difference in the storage capacities for carbohydrate and for fat and its implications in the regulation of body weight. *Ann NY Acad Sci* 1987; 499:104–23. Flatt, J.P. The biochemistry of energy expenditure. In Bray, G., ed. *Recent advances in obesity research II*. London: Libbey, 1980, pp. 211–18. Flatt, J., Ravussin, E., Acheson, K., and Jequier, E. Effects of dietary fat on post-prandial substrate oxidation and carbohydrate and fat balance. *J Clin Invest* 1985; 76:1019–24. Schutz, Y., Flatt, J.P., and Jequier, E. Failure of dietary fat intake to promote fat oxidation: a factor favoring the development of obesity. *Am J Clin Nutr* 1989; 50:307–14.

35. For a good recent review see Augustin, L.S., Faranceschi, S., Jenkins, D.J., et al. Glycemic index in chronic disease: a review. *Eur J Clin Nutr* 2002; 56:1049–71.

36. This is a controversial topic about which exercise physiologists, who actually measure what is happening in the body, are often at odds with nutritional epidemiologists, who study eating habits of large populations. It's important to look at what is happening in the laboratory as well as in the field to come to evidence-based conclusions. The following scientific studies actually measured the amounts and type of fat that are formed with carbohydrate overfeeding. Stuffing people with carbs did not result in carbs being converted to fat but when in excess of total caloric needs (i.e., positive energy balance) does signal the body to store dietary fat as fat. A physiologist may interpret this as fat making you fat and an epidemiologist may see this as carbs making you fat. The lesson here is that eating too many calories of any source causes the body to store fat so any macronutrient consumed in excess will make you fat whether it's carbs, fat, or protein. Remember that the Okinawan traditional diet back in the 1950s had up to 90 percent of its calories derived from carbs (compared to about 45 percent in the United States at present) and it was pretty rare to find an obese Okinawan in those days. Aarsland, A., Chinkes, D., and Wolfe, R.R. Hepatic and whole-body fat synthesis in humans during carbohydrate overfeeding. *Am J Clin Nutr* 1997; 65:1774–82. Acheson, K., Schutz, Y., Bessard, T., et al. Glycogen storage capacity and de novo lipogenesis during massive carbohydrate overfeeding in man. *Am J Clin Nutr* 1988; 48:240–47.

37. These important papers show the risk for insulin resistance, part of the pathway to type-2 diabetes, is facilitated by amylopectin starch, which is present in higher quantities in high GI foods. Hallfrisch, J., and Behall, K.M. Mechanisms of the effects of grains on insulin and glucose responses. *J Am Coll Nutr* 2000; 19(3 Suppl):320S–325S. Higgins, J.A., Brand Miller, J.C., and Denyer, G.S. Development of insulin resistance in the rat is dependent on the rate of glucose absorption from the diet. *J Nutr* 1996; 126:596–602. Wiseman, C.E., Higgins, J.A., Denyer, G.S., and Miller, J.C. Amylopectin starch induces nonreversible insulin resistance in rats. *J Nutr* 1996; 126:410–5.

38. Carbohydrates seem to be the new macronutrient villain, which is quite ironic since "carbohydrate phobia" is loosely based on the carbohydrate research of Dr. David Jenkins and his research group at the University of Toronto, where my brother and I received part of our training in the

early 1990s. Dr. Jenkins is an expert in dietary fiber and quite a fan of a high-carbohydrate diet, provided those carbs are of the low Glycemic Index (GI) variety. He is well known for developing the Glycemic Index—the tool by which the body's glucose response to carbohydrate is measured, which has implications for insulin levels. Dr. Jenkins' research follows the tradition of a long line of carbohydrate-related research at the University of Toronto and Oxford University. The University of Toronto work on the health effects of carbohydrates began in the 1920s and led to the 1923 Nobel prize in Physiology/Medicine awarded to Frederick Banting, C.H. Best, and J.J.R. Macleod for the discovery of insulin, the hormone that packs glucose, the simplest carbohydrate, into the body's cells. Another milestone was reached when a Nobel prize was awarded to Dr. Jenkins' research supervisor at Oxford University, Sir Hans Krebs, for discovering how carbohydrates are converted into energy during the citric acid cycle. The tradition continued with Dr. Jenkins' and Dr. Tom Wolever's development of the Glycemic Index after an elegant series of experiments that began at Oxford University in the 1960s and continued at the University of Toronto in the 1970s. These experiments were published over the next decade in a landmark collection of scientific papers in *The Lancet* and *Nature*. The classic scientific paper that presented the Glycemic Index to the scientific community was published in the *American Journal of Clinical Nutrition* in 1981. See Jenkins, D.J.A., et al. Glycemic index of foods: a physiological basis of carbohydrate exchange. *Am J Clin Nutr* 1981; 34:362–66.

39. Roth, G.S., Lane, M.A., Ingram, D.K., et al. Biomarkers of caloric restriction may predict longevity in humans. *Science* 2002; 297:811.

40. Holt, S.H., Miller, J.C., and Petocz, P. An insulin index of foods: the insulin demand generated by 1000-kj portions of common foods. *Am J Clin Nutr* 1997; 66:1264–76.

41. Koh-Banerjee, P., and Rimm, E.B. Whole grain consumption and weight gain: a review of the epidemiological evidence, potential mechanisms and opportunities for future research. *Proc Nutr Soc* Feb 2003; 62(1):25–9.

42. Pelkman, C.L. Effects of the glycemic index of foods on serum concentrations of high-density lipoprotein cholesterol and triglycerides. *Curr Atheroscler Rep* 2001; 3:456–61.

43. Schwarz, J.-M., Neese, R.A., Turner, S., et al. Short-term alterations in carbohydrate energy intake in humans. *J Clin Invest* 1995; 96:2735–43.

44. Vuksan, V., Jenkins, D.J., Spadafora, P., et al. Konjac-mannan (glucomannan) improves glycemia and other associated risk factors for coronary heart disease in type 2 diabetes. A randomized controlled metabolic trial. *Diabetes Care* 1999; 22:913–9. Chen, H.L., Sheu, W.H., Tai, T.S., et al. Konjac supplement alleviated hypercholesterolemia and hyperglycemia in type 2 diabetic subjects—a randomized double-blind trial. *J Am Coll Nutr* 2003; 22:36–42. Walsh, D.E., Yaghoubian, V., and Behforooz, A. Effect of glucomannan on obese patients: a clinical study. *Int J Obes* 1984; 8:289–93.

45. Recommending a particular percentage of the diet as protein is both difficult and controversial since scientists don't know precisely what happens to humans maintained on very high-protein intake for extended periods. What we do know comes from animal experiments which show that restriction of particular amino acids can lead to a CR-like lifespan increase in rodents, possibly by lowering homocysteine levels. Limited experiments in rodents show that higher than 30 percent of the diet as protein for extended periods increases risk for certain cancers and kidney disease and mildly increases heart disease. In humans we know that very low-protein intakes can lead to disease *(kwashiorkor)* and very high intakes mean our kidneys must work overtime to clear the excess uric acid and other nitrogenous waste products that accumulate from protein breakdown. Too much protein causes an acid load on the body that must be buffered with calcium so can lead to osteoporosis in susceptible populations. We also know that too much can lead to uric acid–type kidney stones, gout, and uric acid deposits in our joints and tissues that cause aches and pains. Protein restriction (but not to deficiency levels) in humans with kidney disease can make the kidneys last significantly longer than they would otherwise. On the positive side higher intake of protein has been associated with lower blood pressure and, if you cut out high–GI carbs and replace them with protein, better triglyceride levels and lower risk for cardiovascular disease. Particularly

impressive is the ability of soy protein to improve blood lipid levels and cardiovascular risk. Finally, getting a variety of amino acids may lower stroke risk. And for dieters we know that protein tends to dull the appetite more than carb or fat. The final point is that in healthy people our kidneys are quite efficient at ridding us of excess protein. Thus the most sage advice we can give is that your percentage depends on your unique health needs and how many calories you need. If you are trying to lose body fat, then cut your calories and increase your physical activity to maintain a set level (0.36 grams/pound body weight) based on your individual requirements. The National Academy of Sciences recommends between 10 and 35 percent of your diet come from protein and that appears to be consistent with what we have seen in our studies of the Okinawans, who have ranged from a low of 8 percent (traditional diet) to a high of 20 percent (current diet of the elders). Bottom line: Plant protein appears healthier than animal protein, get your minimum level whether dieting or not, and don't overdo it. Eating mostly a plant-based diet with lean sources of protein will keep you in the safety zone—an Atkins Diet will not. See Lupton, J.R. Opening Statement. In Food and Nutrition Board, Institute of Medicine, eds. *Dietary reference intakes for energy, carbohydrate, fiber, fat, fatty acids, cholesterol, protein, and amino acids (macronutrients)*. Washington: National Academy of Sciences 2002. Bravata, D., Sanders, L., Huang, J., et al. Efficacy and safety of low-carbohydrate diets: a systematic review. *JAMA* 2003; 289:1837–50; and notes 46–58 for further reading.

46. Eisenstein, J., Roberts, S.B., Dallal, G., and Saltzman, E. High-protein weight-loss diets: are they safe and do they work? A review of the experimental and epidemiologic data. *Nutr Rev* 2002; 60:189–200.

47. Layman, D.K., Boileau, R.A., Erickson, D.J., et al. A reduced ratio of dietary carbohydrate to protein improves body composition and blood lipid profiles during weight loss in adult women. *J Nutr* 2003; 133:411–7.

48. For a good review of recent research and current thinking on protein and cardiovascular risk, see Appel, L.J. The effects of protein intake on blood pressure and cardiovascular disease. *Curr Opin Lipidol* Feb 2003; 14(1):55–9. For recent research on amino acid restriction and longevity see Zimmerman, J.A., Malloy, V., Krajcik, R., and Orentreich, N. Nutritional control of aging. *Exper Gerontol* 2003; 38:47–52. For studies of dementia risk and homocysteine see Leboeuf, R. Homocysteine and Alzheimer's disease. *J Am Diet Assoc* 2003; 103:304–7. Mattson, MP. Will caloric restriction and folate protect against AD and PD? *Neurology* 2003;60:690–5.

49. A study of subjects who ate meat as their main protein source showed that they were nearly three times as likely to become demented as their vegetarian counterparts. See Giem, P., Beeson, W.L., and Fraser, G.E. The incidence of dementia and intake of animal products: preliminary findings from the Adventist Health Study. *Neuroepidemiology* 1993; 12:28–36. Another recent study showed that subjects who adopted a vegan diet had their homocysteine levels drop between 13 percent and 20 percent in just one week. See DeRose, D.J., Charles-Marcel, Z.L., Jamison, J.M., et al. Vegan diet-based lifestyle program rapidly lowers homocysteine levels. *Prev Med* 2000; 30:225–33.

50. The Japanese group in this study consisted of Okinawans only and the study showed that their low homocysteine levels were highly correlated with their low risk for cardiovascular death (coronary heat disease and stroke). See Alfthan, G., Aro, A., and Gey, K.F. Plasma homocysteine and cardiovascular disease mortality. *Lancet* 1997; 349:397.

51. Astrup, A., Astrup, A., Buemann, B., et al. Low-fat diets and energy balance: how does the evidence stand in 2002? *Proc Nutr Soc* 2002; 61:299–309.

52. Samaha, F.F., Iqbal, N., Seshadri, P., et al. A low-carbohydrate as compared with a low-fat diet in severe obesity. *N Engl J Med* 2003; 348:2074–81.

53. Bravata, D., Sanders, L., Huang, J., et al. Efficacy and safety of low-carbohydrate diets: a systematic review. *JAMA* 2003; 289:1837–50. Knight, E.L., Stampfer, M.J., Hankinson, S.E., et al. The impact of protein intake on renal function decline in women with normal renal function or mild renal insufficiency. *Ann Intern Med* 2003; 138:460–67.

54. Ross, M.H., and Bras, G. Dietary preference and diseases of age. *Nature* 1974; 250:263–5.

55. Franz, M.J., Bantle, J.P., Beebe, C.A., et al. Evidence-based nutrition principles and recommendations for the treatment and prevention of diabetes and related complications. *Diabetes Care* 2001; 25:148–91.

56. Atkins, R.C. *Dr. Atkins' New Diet Revolution.* New York: Avon Books, 2001. Eades, M.R., and Eades, M.D. *Protein Power: The High-Protein/Low-Carbohydrate Way to Lose Weight, Feel Fit, and Boost Your Health in Just Weeks!* New York: Bantam Books, 1997. Steward, H.L., Bethea, M.C., Andrews, S.S.M., and Balart, L.A. *Sugar Busters! Cut Sugar to Trim Fat.* New York: Ballantine Books, 1998. Sears, B. *The Zone: Revolutionary Life Plan to Put Your Body in Total Balance for Permanent Weight Loss.* New York: Harper Collins, 1995.

57. For the scientist see Eisenstein, J., Roberts, S.B., Dallal, G., and Saltzman, E. High-protein weight-loss diets: are they safe and do they work? A review of the experimental and epidemiologic data. *Nutr Rev.* Jul 2002; 60(7 Pt 1):189–200. For the scientist and nonscientist alike see American Kidney Fund (AKF) website. "AKF warns about impact of high-protein diets on kidney health." Newsroom American Kidney Fund. 2002. www.akfinc.org/AboutAKF/AboutAKF.htm. For an excellent review for the nonscientist see Lee, T.H. Ask the doctor. In early July, the *New York Times Magazine* published an article that had good things to say about the Atkins high-protein diet. It also claimed that low-fat diets might be harmful. This shocked many of us who have been following a low-fat diet to reduce our risk from heart disease. Have we been barking up the wrong tree all these years? *Harv Health Lett* Nov 2002; 13(3):8.

58. See the excellent workshop report issued by the International Longevity Center: Biomarkers of aging: from primitive organisms to man. *Workshop report.* International Longevity Center–USA. 2000.

59. Willcox, B.J., Willcox, D.C., and Suzuki, M. Defining cardiovascular health in a large population-based study of exceptional survivors. *Circulation Online* June 2003.

60. Suzuki, M. Endocrine function of centenarians. In Tauchi, H., Sato, T., and Watanabe, T., eds. *Japanese centenarians: medical research for the final stages of human aging.* Aichi, Japan: Institute for Medical Science of Aging, 1999, pp. 101–10.

61. Suzuki, M., Akisaka, M., and Inayama, S. Medicobiological studies on centenarians in Okinawa, measuring plasma lipid peroxide, proline, and plasma and intracellular tocopherol. In Beregi, E., Gergely, I.A., Rajczi, K., eds. Recent advances in aging science. *Proceedings of the 15th Congress of International Association of Gerontology;* Bologna, Italy. 1993; 1505–9.

62. Mortality data from the US National Center for Health Statistics: Centers for Disease Control and Prevention, U.S. Department of Health and Human Services. See www.cdc.gov/nchs/about/major/dvs/mortdata.

63. National Heart, Lung and Blood Institute. *Seventh report of the joint national committee on prevention, detection, evaluation, and treatment of high blood pressure (JNC 7).* Bethesda, MD: National Heart, Lung and Blood Institute; 2003.

64. Osler, W., McGovern, J.P., Hinohara, S., and Niki, H. Osler's "a way of life" and other addresses: with commentary and annotations. Durham, N.C.: Duke University Press, 2001.

65. Kris-Etherton, P.M., Hecker, K.D., Bonanome, A., et al. Bioactive compounds in foods: their role in the prevention of cardiovascular disease and cancer. *Am J Med* 2002; 113 Suppl 9B:71S–88S. Lampe, J.W. Isoflavonoid and lignan phytoestrogens as dietary biomarkers. *J Nutr* Mar 2003; 133 Suppl 3:956S–964S.

66. Jenkins, D.J.A., Jenkins, A.L., Kendall, C.W.C., et al. The garden of Eden: implications for cardiovascular disease prevention. *Asia Pacific J Clin Nutr* 2000; 9:S1. Jenkins, D.J., Kendall, C.W., Faulkner, D., et al. A dietary portfolio approach to cholesterol reduction: combined effects of plant sterols, vegetable proteins, and viscous fibers in hypercholesterolemia. *Metabolism* Dec 2002; 51(12):1596–604.

67. Walford, R.L., Mock, D., Verdery, R., and MacCallum, T. Calorie restriction in biosphere 2: alterations in physiologic, hematologic, hormonal, and biochemical parameters in humans restricted for a 2-year period. *J Gerontol A Biol Sci Med Sci* 2002; 57:B211–24.

68. Recent research by former colleagues at Harvard Medical School highlights the intimate link between maintaining low body-fat stores, which lead to lower insulin levels and longer lifespan. These researchers bred mice without insulin receptors in their fat cells and thus the mice were very lean and lived a very long time. See Bluher, M., Kahn, B.B., and Kahn, C.R. Extended longevity in mice lacking the insulin receptor in adipose tissue. *Science* 2003; 299:572–4.

69. Schumaker, S.A., Legault, C., Leon Thai, S., et al. Estrogen plus progestin and the incidence of dementia and mild cognitive impairment in postmenopausal women. *JAMA* 2003; 289:2651–62.

70. Mattison, J.A., Lane, M.A., Roth, G.S., and Ingram, D.K. Calorie restriction in rhesus monkeys. *Exp Gerontol* 2003; 38:35–46.

71. This figure represents males, but similar trends are seen in females. Willcox, B., Willcox, D.C., Suzuki, M. *The Okinawa centenarian study: highlights from a 25-year population-based study of exceptional survival.* Grand Rounds Lecture, Harvard Medical School, Division on Aging, Boston, Mass. March 2001. Data are adapted from Suzuki, M., Hirose, N. Endocrine function of centenarians. In Tauchi, H., Sato, T., Watanabe, T., eds. *Japanese centenarians: medical research for the final stages of human aging.* Aichi, Japan: Institute for Medical Science of Aging, Aichi Medical University, 1999. Greendale, G.A., Edelstein, S., and Barrett-Connor, E. Endogenous sex steroids and bone mineral density in older women and men: The Rancho Bernardo Study. *J Bone Mineral Res* 1997; 12:1833–43.

72. Lanaz, G., Bovina, C., D'Aurelio, M., et al. Role of mitochondria in oxidative stress and aging. *Ann NY Acad Sci* 2002; 959:199–213. Barja, G. Rate of generation of oxidative stress-related damage and animal longevity. *Free Radic Biol Med* 2002; 33:1167–72.

73. Meydani, M. Nutrition interventions in aging and age-associated disease. *Ann NY Acad Sci* 2001; 928:226–35.

74. Yamaza, H., Chiba, T., Higami, Y., and Shimokawa, I. Lifespan extension by caloric restriction: an aspect of energy metabolism. *Microsc Res Tech* 2002; 59:325–30.

75. Tortorella, C., Piazzolla, G., and Antonaci, S. Neutrophil oxidative metabolism in aged humans: a perspective. *Immunopharmacol Immunotoxicol* 2001; 23:565–72.

76. *Okinawa Centenarian Study,* Nutrition Database and chapter 1, note 26.

77. *Okinawa Centenarian Study,* Nutrition and Biochemical Databases.

78. Chung, H.Y., Kim, H.J., Kim, K.W., et al. Molecular inflammation hypothesis of aging based on the anti-aging mechanism of calorie restriction. *Microsc Res Tech* 2002; 59:264–72.

79. Ogura, C., Nakamoto, H., Uema, T., et al. Prevalence of senile dementia in Okinawa, Japan. *Int J Epidemiol* 1995; 24:373–80.

80. Yu, B.P., and Chung, H.Y. Stress resistance by caloric restriction for longevity. *Ann NY Acad Sci* 2001; 928:39–47. Leakey, J.E., Chen, S., Manjgaladze, M., et al. Role of glucocorticoids and "caloric stress" in modulating the effects of caloric restriction in rodents. *Ann NY Acad Sci* 1994; 719:171–94.

81. Longo, V.D., and Finch, C.E. Evolutionary medicine: from dwarf model systems to healthy centenarians? *Science* 2003; 299:1342–6.

82. Guzzetti, S., Costantino, G., and Fundaro, C. Systemic inflammation, atrial fibrillation, and cancer. *Circulation* 2002; 106:40;

83. Simopoulos, A.P. Omega–3 fatty acids in inflammation and autoimmune diseases. *J Am Coll Nutr* 2002; 21:495–505. Tapiero, H., Tew, K.D., Ba, G..N., and Mathe, G., Polyphenols: do they play a role in the prevention of human pathologies? *Biomed Pharmacother* 2002; 56:200–7. SoRelle, R. Inflammation-sensitive proteins: another ingredient in stroke? *Circulation* 2002; 105:9111. Lim, G.P., Chu, T., Yang, F., et al. The curry spice curcumin reduces oxidative damage and amyloid pathology in an Alzheimer transgenic mouse. *J Neurosci* Nov 2001; 21(21):8370–7. Chainani-Wu, N. Safety and anti-inflammatory activity of curcumin: a component of turmeric (Curcuma Longa). *J Altern Complement Med* Feb 2003; 9(1):161–8.

84. Pasanisi, F., Contaldo, F., de Simone, G., and Mancini, M. Benefits of sustained moderate weight loss in obesity. *Nutr Metab Cardiovasc Dis* 2001; 11:401–6.

CHAPTER 3. MAKING CALORIC DENSITY WORK FOR YOU

1. Duncan, K.H., Bacon, J.A., and Weinsier, R.L. The effects of high and low energy density diets on satiety, energy intake, and eating time of obese and nonobese subjects. *Am J Clin Nutr* 1983; 37:763–7. Poppitt, S.D. Energy density of diets and obesity. *International Journal of Obesity* 1995; 19:S20–6.
2. USDA and DHHS, 2000. Nutrition and your health: dietary guidelines for Americans. Fifth Edition. *Home and Garden Bulletin No. 23.*
3. Roth, G.S., Lane, M.A., Ingram, D.K., et al. Biomarkers of caloric restriction may predict longevity in humans. *Science* 2002; 297:811.
4. Bray, G.A. Low-carbohydrate diets and realities of weight loss. *JAMA* 2003; 289:1853–5.
5. Samaha, F.F., Iqbal, N., Seshadri, P., et al. A low-carbohydrate as compared with a low-fat diet in severe obesity. *N Engl J Med* 2003; 348:2074–81.

CHAPTER 4. THE TEN OKINAWA DIET PRINCIPLES
FOR LIFELONG HEALTHY WEIGHT

1. Rolls, B.J., Fedoroff, I.C., Guthrie, J.F., and Laster, L.J. Effects of temperature and mode of presentation of juice on hunger, thirst and food intake in humans. *Appetite* 1990; 15:199–208.
2. Rolls, B.J., Castellanos, V.H., Halford, J.C., et al. Volume of food consumed affects satiety in men. *Am J Clin Nutr* 1998; 67(6):1170–7.
3. USDA and DHHS, 2000. Nutrition and your health: dietary guidelines for Americans. Fifth Edition. *Home and Garden Bulletin No. 23.*
4. Knight, E.L., Stampfer, M.J., Hankinson, S.E., et al. The impact of protein intake on renal function decline in women with normal renal function or mild renal insufficiency. *Ann Intern Med* 2003; 460–467.
5. Kennedy, E., Bowman, S., and Spence, J. Popular diets: correlation to health, nutrition and obesity. *J Am Dietetic Assoc* 2001; 101:411–20. Freedman, M., King, J., and Kennedy, E. Popular diets: a scientific review. *J Obes Res* 2001; 9 Suppl 1:1S–40S.
6. Denke, M. Metabolic effects of high-protein, low-carbohydrate diets. *Am J Card* 2001; 88:59–61.
7. Feskanich, D., Willett, W.C., Stampfer, M.J., and Colditz, G.A. Protein consumption and bone fractures in women. *Am J Epidemiol* 1996; 143:472–9.
8. A problem with animal protein is that animal foods tend to have higher methionine:cysteine ratio, which favors the production of homocysteine. High levels of homocysteine are associated with increased risk for cardiovascular disease, cancer (e.g., renal cell cancer) and dementia. See *USDA Nutrient Database for Standard Reference, Release 14.* U.S. Department of Agriculture, Washington, D.C.: 2000 for more information on methionine:cysteine levels in particular foods. Protein itself has also been linked to higher levels of insulin-like growth factor–1, a natural growth-promoting hormone linked to higher risk for breast, prostate, and colon cancers. Cooking methods for meat, for example, barbecuing red meat, have been linked to production of heterocyclic amines, which may increase risk for cancers of the GI tract, such as stomach or colon cancers. The news is not all bad, however, as replacing high-GI carbohydrates (e.g., white bread) with lean protein (e.g., omega–3 rich fish), may actually lower risk for certain cancers, because of lower production of insulin and its associated growth factors. For further reading see chapter 2, note 45.
9. Fraser, G.E., Sabate, J., Beeson, W.L., and Strahan, T.M. A possible protective effect of nut consumption on risk of coronary heart disease. The Adventist Health Study. *Arch Intern Med* 1992; 152(7):1416–24.
10. Ellsworth, J.L., Kushi, L.H., and Folsom, A.R. Frequent nut intake and risk of death from coronary heart disease and all causes in postmenopausal women: the Iowa Women's Health Study. *Nutr Metab Cardiovasc Dis* 2001; 11(6):372–7.

11. Hu, F.B., Stampfer, M.J., Manson, J.E., et al. Dietary protein and risk of ischemic heart disease in women. *Am J Clin Nutr* 1999; 70:221–7.

12. Curb, J.D., Wergowske, G., Dobbs, J.C., et al. Serum lipid effects of a high-monounsaturated fat diet based on macadamia nuts. *Arch Intern Med* 2000; 160(8):1154–8.

13. Lemaitre, R.N., King, I.B., Mozaffarian, D., et al. N–3 Polyunsaturated fatty acids, fatal ischemic heart disease, and nonfatal myocardial infarction in older adults: the Cardiovascular Health Study. *Am J Clin Nutr* 2003; 77(2):319–25. Rosenberg, I.H. Fish—food to calm the heart. *N Engl J Med* Apr 2002; 346(15):1102–3.

14. Simopoulos, A.P. Omega–3 fatty acids in health and disease and in growth and development. *Am J Clin Nutr* 1991; 54(3):438–63. Calder, P.C., Grimble, R.F. Polyunsaturated fatty acids, inflammation and immunity. *Eur J Clin Nutr* 2002; 56 Suppl 3:S14–9.

15. Kromhout, D. Diet and cardiovascular diseases. *J Nutr Health Aging* 2001; 5(3):144–9. Jacobs, D.R. Jr., and Murtaugh, M.A. It's more than an apple a day: an appropriately processed, plant-centered dietary pattern may be good for your health. *Am J Clin Nutr* 2000; 72:899–900. Willett, W.C. Diet and health: What should we eat? *Science* 1994; 264:532–37.

16. Okinawa Centenarian Study database. 2000. Willcox, B.J., Willcox, D.C., Suzuki, M., et al. Isoflavone intake in Japanese and Japanese-Canadians. *Am J Clin Nutr* 1995; 61:901.

17. Messina, M. Legumes and soybeans: overview of their nutritional profiles and health effects. *Am J Clin Nutr* 1999; 70(3):439S–50S.

18. Barnes, S. Rationale for the use of genistein containing soy matrices in chemo-prevention trials for breast and prostate cancer. *J Cellular Biochemistry* 1995; 22:181–87. Messina, M., and Barnes, S. The role of soy products in reducing risk of cancer. *J National Cancer Inst* 1991; 83:541–46. Messina, M.J., Persky, V., Setchell, K.D.R., et al. Soy intake and cancer risk: a review of the in vitro and in vivo data. *Nutr Cancer* 1994; 21(2):113–31. Moyad, M.A. Soy, disease prevention and prostate cancer. *Seminars in Urologic Oncology* 1999; 17(2):97–102. Erdman, J.W. Jr., Stillman, R.J., and Boileau, R.A. Provocative relation between soy and bone maintenance. Editorial. *Am J Clin Nutr* 2000; 72:679–80. Kris-Etherton, P.M., Hecker, K.D., Bonanome, A., et al. Bioactive compounds in foods: their role in the prevention of cardiovascular disease and cancer. *Am J Med* Dec 2002;113 Suppl 9B:71S–88S.

19. Bonita, R. Cardiovascular disease in Okinawa. *Lancet* 1993; 341(8854):1185.

20. Gallagher, R.P., and Kutynec, C.L. Diet, micronutrients and prostate cancer: a review of the evidence. *Can J Urol* 1997; 4(2 Supp 1):22–27.

21. Suzuki, M., Willcox, B.J., and Willcox, D.C. Implications from and for food cultures for cardiovascular disease: longevity. *Asia Pacific J Clin Nutr* 2001; 10:165–71.

22. Takeya, Y., Popper, J.S., Shimizu, Y., et al. Epidemiologic studies of coronary heart disease and stroke in Japanese men living in Japan, Hawaii and California: incidence of stroke in Japan and Hawaii. *Stroke* 1984; 15(1):15–23. Benfante, R. Studies of cardiovascular disease and cause-specific mortality trends in Japanese-American men living in Hawaii and risk factor comparisons with other Japanese populations in the Pacific region: a review. *Hum Biol* 1992; 64(6):791–805. Curb, J.D. and Kodama, K. The Ni-Hon-San Study. *J Epidemiol* 1996; 6(4 suppl.):S197–201. Mizushima, S., Moriguchi, E., Nakada, Y., et al. The relationship of dietary factors to cardiovascular diseases among Japanese in Okinawa and Japanese immigrants, originally from Okinawa, in Brazil. *Hyperten Res* 1992; 15:45–55.

23. Food labeling: Health claims; soy protein and coronary heart disease. Food and Drug Administration, HHS. Final rule. *Fed Regist* 64, no. 206 (October 26, 1999):57700–33.

24. Rolls, B.J. The role of energy density in the overconsumption of fat. *J Nutr* 2000; 130(2S Suppl):268S–271S. Blundell, J.E., and MacDiarmid, J.I. Fat as a risk factor for overconsumption: satiation, satiety, and patterns of eating. *J Am Diet Assoc* 1997; 97(7 Suppl):S63–69.

25. Ascherio, A. Epidemiologic studies on dietary fats and coronary heart disease. *Am J Med* 2002; 113 Suppl 9B:9S–12S. Jenkins, D.J.A., Kendall, C., and Marchie, A. Dose response of almonds on coronary heart disease risk factors: blood lipids, oxidized low-density lipoproteins, lipopro-

tein(a), homocysteine, and pulmonary nitric oxide. *Circulation* 2002; 106:1327–32. Hung, T., Sievenpiper, J.L., Marchie, A., et al. Fat versus carbohydrate in insulin resistance, obesity, diabetes and cardiovascular disease. *Curr Opin Clin Nutr Metab Care* Mar 2003; 6(2):165–76. Cholesterol and all-cause mortality in elderly people from the Honolulu Heart Program: a cohort study. *Lancet.* 2001; 358:351–5. For a good review for the nonscientist see Bad fats, good fats: new insights into diet and health. *Harv Mens Health Watch* 2000; 4:1–6.

26. McNamara, D.J. Dietary cholesterol and atherosclerosis. *Biochim Biophys Acta* 2000; 1529(1–3):310–20.

27. Gordon, T., and Kannel, W.B. Premature mortality from coronary heart disease. The Framingham Study. *JAMA* 1971; 215:1617–25. Castelli, W.P., Kannel, W.B., Castelli, W.P., et al. Serum cholesterol, lipoproteins, and the risk of coronary heart disease. The Framingham Study. *Ann Intern Med* 1971; 74(1):1–12. Castelli, W.P. Cholesterol and lipids in the risk of coronary artery disease—The Framingham Heart Study. *Can J Cardiol* 1988; 4:5A–10A.

28. Ornish, D., Brown, S.E., Scherwitz, L.W., et al. Can lifestyle changes reverse coronary heart disease? The lifestyle heart trial. *Lancet* 1990; 336(8708):129–33. Hu, F.B., and Willett, W.C. Optimal diets for prevention of coronary heart disease. *JAMA* 2002; 288(20):2569–78.

29. *Third report of the expert panel on detection, evaluation, and treatment of high blood cholesterol in adults (adult treatment panel III).* National Heart, Lung, and Blood Institute, National Cholesterol Education Program: 2002. National Cholesterol Education Program. *Second report of the expert panel on detection, evaluation, and treatment of high blood cholesterol in adults (adult treatment panel II).* National Heart, Lung, and Blood Institute. Publication NIH 1993; 93–3095.

30. Willcox, B.J., Willcox, D.C., and Suzuki, M. Defining cardiovascular health in a large population-based study of exceptional survivors. *Circulation* 2003. In press.

31. Zock, P.L., and Katan, M.B. Trans fatty acids, lipoproteins, and coronary risk. *Can J Physiol Pharmacol* 1997; 75(3):211–6. Lichtenstein, A.H. Dietary trans farry acids. *J Cardiopulm Rehabil* 2000; 20(3):143–6. Wilson, T.A., McIntyre, M., and Nicolosi, R.J. Trans fatty acids and cardiovascular risk. *Nutr Health Aging* 2001; 5(3):184–7. Lichtenstein, A.H., Ausman. L.M., Jalbert, S.M., and Schaefer, E.J. Effects of different forms of dietary hydrogenated fats on serum lipoprotein cholesterol levels. *N Engl J Med* 1999; 340(25):1933–40. Ascherio, A., Katan, M.B., Zock, P.L., et al. Trans fatty acids and coronary heart disease. *N Engl J Med* 1999; 340(25):1994–8.

32. Coulston, A.M. The role of dietary fats in plant-based diets. *Am J Clin Nutr* 1999; 70(3 Suppl):512S–515S. Nestel, P.J. Adulthood—prevention: Cardiovascular disease. *Med J Aust* 2002; 176(11 Suppl):S118–9.

33. Blackburn, G. Fats: the good, the bad, the trans. *Health News* July 1999; 5(9):1–2. Sinclair, H.M. Food fats, good and bad. *Br J Clin Pract* 1987; 41(12):1033–6.

34. Mensink, R.P., Zock, P.L., Kester, A.D., and Katan, M.B. Effects of dietary fatty acids and carbohydrates on the ratio of serum total to HDL cholesterol and on serum lipids and apolipoproteins: a meta-analysis of 60 controlled trials. *Am J Clin Nutr* 2003; 77(5):1146–55. Williams, C.M., Francis-Knapper, J.A., Webb, D., et al. Cholesterol reduction using manufactured foods high in monounsaturated fatty acids: a randomized crossover study. *Br J Nutr* 1999; 81(6):439–46. Kris-Etherton, P.M., Pearson, T.A., Wan, Y., et al. High-monounsaturated fatty acid diets lower both plasma cholesterol and triacylglycerol concentrations. *Am J Clin Nutr* 1999; 70(6):1009–15. Foley, M., Ball, M., Chisholm, A., et al. Should mono- or polyunsaturated fats replace saturated fat in the diet? *Eur J Clin Nutr* Jun 1992; 46(6):429–36. Katan, M.B., Zock, P.L., Mensink, R.P. Effects of fats and fatty acids on blood lipids in humans: an overview. *Am J Clin Nutr* 1994; 60(6 Suppl):1017S–1022S.

35. *American Heart Association Dietary Guidelines,* October 2000. For further information see www.americanheart.org. Lauber, R.P., and Sheard, N.F. American Heart Association. The American Heart Association Dietary Guidelines for 2000: a summary report. *Nutr Rev* 2001; 59(9):298–306.

36. Hu, F.B., and Willett, W.C. Diet and coronary heart disease: findings from the Nurses' Health Study and Health Professionals' Follow-up Study. *J Nutr Health Aging* 2001; 5(3):132–8.

37. Hu, F.B., Stampfer, M.J., Manson, J.E., et al. Dietary fat intake and the risk of coronary heart disease in women. *N Engl J Med* 1997; 337(21):1491–9.

38. Nakamura, T., Azuma, A., Kuribayashi, T., et al. Serum fatty acid levels, dietary style and coronary heart disease in three neighbouring areas in Japan: the Kumihama study. *Br J Nutr* 2003; 89(2):267–72. Bucher, H.C., Hengstler, P., Schindler, C., and Meier, G. N–3 polyunsaturated fatty acids in coronary heart disease: a meta-analysis of randomized controlled trials. *Am J Med* 2002; 112(4):298–304. O'Keefe, J.H., Jr., and Harris, W.S. From Inuit to implementation: Omega–3 fatty acids come of age. *Mayo Clinic Proc* 2000; 75(6):607–614. Marchioli, R., Barzi, F., Bomba, E., et al. Early protection against sudden death by n–3 polyunsaturated fatty acids after myocardial infarction: time-course analysis of the results of the Gruppo Italiano per lo Studio della Sopravvivenza nell'Infarto Miocardico (GISSI)-Prevenzione. *Circulation* 2002; 105(16):1897–903. Marchioli, R., Schweiger, C., Tavazzi, L., and Valagussa, F. Efficacy of n–3 polyunsaturated fatty acids after myocardial infarction: results of GISSI-Prevenzione trial. *Lipids* 2001; 36 Suppl:S119–26.

39. Dietary supplementation with n–3 polyunsaturated fatty acids and vitamin E after myocardial infarction: results of the GISSI-Prevenzione trial. *Lancet* 1999; 354:447–55.

40. Kris-Etherton, P.M., Harris, W.S., and Appel, L.J. Fish consumption, fish oil, omega–3 fatty acids, and cardiovascular disease. *Circulation* 2002; 106:2747–57.

41. Okinawa Centenarian Study, Nutrition Database; U.S. National Archives. 1949; Department of Ecology and Welfare. Prefectural Nutrition Survey for Year 1994. Okinawa, Japan: Prefecture of Okinawa: 1996.

42. Rose, D.P., Connolly, J.M., and Coleman, M. Effect of omega–3 fatty acids on the progression of metastases after the surgical excision of human breast cancer cell solid tumors growing in nude mice. *Clin Cancer Res* 1996; 2(10):1751–6. Cave, W.T. Jr. Dietary omega–3 polyunsaturated fats and breast cancer. *Nutrition* 1996; 12(1 Suppl):S39–42.

43. A recent large study of diet and breast cancer suggests saturated fat may be an important risk factor for breast cancer. This finding may have been previously overlooked by relying too heavily on food frequency questionnaires rather than food records (more accurate) to gauge fat intake in large research studies. See Are imprecise methods obscuring a relation between fat and breast cancer. *Lancet* 2003; 362(9379):212–14. Blackburn, G.L., Copeland, T., Khaodhiar, L., and Buckley, R.B. Diet and breast cancer. *J Womens Health (Larchmt)* 2003; 12(2):183–92. Huncharek, M., and Kupelnick, B. Dietary fat intake and risk of epithelial ovarian cancer: a meta-analysis of 6,689 subjects from 8 observational studies. *Nutr Cancer* 2001; 40(2):87–91. Newcomer, L.M., King, I.B., Wicklund, K.G., and Stanford, J.L. The association of fatty acids with prostate cancer risk. *Prostate* 2001; 47(4):262–8. Steinmaus, C.M., Nunez, S., and Smith, A.H. Diet and bladder cancer: a meta-analysis of six dietary variables. *Am J Epidemiol* 2000; 151(7):693–702.

44. Simonsen, N.R., Fernandez-Crehuet Navajas, J., Martin-Moreno, J.M., et al. Tissue stores of individual monounsaturated fatty acids and breast cancer: the EURAMIC study. European Community Multicenter Study on Antioxidants, Myocardial Infarction, and Breast Cancer. *Am J Clin Nutr* 1998; 68(1):134–41.

45. Giovannucci, E. Diet, body weight, and colorectal cancer: a summary of the epidemiologic evidence. *J Womens Health* (Larchmt) 2003; 12(2):173–82. Chiu, B.C., Ji, B.T., Dai, Q., et al. Dietary factors and risk of colon cancer in Shanghai, China. *Cancer Epidemiol Biomarkers Prev* 2003; 12(3):201–8.

46. Michaud, D.S., Augustsson, K., Rimm, E.B., et al. A prospective study on intake of animal products and risk of prostate cancer. *Cancer Causes Control* 2001; 12(6):557–67. Giovannucci, E., Rimm, E,B,, Colditz, G.A., et al. A prospective study of dietary fat and risk of prostate cancer. *J Natl Cancer Inst* 1993; 85(19):1571–9.

47. Tonstad, S., Strom, E.C., Bergei, C.S., et al. Serum cholesterol response to replacing butter with a new trans-free margarine in hypercholesterolemic subjects. *Nutr Metab Cardiovasc Dis* 2001;

11(5):320–6. Valenzuela, A., and Morgado, N. Trans fatty acid isomers in human health and in the food industry. *Biol Res* 1999; 32(4):273–87.

48. November 17, 1999 Federal Register Notice: Food labeling: trans fatty acids in nutrition labeling, nutrient content claims, and health claims; proposed rule. Scarbrough FE. Some Food and Drug Administration perspectives of fat and fatty acids. *Am J Clin Nutr.* 1997; 65(5 Suppl):1578S–1580S.

49. Hu, F.B., Stampfer, M.J., Rimm, E.B., et al. A prospective study of egg consumption and risk of cardiovascular disease in men and women. *JAMA* 1999; 281(15):1387–94.

50. Lewis, N.M., Seburg, S., and Flanagan, N.L. Enriched eggs as a source of N–3 polyunsaturated fatty acids for humans. *Poult Sci* 2000; 79(7):971–74.

51. Pereira, M.A., and Liu, S. Types of carbohydrates and risk of cardiovascular disease. *J Womens Health (Larchmt)* 2003; 12(2):115–22. Slavin, J. Why whole grains are protective: biological mechanisms. *Proc Nutr Soc* 2003; 62(1):129–34.

52. Wurtman, R.J., and Wurtman, J.J. Do carbohydrates affect food intake via neurotransmitter activity? *Appetite* 1988; 11 Suppl 1:42–7.

53. Felber, J.P., and Golay, A. Pathways from obesity to diabetes. *Int J Obes Relat Metab Disord* Sep 2002; 26 Suppl 2:S39–45.

54. Hu, F.B., Manson, J.E., Stampfer, M.J., et al. Diet, lifestyle, and the risk of type 2 diabetes mellitus in women. *N Engl J Med* 2001; 345(11):790–7. Reusch, J.E. Focus on insulin resistance in type 2 diabetes: therapeutic implications. *Diabetes Educ* 1998; 24(2):188–93. Bell, P.M. Dietary and lifestyle factors contributing to insulin resistance. *Proc Nutr Soc* 1997; 56(1B):263–72.

55. Wolever, T.M. The glycemic index. *World Rev Nutr Diet* 1990; 62:120–85. Foster-Powell, K., and Miller, J.B. International tables of glycemic index. *Am J Clin Nutr* 1995; 62(4):871S–890S. Truswell, A.S. Glycaemic index of foods. *Eur J Clin Nutr* 1992; 46 Suppl 2:S91–101.

56. Jenkins, D.J., Kendall, C.W., Augustin, L.S, et al. Glycemic index: overview of implications in health and disease. *Am J Clin Nutr* 2002; 76(1):266S–73S. Leeds, A.R. Glycemic index and heart disease. *Am J Clin Nutr* 2002; 76(1):286S–9S. Morris, K.L., and Zemel, M.B. Glycemic index, cardiovascular disease, and obesity. *Nutr Rev* 1999; 57(9 Pt 1):273–6. Ludwig, D.S. The glycemic index: physiological mechanisms relating to obesity, diabetes, and cardiovascular disease. *JAMA* 2002; 287(18):2414–23.

57. Holt, S.H., Miller, J.C., and Petocz, P. An insulin index of foods: the insulin demand generated by 1000-kj portions of common foods. *Am J Clin Nutr* 1997; 66:1264–76. Pi-Sunyer, F.X. Glycemic index and disease. *Am J Clin Nutr* 2002; 76(1):290S–8S.

58. Miller, J.B., Pang, E., and Bramall, L. Rice: a high or low glycemic index food? *Am J Clin Nutr* 1992; 56(6):1034–6.

59. Meydani, M. Effect of functional food ingredients: vitamin E modulation of cardiovascular diseases and immune status in the elderly. *Am J Clin Nutr* 2000; 71(6):1665S–8S; discussion 1674S–5S. Wargovich, M.J. Nutrition and cancer: the herbal revolution. *Curr Opin Clin Nutr Metab Care* 1999; 2(5):421–4. Liu, S., Lee, I.M., Ajani, U., et al. Intake of vegetables rich in carotenoids and risk of coronary heart disease in men: the Physicians' Health Study. *Int J Epidemiol* 2001; 30(1):130–5. Liu, S., Manson, J.E., Lee, I.M., et al. The effect of fruit and vegetable intake on risk for coronary heart disease. *Ann Intern Med* 2001; 134(12):1106–14. Van Duyn, M.A., and Pivonka, E. Overview of the health benefits of fruit and vegetable consumption for the dietetics professional: selected literature. *J Am Diet Assoc* 2000; 100(12):1511–21. Ford, E.S., and Mokdad, A.H. Fruit and vegetable consumption and diabetes mellitus incidence among U.S. adults. *Prev Med* 2001; 32(1):33–9.

60. Anderson, J.W., Smith, B.M., and Gustafson, N.J. Health benefits and practical aspects of high-fiber diets. *Am J Clin Nutr* 1994; 59(5):1242S–1247S.

61. Slavin, J. Why whole grains are protective: biological mechanisms. *Proc Nutr Soc* 2003; 62(1):129–34. Liu, S. Intake of refined carbohydrates and whole grain foods in relation to risk of type 2 diabetes mellitus and coronary heart disease. *J Am Coll Nutr* 2002; 21(4):298–306. McKeown, N.M., and Jacques, P. Whole grain intake and risk of ischemic stroke in women. *Nutr Rev* 2001; 59(5):149–52. Jacobs, D.R. Jr, Meyer, H.E., and Solvoll, K. Reduced mortality

among whole grain bread eaters in med and women in the Norwegian County Study. *Eur J Clin Nutr* 2001; 55(2):137–43. Jacobs, D.R., Pereira, M.A., Meyer, K.A., and Kushi, L.H. Fiber from whole grains, but not refined grains, is inversely associated with all-cause mortality in older women: the Iowa Women's Health Study. *J Am Coll Nutr* 2000; 19(3):326S–330S. Jacobs, D.R. Jr, Meyer, K.A., Kushi, L.H., and Folsom, A.R. Is whole grain intake associated with reduced total and cause-specific death rates in older women? The Iowa Women's Health Study. *Am J Public Health* 1999; 89(3):322–9. Slavin, J., Jacobs, D., and Marquart, L. Whole-grain consumption and chronic disease: protective mechanisms. *Nutr Cancer* 1997; 27(1):14–21. Anderson, J.W. Whole grains protect against atherosclerotic cardiovascular disease. *Proc Nutr Soc* 2003; 62(1):135–42. Slavin, J.L., Jacobs, D., Marquart, L., and Wierner, K. The role of whole grains in disease prevention. *J Am Diet Assoc* 2001; 101(7):780–5.

62. Soh, N.L., and Brand-Miller, J. The glycaemic index of potatoes: the effect of variety, cooking method and maturity. *Eur J Clin Nutr* 1999; 53(4):249–54. Bjorck, I, Liljeberg, H., and Ostman, E. Low glycaemic-index foods. *Br J Nutr* 2000; 83(1):S149–55.

63. Ferguson, L.R., Roberton, A.M., Watson, M.E., et al. The effects of a soluble-fibre polysaccharide on the adsorption of carcinogens to insoluble dietary fibres. *Chem Biol Interact* 1995; 95(3):245–55. Harris, P.J., Roberton, A.M., Watson, M.E., et al. The effects of soluble-fiber polysaccharides on the adsorption of a hydrophobic carcinogen to an insoluble dietary fiber. *Nutr Cancer* 1993; 19(1):43–54. McIntosh, G.H., Jorgensen. L., and Royle, P. The potential of an insoluble dietary fiber-rich source from barley to protect from DMH-induced intestinal tumors in rats. *Nutr Cancer* 1993; 19(2):213–21.

64. Jenkins, D.J., Kendall, C.W., Vuksan, V., et al. Soluble fiber intake at a dose approved by the U.S. Food and Drug Administration for a claim of health benefits: serum lipid risk factors for cardiovascular disease assessed in a randomized controlled crossover trial. *Am J Clin Nutr* 2002; 75(5):834–9. Jenkins, D.J., Wolever, T.M., Rao, A.V., et al. Effect on blood lipids of very high intakes of fiber in diets low in saturated fat and cholesterol. *N Engl J Med* 1993; 329(1):21–6. Moriceau, S., Besson, C., Levrat, M.A., et al. Cholesterol-lowering effects of guar gum: changes in bile acid pools and intestinal reabsorption. *Lipids* 2000; 35(4):437–44.

65. Aldoori, W., and Ryan-Harshman, M. Preventing diverticular disease. Review of recent evidence on high-fibre diets. *Can Fam Physician* 2002; 48:1632–7. Aldoori, W.H., Giovannucci, E.L., Rockett, H.R., et al. A prospective study of dietary fiber types and symptomatic diverticular disease in men. *J Nutr* 1998; 128(4):714–9.

66. Behall, K.M. Dietary fiber: nutritional lessons for macronutrient substitutes. *Ann N Y Acad Sci* 1997; 819:142–54. Dongowski, G., Huth, M., Gebhardt, E., and Flamme, W. Dietary fiber-rich barley products beneficially affect the intestinal tract of rats. *J Nutr* 2002; 132(12):3704–14. Chandalia, M., Garg, A., and Lutjohann, D. Beneficial effects of high dietary fiber intake in patients with type 2 diabetes mellitus. *N Engl J Med* 2000; 342(19):1392–8. Tabatabai, A., and Li. S. Dietary fiber and type 2 diabetes. *Clin Excell Nurse Pract* 2000; 4(5):272–6. Moriceau, S., Besson, C., Levrat, M.A., et al. Cholesterol-lowering effects of guar gum: changes in bile acid pools and intestinal reabsorption. *Lipids* 2000; 35(4):437–44.

67. Tabatabai, A., and Li, S. Dietary fiber and type 2 diabetes. *Clin Excell Nurse Pract* 2000; 4(5):272–6. Meyer, K.A., Kushi, L.H., Jacobs, D.R. Jr, et al. Carbohydrates, dietary fiber, and incident type 2 diabetes in older women. *Am J Clin Nutr* 2000; 71(4):921–30.

68. Yao, M., and Roberts, S.B. Dietary energy density and weight regulation. *Nutr Rev* 2001; 59(8):247–58. Howarth, N.C., Saltzman, E., and Roberts, S.B. Dietary fiber and weight regulation. *Nutr Rev* 2001; 59(5):129–39. Birketvedt, G.S., Aaseth, J., Florholmen, J.R., and Ryttig, K. Long-term effect of fibre supplement and reduced energy intake on body weight and blood lipids in overweight subjects. *Acta Medica* 2000; 43(4):129–32.

69. U.S. Department of Health and Human Services Public Health Service DHHS (PHS) 1988; Publication No. 88–50211. Marlett, J.A., McBurney, M.I., and Slavin, J.L.; American Dietetic Association. Position of the American Dietetic Association: health implications of dietary fiber.

J Am Diet Assoc 2002; 102(7):993–1000. *U.S. Dietary Guidelines for Americans. Nutrition and Your Health: Dietary Guidelines for Americans, 2000, 5th Edition,* USDA.

70. Rolls, B.J., Bell, E.A., and Thorwart, M.L. Water incorporated into a food but not served with a food decreases energy intake in lean women. *Am J Clin Nutr* 1999; 70(4):448–55.

71. Danbrot, M. *The New Cabbage Soup Diet.* New York: St. Martin's, 1997

72. Water Quality Association. *January Legislative Update, June 18, 2003.* International Headquarters & Laboratory, 4151 Naperville Road Lisle, IL 60532–1088 info@wga.org, www.wga.org.

73. Anti, M., Pignataro, G., and Armuzzi, A. Water supplementation enhances the effect of high-fiber diet on stool frequency and laxative consumption in adult patients with functional constipation. *Hepatogastroenterology* 1998; 45(21):727–32.

74. Borghi, L., Meschi, T., Schianchi, T., et al. Urine volume: stone risk factor and preventive measure. *Nephron* 1999; 81(1):31–7. Goldfarb, S. The role of diet in the pathogenesis and therapy of nephrolithiasis. *Endocrinol Metab Clin North Am* 1990; 19(4):805–20. Kleiner, S.M. Water: an essential but overlooked nutrient. *J Am Diet Assoc* 1999; 99(2):200–6.

75. Michaud, D.S., Spiegelman, D., and Clinton, S.K. Fluid intake and the risk of bladder cancer in men. *N Engl J Med* 1999; 340(18);1390–7. Kleiner, S.M.. Water: an essential but overlooked nutrient. *J Am Diet Assoc* 1999; 99(2):200–6.

76. Slattery, M.L., Caan, B.J., Anderson, K.E., and Potter, J.D. Intake of fluids and methylxanthine-containing beverages: association with colon cancer. *Int J Cancer* 1999; 81(2):199–204. Shannon, J., White, E., Shattuck, A.L., and Potter, J.D. Relationship of food groups and water intake to colon cancer risk. *Cancer Epidemiol Biomarkers Prev* 1996; 5(7):495–502.

77. National Research Council. Food and Nutrition Board. National Academy of Science. Washington, D.C.: National Academy Press, 1989. Valtin, H. "Drink at least eight glasses of water a day." Really? Is there scientific evidence for "8 x 8?" *Am J Physiol Regul Integr Comp Physiol* 2002; 283(5):R993–1004.

78. Asfar, S., Abdeen, S., Dashti, H., et al. Effect of green tea in the prevention and reversal of fasting-induced intestinal mucosal damage. *Nutrition* 2003; 19(6):536–40. Demeule, M., Michaud-Levesque, J., Annabi, B., et al. Green tea catechins as novel antitumor and antiangiogenic compounds. *Curr Med Chem Anti-Canc Agents* 2002; 2(4):441–63. McKay, D.L., and Blumberg, J.B. The role of tea in human health: an update. *J Am Coll Nutr* 2002; 21(1):1–13. Sueoka, N., Suganuma, M., Sueoka, E., et al. A new function of green tea: prevention of lifestyle-related diseases. *Ann N Y Acad Sci* 2001; 928:274–80. Kris-Etherton, P.M., and Keen, C.L. Evidence that the antioxidant flavonoids in tea and cocoa are beneficial for cardiovascular health. *Curr Opin Lipidol* 2002; 13(1):41–9.

79. Rylander, R., Bonevik, H., and Rubenowitz, E. Magnesium and calcium in drinking water and cardiovascular mortality. *Scand J Work Environ Health* 1991; 17(2):91–4. Yang, C.Y., and Hung, C.F. Colon cancer mortality and total hardness levels in Taiwan's drinking water. *Arch Environ Contam Toxicol* 1998; 35(1):148–51. Yang, C.Y., Chiu, H.F., Tsai, S.S., et al. Calcium and magnesium in drinking water and risk of death from prostate cancer. *J Toxicol Environ Health A* 2000; 60(1):17–26. Yang, C.Y., Chiu, H.F., Cheng, M.F., et al. Pancreatic cancer mortality and total hardness levels in Taiwan's drinking water. *J Toxicol Environ Health A* 1999; 56(5):361–9. Yang, C.Y., Chiu, H.F., Cheng, M.F., et al. Calcium and magnesium in drinking water and the risk of death from breast cancer. *J Toxicol Environ Health A* 2000; 60(4):231–41.

80. Akisaka, M., Asato, L., Chan, Y.C., et al. Energy and nutrient intakes of Okinawan centenarians. *J Nutr Sci Vitaminol* 1996; 42:241–48.

81. Willcox, B.J., Willcox, D.C., and Suzuki, M. *The Okinawa Program: How the World's Longest-Lived People Achieve Everlasting Health and How You Can Too.* New York: Clarkson Potter, 2001.

82. Leclerc, H., Schwartzbrod, L., and Dei-Cas, E. Microbial agents associated with waterborne diseases. *Crit Rev Microbiol* 2002; 28(4):371–409. Lee, S.H., Levy, D.A., Craun, G.F., et al. Surveillance for waterborne-disease outbreaks—United States, 1999–2000. *MMWR Surveill Summ* 2002; 51(8):1–47. Schvoerer, E., Bonnet, F., Dubois, V., et al. A hospital outbreak of gastroenteritis pos-

sibly related to the contamination of tap water by a small round structured virus. *J Hosp Infect* 1999; 43(2):149–54. Cunney, R.J., Costigan, P., McNamara, E.B., et al. Investigation of an outbreak of gastroenteritis caused by Norwalk-like virus, using solid phase immune electron microscopy. *J Hosp Infect* 2000; 44(2):113–8.

83. Dragland, S., Senoo, H., Wake, K., et al. Several culinary and medicinal herbs are important sources of dietary antioxidants. *J Nutr* 2003; 133(5):1286–90. Warren, C.P. Antioxidant effects of herbs. *Lancet* 1999; 353(9153):676. Craig, W.J.. Health-promoting properties of common herbs. *Am J Clin Nutr* 1999; 70(3):491S–499S.

84. Jenkins, D.J., Wolever, T.M., Vuksan, V., et al. Nibbling versus gorging: metabolic advantages of increased meal frequency. *N Engl J Med* 1989; 321(14):929–34.

85. Haines, P.S., Guilkey, D.K., and Popkin, B.M. Trends in breakfast consumption of U.S. adults between 1965–1991. *J Am Diet Assoc* 1996; 96(5):464–70.

86. Wyatt, H.R., Grunwald, G.K., Mosca, C.L., et al. Long-term weight loss and breakfast in subjects in the National Weight Control Registry. *Obes Res* 2002; 10(2):78–82.

87. Nielson, S.J., and Popkin, B.M. Patterns and trends in food portion sizes, 1977–1998. *JAMA* 2003; 289(4):450–3. Young, L.R., and Nestle, M. The contribution of expanding portion sizes to the US obesity epidemic. *Am J Public Health* 2002; 92(2):246–9.

88. Marmot, M.G. Alcohol and coronary heart disease. *Int J Epidemiol* 2001; 30(4):724–9. Thun, M.J., Peto, R., Lopez, A.D., et al. Alcohol consumption and mortality among middle-aged and elderly U.S. adults. *N Engl J Med* 1997; 337(24):1705–14. Kromhout, D., Menotti, A., Kesteloot, H., and Sans, S. Prevention of coronary heart disease by diet and lifestyle: evidence from prospective cross-cultural, cohort, and intervention studies. *Circulation* 2002; 105(7):893–8.

89. Criqui, M.H., and Ringel, B.L. Does diet or alcohol explain the French paradox? *Lancet* 1994; 344(8939–8940):1719–23.

90. World Health Organization (WHO). The World Health Report Geneva, 1997.

91. Huang, W.Y., Winn, D.M., Brown, L.M., et al. Alcohol concentration and risk of oral cancer in Puerto Rico. *Am J Epidemiol* 2003; 157(10)881–7.

92. Zhang, S., Hunter, D.J., Hankinson, S.E., et al. A prospective study of folate intake and the risk of breast cancer. *JAMA* 1999; 281(17):1632–7. La Vecchia, C., Negri, E., Pelucchi, C., and Franceschi, S. Dietary folate and colorectal cancer. *Int J Cancer* 2002; 102(5):545–7; Su, L.J., and Arab, L. Nutritional status of folate and colon cancer risk: evidence from NHANES I epidemiologic follow-up study. *Ann Epidemiol* 2001; 11(1):65–72. Giovannucci, E. Insulin, insulin-like growth factors and colon cancer: a review of the evidence. *J Nutr* 2001; 131(11 suppl.):3109S–20S.

93. van de Berg, H., van der Gaag, M., and Hendriks, H. Influence of lifestyle on vitamin bioavailability. *Int J Vitam Nutr Res* 2002; 72(1):53–9. Gloria. L., Cravo, M., Camilo, M.E., et al. Nutritional deficiencies in chronic alcoholics: relation to dietary intake and alcohol consumption. *Am J Gastroesterol* 1997; 92(3):485–9.

94. World, M.J., Ryle, P.R., snf Thomson, A.D. Alcoholic malnutrition and the small intestine. *Alcohol Alcohol* 1985; 20(2):89–124. Falck-Ytter, Y., and McCullough, A.J. Nutritional effects of alcoholism. *Curr Gastroenterol Rep* 2000; 2(4):331–6.

95. Levine, J.A., Harris, M.M., and Morgan, M.Y. Energy expenditure in chronic alcohol abuse. *Eur J Clin Invest* 2000; 30(9):779–86.

96. van Velden, D.P., Mansvelt, E.P., Fourie, E., et al. The cardioprotective effect of wine on human blood chemistry. *Ann N Y Acad Sci* 2002; 957:337–40. Aviram, M., and Fuhrman, B. Wine flavanoids protect against LDL oxidation and atherosclerosis. *Ann N Y Acad Sci* 2002; 957:146–5. Rosenkranz, S., Knirel, D., Dietrich, H., et al. Inhibition of the PDGF receptor by red wine flavonoids provides a molecular explanation for the "French paradox." *FASEB J* 2002; 16(14):1958–60. Folts, J.D. Potential health benefits from the flavonoids in grape products on vascular disease. *Adv Exp Med Biol* 2002; 505:95–111. Sato, M., Maulik, N., and Das, D.K.

Cardioprotection with alcohol: role of both alcohol and polyphenolic antioxidants. *Ann N Y Acad Sci* 2002; 957:122–35. Burns, J., Crozier, A., and Lean, M.E. Alcohol consumption and mortality: is wine different from other alcoholic beverages? *Nutr Metab Cardiovasc Dis* 2001; 11(4):249–58.

97. Howitz, K.T., Bitterman, K.J., Sinclair, D.A., et al. Small molecule activators of sirtuins extend Saccharomyces cerevisiae lifespan. *Nature* 2003; 425(6954):191–6.

98. Pelchat, M.L. Of human bondage: food craving, obsession, compulsion, and addiction. *Physiol Behav* 2002; 76(3):347–52. Ramirez, I. Why do sugars taste good? *Neurosci Biobehav Rev* 1990;14(2):125–34.

99. Davenport, R.J. Taste research. New gene may be key to sweet tooth. *Science* 2001; 27;292(5517):620. Montmayeur, J.P., Liberles, S.D., Matsunami, H., and Buck, L.B. A candidate taste receptor gene near a sweet taste locus. *Nat Neurosci* 2001; 4(5):492–8. Max, M., Shanker, Y.G., Huang, L., et al. Tast1r3, encoding a new candidate taste receptor, is allelic to the sweet responsiveness locus Sac. *Nat Genet* 2001; 28(1):58–63.

100. Bartoshuk, L.M., Duffy, V.B., Lucchina, L.A, et al. PROP (6-n-propylthiouracil) supertasters and the saltiness of NaCl. *Ann N Y Acad Sci* 1998; 855:793–6.

CHAPTER 5. THE POWER FOODS OF OKINAWA

1. From our analysis of the Unified Dietary Guidelines below, you can see that Okinawan elders meet or exceed the recommendations for every single category (except salt intake) for the type of diet recommended by nutritional scientists and medical authorities for minimizing risk for debilitating diseases, such as obesity, diabetes, cardiovascular disease, cancer, and other age-related diseases. If there ever was a diet that might lead to better lifetime weight control, lower insulin levels, and result in slower aging, this would be it. The only place they have room for improvement is their salt intake, which admittedly could be a little lower. The table below was calculated from the 1998 Okinawa Prefecture Dept. of Health and Welfare Nutrition and Health Survey, The Okinawa Centenarian Study Database and the USDA 1994–96 Continuing Survey of Food Intakes by Individuals. The Unified Dietary Guidelines are a set of nutritional guidelines designed to resolve public confusion regarding healthy eating habits and were set forth by the National Cancer Institute, the American Heart Association, the American Dietetic Association and the National Institutes of Health. See Goldman, E. Unified dietary guidelines target four key killers. *Intern Med News* 1999; 32:14; Deckelbaum, R.J., et al. Summary of a scientific conference on preventive nutrition: Pediatrics to geriatrics. *Circulation* 1999; 100:450–56.

UNIFIED GUIDELINES VERSUS THE OKINAWAN ELDERS' AND THE U.S. DIET

	Unified Guidelines	Okinawa Elders*	U.S.
Carbohydrates	≥ 55%	57.4	51.8
Protein	10–20%	17.2	15.4
Total fat	≤ 30%	25.4	32.8
Saturated fat	< 10% (1)	7	11.3
Monounsaturated fat	≤ 15% (1.5)	12	12.5
Polyunsaturated fat	≤ 10% (1)	5	6.4
Cholesterol	≤ 300 mg/day	205	256
Salt intake	< 6 g/day	6.8	6.5

*Okinawan elders are defined here as aged 80 years and over.

2. For more information on the importance of the sweet potato to the traditional diet see Sho, H. History and characteristics of Okinawan longevity food. *Asia Pacific J Clin Nutr* 2001; 10(2):159–164.

3.   In vitro, carotenoids exert antioxidant functions and inhibit carcinogen-induced cancer transformation as well as inhibit plasma membrane lipid oxidation. These in vitro results suggest that carotenoids may have intrinsic cancer chemopreventive actions in humans, although the clinical trials have been inconclusive. For recent reviews, see Gescher, A. J. Sharma, R. A., Steward, W. P., et al. Cancer chemoprevention by dietary constituents: a tale of failure and promise. *Lancet Oncol* 2001; 2(6):371–9. Nishino, H., Tokuda, H., Murakoshi, M., et al. Cancer prevention by natural carotenoids. *Biofactors* 2000; 13:89–94. Johnson, E. The role of carotenoids in human health. *Nutr Clin Care* 2002; 5(2):56–6. Similarly, the major storage proteins of sweet potatoes have been shown to act as proteinase inhibitors and may have other anti-cancer properties. Japanese researchers have recently speculated that higher serum levels of carotenoids such as alpha- and beta-carotenes may play a role in preventing death from lung cancer among Japanese. See Ito, Y., Wakai, K., Suzuki, K. Serum carotenoids and mortality from lung cancer: a case-control study nested in the Japan Collaborative Cohort (JACC) Study. *Cancer Sci* 2003; 94(1):57–63.

4.   The hypoglycemic effects of goya (Momordica charantia) have been explored in vitro and in some clinical trials with promising results. However, more adequately powered, randomized, and placebo-controlled trials are needed to properly assess safety and efficacy before bitter melon can be routinely recommended for those with blood sugar problems. For examples of research, see Sarkar, S., Pranava, M., and Marita, R. Demonstration of the hypoglycemic action of Momordica Charantia in a validated animal model of diabetes. *Pharmacol Res* 1996; 33(1):1–4. Leatherdale, B.A., Panesar, R.K., Singh, G, et al. Improvement in glucose tolerance due to Momordica charantia (karela). *BMJ* 1981; 282:1823–1824. Raman, A., and Lau, C. Antidiabetic properties and phytochemistry of Momordica charantia L. (Cucurbitaceae). *Phytomedicine* 1996; 2:349–362. Srivastava, Y., Venkatakrishna-Bhatt, H., Verma, Y., et al. Antidiabetic and adaptogenic properties of Momordica-charantia extract: an experimental and clinical evaluation. *Phytother Res* 1993; 7:285–289. Ali, L., Khan, A.K., Mamum, M.I., et al. Studies on hypoglycemic effects of fruit pulp, seed, and whole plant of Momordica Charantia on normal and diabetic model rats. *Planta Med* 1993; 59(5):408–12. Welihinda, J., Karunanayake, E.H., Sheriff, M.H.R., et al. Effect of Momordica charantia on the glucose tolerance in maturity onset diabetes. *J Ethnopharmacol* 1986; 17:277–282.

5.   Researchers reported rats fed a high-fat diet in combination with freeze-dried bitter melon juice exhibited improved oral glucose tolerance. They also reported that rats taking the supplement had less visceral fat mass than rats taking a high-fat diet alone. Rats habitually fed a high-fat diet either continued to consume the diet (control group) or were switched to one of three diets: (1) high-fat plus bitter melon; (2) low-fat; or (3) low-fat plus bitter melon. After seven weeks, rats that were switched to the high-fat, bitter melon diet gained less weight and had less visceral fat than the rats on the high-fat diet alone. Researchers noted that adding bitter melon did not change apparent fat absorption, although it did improve insulin resistance, lower serum insulin and leptin levels, and raise serum free fatty acid concentration. They concluded bitter melon reduced body fat and appeared to have multiple influences on glucose and lipid metabolism that counteracted the negative effects of the high-fat diet. See Chen, Q., Chan, L.L., and Li, E.T. Bitter melon (Momordica charantia) reduces adiposity, lowers serum insulin and normalizes glucose tolerance in rats fed a high-fat diet. *J Nutr* 2003; 133(4):1088–93.

6.   Marzio, L., Del Bianco, R., and Donne, M.D. Mouth-to-cecum transit time in patients affected by chronic constipation: effect of glucomannan. *Am J Gastroenterol* 1989; 84(8):888–9; Staiano, A., Simeone, D., Del Giudice, E. et al. Effect of the dietary fiber glucomannan on chronic constipation in neurologically impaired children. *J Pediatr* 2000; 136(1):41–5. Durrington, P.N., Manning, A.P., Bolton, C.H., and Hartog M. Effect of pectin on serum Lipids and lipoproteins, whole gut transit time and stool weight. *Lancet* 1976; 2:394–396.

7.   Gallaher, D.D., Gallaher, C.M., and Mahrt, G.J. A glucomannan and chitosan fiber supplement decreases plasma cholesterol and increases cholesterol excretion in overweight normocholesterolemic humans. *J Am Coll Nutr* 2002; 21(5):428–33. Arvill, A., Bodin, L. Effect of short-

term ingestion of konjac glucomannan on serum cholesterol in healthy men. *Am J Clin Nutr* 1995; 61(3):585–9.

8. Vuksan, V., Sievenpiper, J.L., and Owen, R. et al. Beneficial effects of viscous dietary fiber from Konjac-mannan in subjects with the insulin resistance syndrome: results of a controlled metabolic trial. *Diabetes Care* 2000; 23(1):9–14. Doi, K., Matsuura, M., Kawara, A., and Baba, S. Treatment of diabetes with glucomannan (konjac mannan). *Lancet.* 1979;1(8123):987–8.

9. Shimada, Y., Morita, T., and Sugiyama, K. Dietary eritadenine and ethanolamine depress fatty acid desaturase activities by increasing liver microsomal phosphatidylethanolamine in rats. *J Nutr* 2003; 133(3):758–65. Sugiyama, K., Akachi, T., and Yamakawa, A. Hypocholesterolemic action of eritadenine is mediated by a modification of hepatic phospholipid metabolism in rats. *J Nutr* 1995; 125(8):2134–44. Kabir, Y., Yamaguchi, M., and Kimura, S. Effect of shiitake (Lentinus edodes) and maitake (Grifola frondosa) mushrooms on blood pressure and plasma lipids of spontaneously hypertensive rats. *J Nutr Sci Vitaminol* 1987; (Tokyo) 33(5):341–6.

10. Yang, B.K., Kim, D.H., Jeong, S.C. Hypoglycemic effect of a Lentinus edodes exo-polymer produced from a submerged mycelial culture. *Biosci Biotechnol Biochem* 2002; 66(5):937–42.

11. One of shiitake's key constituents is a polysaccharide called *lentinan*. A highly purified, intravenous form of lentinan is approved for use in Japan as an anti-cancer drug and has been reported to increase survival in people with cancer of the stomach or pancreas, particularly when used in combination with chemotherapy. See Taguchi, I. Clinical efficacy of lentinan on patients with stomach cancer: End point results of a four-year follow-up survey. *Cancer Detect Prevent Suppl* 1987; 1:333–49; Matsuoka, H., Seo, Y., Wakasugi, H., et al. Lentinan potentiates immunity and prolongs survival time of some patients. *Anticancer Res* 1997; 17:2751–6. Purified lentinan is considered a drug in Japan and is not currently available as an herbal supplement in North America, although clinical tests are underway, see Gordon, M., Bihari, B., Goosby, E., et al. A placebo-controlled trial of the immune modulator, lentinan, in HIV-positive patients: a phase I/II trial. *J Med* 1998; 29(5–6):305–30.

12. Lin, S.C., Lin, C.H., and Lin, C.C. Hepatoprotective effects of Arctium lappa Linne on liver injuries induced by chronic ethanol consumption and potentiated by carbon tetrachloride. *J Biomed Sci* 2002; 9(5):401–9. Lin, C.C., Lin, J.M., Yang, J.J., et al. Anti-inflammatory and radical scavenge effects of *Arctium lappa. Am J Chin Med* 1996; 24:127–37.

13. Sipos, P., Hagymasi, K., and Lugasi, A. Effects of black radish root (Raphanus sativus L. var niger) on the colon mucosa in rats fed a fat-rich diet. *Phytother Res* 2002; 16(7):677–9.

14. Funahashi, H., Imai, T., Mase, T., et al. Seaweed prevents breast cancer? *Jpn J Cancer Res* 2001; 92(5):483–7. Tokudome, S., Kuriki, K., and Moore, MA.. Seaweed and cancer prevention. *Jpn J Cancer Res* 2001; 92(9):1008–9. Maruyama, H. and Yamamoto, I. Suppression of 125I-uptake in mouse thyroid by seaweed feeding: possible preventative effect of dietary seaweed on internal radiation injury of the thyroid by radioactive iodine. *Kitasato Arch Exp Med* 1992; 65(4):209–16.

15. Sato, T., Koike, L., Miyata, Y., et al. Inhibition of activator protein–1 binding activity and phosphatidylinositol 3-kinase pathway by nobiletin, a polymethoxy flavonoid, results in augmentation of tissue inhibitor of metalloproteinases–1 production and suppression of production of matrix metalloproteinases–1 and –9 in human fibrosarcoma HT–1080 cells. *Cancer Res* 2002; 62(4):1025–9. Minagawa, A., Otani, Y., Kubota, T., et al. The citrus flavonoid, nobiletin, inhibits peritoneal dissemination of human gastric carcinoma in SCID mice. *Jpn J Cancer Res* 2001; 92(12):1322–8. Isawa, J., Sato, T., Mimaki, Y., et al. A citrus flavonoid, nobiletin, suppress production and gene expression of matrix metaroproteinase 9/gelatinase B in Rabbit synovial fibroblast B. *J Rheumatol* 2000; 27:20–25.

16. Rooprai, H.K., Kandanearatchi, A., Maidment, S.L., et al. Evaluation of the effects of swainsonine, captopril, tangeretin and nobiletin on the biological behaviour of brain tumour cells in vitro. *Neuropathol Appl Neurobiol* 2001; 27(1):29–39. Pan, M.H., Chen, W.J., Lin-Shiau, S.Y., et al.Tangeretin induces cell-cycle G1 arrest through inhibiting cyclin-dependent kinases 2 and

4 activities as well as elevating Cdk inhibitors p21 and p27 in human colorectal carcinoma cells. *Carcinogenesis* 2002; 23(10):1677–84. Hirano, T., Abe, K., Gotoh, M., et al. Citrus flavone tangeretin inhibits leukaemic HL–60 cell growth partially through induction of apoptosis with less cytotoxicity on normal lymphocytes. *Br J Cancer* 1995; 72(6):1380–8. Kohno, H., Yoshitani, S., and Tsukio, Y. Dietary administration of citrus nobiletin inhibits azoxymethane-induced colonic aberrant crypt foci in rats. *Life Sci* 2001; 69(8):901–13.

17. For example, see Walker, A.F., Bundy, R., Hicks, S.M., et al. Bromelain reduces mild acute knee pain and improves well-being in a dose-dependent fashion in an open study of otherwise healthy adults. *Phytomedicine* 2002; 9(8):681–6.

18. Flavonoids found in legumes (particularly soy products) have seen much attention by researchers in the past decade or so. The isoflavones in soy, primarily genistein and daidzein, have been well researched by scientists for their *antioxidant* and phytoestrogenic properties. Saponins have been found to enhance *immune function* and bind to cholesterol to limit its absorption in the intestine. Phytosterols and other components of soy have been reported to lower *cholesterol levels* in vivo and in vitro. Human clinical intervention trials also have shown that soy product consumption reduces levels of total cholesterol and low-density lipoprotein cholesterol. This effect appears to be more pronounced in individuals with elevated cholesterol. Soy and its associated isoflavones also reduce LDL oxidation and improve vascular reactivity. A review of 38 studies revealed that soy consumption reduced *cholesterol* levels in 89 percent of the studies. A meta-analysis of these studies indicated that eating soy resulted, on average, in a cholesterol reduction of 23 mg per deciliter. See Anderson, J.W., Johnstone, B.M., and Cook-Newell, M.E. Meta-analysis of the effects of soy protein intake on serum lipids. *N Engl J Med* 1995; 333:276–82. Exactly how soy lowers cholesterol remains in debate, although isoflavones appear to be one key component. The wealth of studies on soy and its constituents (such as isoflavones) has resulted in the US Food and Drug Administration approving a health claim for the relationship between consumption of soy protein and reduced risk of coronary heart disease. For an overview of the cardiovascular effects of various soy products, including their effects on blood lipids, LDL cholesterol oxidation, blood pressure, and vascular reactivity and a good discussion of potential mechanisms of action that centers on human clinical intervention trials see Hasler, C.M. The cardiovascular effects of soy products. *J Cardiovasc Nurs* July 2002;16(4):50–63. Messina, M., Gardner, C., and Barnes, S. Gaining insight into the health effects of soy but a long way still to go: commentary on the fourth International Symposium on the Role of Soy in Preventing and Treating Chronic Disease. *J Nutr* Mar 2002; 132(3):547S–551S. Clarkson, T.B. Soy, soy phytoestrogens and cardiovascular disease. *J Nutr* Mar 2002; 132(3):566S–569S.

19. Research has suggested that soy may reduce the risk of osteoporosis in peri- and postmenopausal women, pariculary those not on hormone replacement therapy. For a recent example, see Arjmandi, B.H., Khalil, D.A, Smith, B.J, et al. Soy protein has a greater effect on bone in postmenopausal women not on hormone replacement therapy, as evidenced by reducing bone resorption and urinary calcium excretion. *J Clin Endocrinol Metab* Mar 2003; 88(3):1048–54. For recent reviews of studies on the effects of soy and soy isoflavones on bone health, see: Brynin, R. Soy and its isoflavones: A review of their effects on bone density. *Altern Med Rev* Aug 2002; 7(4):317–27. Messina, M., Messina, V. Soyfoods, soybean isoflavones, and bone health: A brief overview. *J Ren Nutr* Apr 2000; 10(2):63–8. Scheiber, M.D., and Rebar, R.W. Isoflavones and postmenopausal bone health: A viable alternative to estrogen therapy? *Menopause* 1999; 6(3):233–41.

20. Burke, G.L., Legault, C., Anthony, M., et al. Soy protein and isoflavone effects on vasomotor symptoms in peri- and postmenopausal women: The Soy Estrogen Alternative Study. *Menopause* 2003; 10(2):147–53. Upmalis, D.H., Lobo, R., Bradley, L., et al. Vasomotor symptom relief by soy isoflavone extract tablets in postmenopausal women: a multicenter, double-blind, randomized, placebo-controlled study. *Menopause* 2000; 7(4):236–42. Albertazzi, P., Pansini, F., Bonaccorsi, G., et al. The effect of dietary soy supplementation on hot flushes. *Obstet Gynecol* 1998; 91:6–11.

21. Murkies, A., Dalais, F.S., Briganti, E.M., et al. Phytoestrogens and breast cancer in post-menopausal women: a case control study. *Menopause* 2000; 7(5):289–96.

22. Studies of soy and cancer have revealed promising but mixed results. A 1994 review found that 65 percent of twenty-six in vitro, animal, and epidemiological studies showed a protective effect of soy or soy isoflavones. See Messina, M.J., Persky, V., Setchell, K.D., and Barnes, S. Soy intake and cancer risk: a review of the in vitro and in vivo data. *Nutr Cancer* 1994; 21:113–3. A more recent review of studies on cancer and soy intake concluded that a soy-containing diet may be slightly protective against breast cancer if initiated before puberty or during adolescence. These findings seem to be supported by conclusions of studies of immigrants and other epidemiological studies. The review also found that in one case-control study and one prospective study, a low-lignan diet increased the risk of breast cancer. Experimental evidence also exists for an inhibitory effect of soy and rye bran on prostate-cancer growth and for rye bran or isolated lig-nans on colon cancer. However, whether these observed protective effects are caused by the presence of dietary phyto-oestrogens, or whether they are merely indicators of a healthy diet in general, has not been established. See Adlercreutz, H. Phyto-oestrogens and cancer. *Lancet Oncol* 2002; 3(6):364–73. Finally, although most research has shown *anti-cancer* effects of soy consumption occasional studies have reported potential cancer enhancing effects. For example, one study showed that when premenopausal women were given soy isoflavones, an increase in breast secretions resulted—an effect thought to *elevate* the risk of breast cancer. See Petrakis, N.L., Barnes, S., King, E.B., et al. Stimulatory influence of soy protein isolate on breast secretion in pre- and postmenopausal women. *Cancer Epidemiol Biomarkers Prev* 1996; 5:785–94.

23. Ishihara, K, Oyaizu, S., Fukuchi, Y., et al. A soybean peptide isolate diet promotes postprandial carbohydrate oxidation and energy expenditure in type II diabetic mice. *J Nutr* 2003; 133(3):752–7. Aoyama, T., Fukui, K., et al. Soy protein isolate and its hydrolysate reduce body fat of dietary obese rats and genetically obese mice (yellow KK). *Nutrition* 2000; 16(5):349–54. Aoyama, T., Fukui, K., Nakamori, T., et al. Effect of soy and milk whey protein isolates and their hydrolysates on weight reduction in genetically obese mice. *Biosci Biotechnol Biochem* 2000; 64(12):2594–600. Hurley, C., Richard, D., Deshaies, Y., and Jacques, H. Soy protein isolate in the presence of cornstarch reduces body fat gain in rats. *Can J Physiol Pharmacol* 1998; 76(10–11):1000–7. Kawano-Takahashi, Y., et al. Effect of soya saponins on gold thioglucose (GTG)-induced obesity in mice. *Int J Obes* 1986; 10(4):293–302.

24. Moeller, L.E., Peterson, C.T., Hanson, K.B., et al. Isoflavone-rich soy favorably affects regional fat and lean tissue in menopausal women. Proceedings of the Experimental Biology 2000 Meeting, San Diego, CA, April 15–18, 2000.

25. Yokogoshi, H., and Oda, H. Dietary taurine enhances cholesterol degradation and reduces serum and liver cholesterol concentrations in rats fed a high-cholesterol diet. *Amino Acids* 2002; 23(4):433–9. Balkan, J., Kanbagli, O., Hatipoglu, A., et al. Improving effect of dietary taurine supplementation on the oxidative stress and lipid levels in the plasma, liver and aorta of rabbits fed on a high-cholesterol diet. *Biosci Biotechnol Biochem* 2002; 66(8):1755–8. Murakami, S., Kondo, Y., and Nagate, T. Effects of long-term treatment with taurine in mice fed a high-fat diet: improvement in cholesterol metabolism and vascular lipid accumulation by taurine. *Adv Exp Med Biol* 2000; 483:177–86.

26. Although younger persons are certainly consuming more of it than the older people, the Oki-nawans' tradition of consuming pork on religious occasions has led to some lively debates about pork as a "longevity food." When Okinawan life expectancy skyrocketed after World War II, so did their standard of living, and thus they began to eat more pork. As we have seen, only limited amounts had been consumed before the war—mostly on religious occasions—with the result that the Okinawan elders have consumed very little meat over the course of their lives. As we pointed out, their prewar diet, like that of the mainland Japanese, was too high in salt content, which pre-disposed both populations to higher stroke and stomach cancer rates than we see in the West. One theory is that too little fat and protein intake in mainland Japan led to extremely low blood

cholesterol levels, which weakens artery walls (too low levels of cholesterol have been implicated in higher stroke levels), exacerbating the tendency for higher stroke levels. It may have been the case that the occasional bite of pork in Okinawa helped balance out protein and fat intakes compared to mainland Japan in the days when the diet was made up almost entirely of carbohydrate. Whatever the exact mechanism, it is clear that when they began to eat a more balanced diet—less salt, a wider variety of vegetables, fruit, grains, fish, and limited dairy and meat products—the stroke rate plummeted and life expectancy increased. Many in Okinawa concluded that eating more pork, their traditional ceremonial food, had lengthened their lives. In reality, their lives were lengthened by getting the right balance, as outlined in the Unified Dietary Guidelines, and there is no doubt that we too would benefit greatly by adhering to the same guidelines.

27. Yoshioka, M., St-Pierre, S., Drapeau, V., et al. Effects of red pepper on appetite and energy intake. *Br J Nutr* 1999; 82:115–23.

28. Yoshioka, M., St-Pierre, S., Suzuki, M., and Tremblay, A. Effects of red pepper added to high-fat and high-carbohydrate meals on energy metabolism and substrate utilization in Japanese women. *Br J Nutr* 1998; 80:503–10.

29. Ahsan, H., Parveen, N., Khan, N.U., and Hadi, S.M. Pro-oxidant, anti-oxidant and cleavage activities on DNA of curcumin and its derivatives demethoxycurcumin and bisdemethoxycurcumin. *Chem Biol Interact* 1999; 121(2):161–75. Selvam, R., Subramanian, L., Gayathri, R., and Angayarkanni, N. The anti-oxidant activity of turmeric *(Curcuma longa)*. *J Ethnobotany* 1995; 47:59–67. Cohly, H.H., Taylor, A., Angel, M.F., and Salahudeen, A.K. Effect of turmeric, turmerin and curcumin on H2O2-induced renal epithelial (LLC-PK1) cell injury. *Free Radic Biol Med* 1998; 24(1):49–54. Shalini, V.K., Srinivas, L. Lipid peroxide induced DNA damage: Protection by turmeric (Curcuma longa). *Mol Cell Biochem* 1987; 77(1):3–10.

30. Aggarwal, B.B., Kumar, A., and Bharti, A.C. Anticancer potential of curcumin: Preclinical and clinical studies. *Anticancer Res* 2003; 23(1A):363–98. Devasena, T., Rajasekaran, K.N., Gunasekaran, G., et al. Anticarcinogenic effect of bis–1,7-(2-hydroxyphenyl)-hepta–1,6-diene–3,5-dione a curcumin analog on DMH-induced colon cancer model. *Pharmacol Res* Feb 2003; 47(2):133–40. Stoner, G.D., and Mukhtar, H. Polyphenols as cancer chemoprotective agents. *J Cell Biochem* 1995; 22(suppl):169–180. Ruby, A.J., Kuttan, G., Babu, K.D., et al. Anti-tumour and antioxidant activity of natural curcuminoids. *Cancer Lett* 1995; 94(1):79–83. Leu, T.H., Maa, M.C. The molecular mechanisms for the antitumorigenic effect of curcumin. *Curr Med Chem Anti-Canc Agents* 2002; 2(3):357–70. Ramsewak, R.S., DeWitt, D.L., and Nair, M.G. Cytotoxicity, antioxidant and anti-inflammatory activities of curcumins I-III from Curcuma longa. *Phytomedicine* 2000; 7(4):303–8.

31. Rafatullah, S., Tariq, M., Al-Yahya, M.A., et al. Evaluation of turmeric *(Curcuma longa)* for gastric and duodenal antiulcer activity in rats. *J Ethnobotany* 1990; 29:25–34. Thamlikitkul, V., Bunyapraphathara, N., Dechatiwongse, T., et al. Randomized double-blind study of *Curcuma domestica* Val for dyspepsia. *J Med Assoc Thai* 1989; 72:613–20. Van Dau, N., Ngoc Ham, N., Huy Khac, D., et al. The effects of traditional drug, turmeric *(Curcuma longa),* and placebo on the healing of duodenal ulcer. *Phytomedicine* 1998; 5:29–34. Kositchaiwat, C., Kositchaiwat, S., and Havanondha, J. *Curcuma longa* Linn in the treatment of gastric ulcer comparison to liquid antacid: A controlled clinical trial. *J Med Assoc Thai* 1993; 76:601–5.

32. Lal, B., Kapoor, A.K., Agrawal, P.K., et al. Role of curcumin in idiopathic inflammatory orbital pseudotumours. *Phytother Res* 2000; 14(6):443–7. Satoskar, R.R., Shah, S.J., and Shenoy, S.G. Evaluation of anti-inflammatory property of curcumin (diferuloyl methane) in patients with postoperative inflammation. *Int J Clin Pharmacol Ther Toxicol* 1986; 24:651–4. Rao, T.S., Basu, N., and Siddiqui, H.H. Anti-inflammatory activity of curcumin analogues. *Indian J Med Res* 1982; 75:574–8. Deodhar, S.D., Sethi, R., and Srimal, R.C. Preliminary studies on antirheumatic activity of curcumin (diferuloyl methane). *Ind J Med Res* 1980; 71:632–4.

33. Deters, M., Klabunde, T., Meyer, H., et al. Effects of curcumin on cyclosporine-induced cholestasis and hypercholesterolemia and on cyclosporine metabolism in the rat. *Planta Med* 2003;

69(4):337–43. Rukkumani, R., Sri Balasubashini, M., Vishwanathan, P., and Menon, V.P. Comparative effects of curcumin and photo-irradiated curcumin on alcohol- and polyunsaturated fatty acid-induced hyperlipidemia. *Pharmacol Res* 2002; 46(3):257–64. Kempaiah, R.K., and Srinivasan, K. Integrity of erythrocytes of hypercholesterolemic rats during spices treatment. *Mol Cell Biochem* 2002; 236(1–2):155–61. Ramirez-Tortosa, M.C., Mesa, M.D., Aguilera, M.C., et al. Oral administration of a turmeric extract inhibits LDL oxidation and has hypocholesterolemic effects in rabbits with experimental atherosclerosis. *Atherosclerosis* 1999; 147(2):371–8. Soni, K.B., and Kuttan, R. Effect of oral curcumin administration on serum peroxides and cholesterol levels in human volunteers. *Indian J Physiol Pharmacol* 1992; 36(4):273–5.

34. Curcumin, the active active component of turmeric, has showed promise against HIV in vitro but clinical trials have yet to provide enough evidence to warrant clinical use for AIDS patients. See Barthelemy, S., Vergnes, L., Moynier, M., et al. Curcumin and curcumin derivatives inhibit Tat-mediated transactivation of type 1 human immunodeficiency virus long terminal repeat. *Res Virol* 1998; 149:43–52. Mazumder, A., Raghavan, K., Weinstein, J., et al. Inhibition of human immunodeficiency virus type–1 integrase by curcumin. *Biochem Pharmacol* 1995; 18;49(8):1165–70. Sui, Z., Salto, R., Li, J., et al. Inhibition of the HIV–1 and HIV–2 proteases by curcumin and curcumin boron complexes. *Bioorg Med Chem* 1993; 1(6):415–22. Curcumin: clinical trial finds no antiviral effect. James JS. *AIDS Treat News* 1996; 242:1–2.

35. Lim, K., Yoshioka, M., Kikuzato, S., et al. Dietary red pepper ingestion increases carbohydrate oxidation at rest and during exercise in runners. *Med Sci Sports Exerc* 1997; 29(3):355–61. Yoshioka, M., St-Pierre, S., Suzuki, M., and Tremblay, A. Effects of red pepper added to high-fat and high-carbohydrate meals on energy metabolism and substrate utilization in Japanese women. *Br J Nutr* 1998; 80:503–10. Hoeger, W.W., Harris, C., Long, E.M., and Hopkins, D.R. Four-week supplementation with a natural dietary compound produces favorable changes in body composition. *Adv Ther* 1998;15(5):305–14.

36. Rosa, A., Deiana, M., Casu, V., et al. Antioxidant activity of capsinoids. *J Agric Food Chem* 2002; 4;50(25):7396–401. Shobanay, S., and Naidu, K.A. Antioxidant activity of selected Indian spices. *Prostaglandins Leukot Essent Fatty Acids* 2000; 62(2):107–10. Okada, Y., Okajima, H. Antioxidant effect of capsaicin on lipid peroxidation in homogeneous solution, micelle dispersions and liposomal membranes. *Redox Rep* 2001; 6(2):117–22.

37. Forst, T., Pohlmann, T., Kunt, T., et al. The influence of local capsaicin treatment on small nerve fibre function and neurovascular control in symptomatic diabetic neuropathy. *Acta Diabetol* 2002; 39(1):1–6. McCarty, D.J., Csuka, M., McCarthy, G., et al. Treatment of pain due to fibromyalgia with topical capsaicin: A pilot study. *Semin Arth Rhem* 1994; 23:41–7. Watson, C.P., Tyler, K.L., Bickers, D.R., et al. A randomized vehicle-controlled trial of topical capsaicin in the treatment of postherpetic neuralgia. *Clin Ther* 1993; 15:510–26. Watson, C.P., Evans, R.J., Watt, V,R. Postherpetic neuralgia and topical capsaicin. *Pain* 1988; 33:333–40. Bernstein, J.E., Parish, L.C., Rapaport, M., et al. Effects of topically applied capsaicin on moderate and severe psoriasis vulgaris. *J Am Acad Dermatol* 1986; 15:504–7.

38. Delargy, H.J., O'Sullivan, K.R., Fletcher, R.J., and Blundell, J.E. Effects of amount and type of dietary fibre (soluble and insoluble) on short-term control of appetite. *Int J Food Sci Nutr* 1997; 48(1):67–77. Turnbull, W.H., and Thomas, H.G. The effect of a Plantago ovata seed containing preparation on appetite variables, nutrient and energy intake. *Int J Obes Relat Metab Disord* 1995; 19(5):338–42. Bergmann, J.F., Chassany, O., Petit, A., et al. Correlation between echographic gastric emptying and appetite: influence of psyllium. *Gut* 1992; 33(8):1042–3.

39. Jenkins, D.J., Kendall, C.W., Vuksan, V., et al. Soluble fiber intake at a dose approved by the US Food and Drug Administration for a claim of health benefits: serum lipid risk factors for cardiovascular disease assessed in a randomized controlled crossover trial. *Am J Clin Nutr* 2002; 75(5):834–9. Anderson, J.W., Allgood, L.D., Turner, J., et al. Effects of psyllium on glucose and serum lipid response in men with type 2 diabetes and hypercholesterolemia. *Am J Clin Nutr* 1999; 70:466–73. Anderson, J.W., Davidson, M.H., and Blonde, L., Long-term cholesterol-

lowering effects of psyllium as an adjunct to diet therapy in the treatment of hypercholes-terolemia. *Am J Clin Nutr* 2000; 71(6):1433–8. Chang, E.K., and Schroeder, D.J. Psyllium in hypercholesterolemia. *Ann Pharmacother* 1995; 29(6):625–7.

40. Sierra, M., Garcia, J.J., Fernandez, N., et al. Therapeutic effects of psyllium in type 2 diabetic patients. *Eur J Clin Nutr* 2002; 56(9):830–42. Rodriguez-Moran, M., Guerrero-Romero, F., Lazcano-Burciaga, G. Lipid- and glucose-lowering efficacy of Plantago Psyllium in type II dia-betes. *J Diabetes Complications* 1998; 12(5):273–8. Effects of psyllium on glucose and serum lipid responses in men with type 2 diabetes and hypercholesterolemia. *Am J Clin Nutr* 1999; 70(4):466–73. Pastors, J.G., Blaisdell, P.W., Balm, T.K., et al. Psyllium fiber reduces rise in post-prandial glucose and insulin concentrations in patients with non-insulin-dependent diabetes. *Am J Clin Nutr* 1991; 53(6):1431–5.

41. Fernandez-Banares, F., Hinojosa, J., and Sanchez-Lombrana, J.L. Randomized clinical trial of Plantago ovata seeds (dietary fiber) as compared with mesalamine in maintaining remission in ulcerative colitis. Spanish Group for the Study of Crohn's Disease and Ulcerative Colitis (GETECCU). *Am J Gastroenterol* 1999; 94(2):427–33.

42. Pieroni, A., Janiak, V., Durr, C.M., et al. In vitro antioxidant activity of non-cultivated vegeta-bles of ethnic Albanians in southern Italy. *Phytother Res* 2002; 16(5):467–73. Budzianowski, J., Pakulski, G., Robak, J. Studies on antioxidative activity of some C-glycosylflavones. *Pol J Phar-macol Pharm* 1991; 43(5):395–401. Ruberto, G., Baratta, M.T., Deans, S.G., and Dorman, H.J. Antioxidant and antimicrobial activity of Foeniculum vulgare and Crithmum maritimum essen-tial oils. *Planta Med* 2000; 66(8):687–93.

43. Forster, H., Niklas, H., and Lutz, S. Antispasmodic effects of some medicinal plants. *Planta Med* 1980; 40:303–19.

44. Hare, H., Caspari, C., and Rusby, H. *The National Standard Dispensatory.* Philadelphia: Lea and Febiger, 1916; 63:1129.

45. El Bardai, S., Lyoussi, B., Wibo, M., and Morel, N. Pharmacological evidence of hypotensive activity of Marrubium vulgare and Foeniculum vulgare in spontaneously hypertensive rat. *Clin Exp Hypertens* 2001; 23(4):329–43.

46. Namavar Jahromi, B., Tartifizadeh, A., and Khabnadidch, S. Comparison of fennel and mefe-namic acid for the treatment of primary dysmenorrhea. *Int J Gynaecol Obstet* Feb 2003; 80(2):153–7.

47. Ruberto, G., Baratta, M.T., Deans, S.G., and Dorman, H.J. Antioxidant and antimicrobial activity of Foeniculum vulgare and Crithmum maritimum essential oils. *Planta Med* 2000; 66(8):687–93. Kwon, Y.S., Choi, W.G., Kim, W.J., et al. Antimicrobial constituents of Foenicu-lum vulgare. *Arch Pharm Res* 2002; 25(2):154–7.

48. Albert-Puleo, M. Fennel and anise as estrogenic agents. *J Ethnopharmacol* 1980; 2(4):337–44.

49. Peters, U., Poole, C., and Arab, L. Does tea affect cardiovascular disease? A meta-analysis. *Am J Epidemiol* 2001; 154(6):495–503. Geleijnse, J.M., Launer, L.J., Van der Kuip, D.A., et al. Inverse association of tea and flavonoid intakes with incident myocardial infarction: The Rotterdam Study. *Am J Clin Nutr* 2002; 75(5):880–6. Mukamal, K.J., Maclure, M., Muller, J.E., et al. Tea consump-tion and mortality after acute myocardial infarction. *Circulation* 2002; 105(21):2476–81.

50. Hegarty, V.M., May, H.M., and Khaw, K.T. Tea drinking and bone mineral density in older women. *Am J Clin Nutr* Apr 2000; 71(4):1003–7. Wu, C.H., Yang, Y.C., Yao, W.J., et al. Epi-demiological evidence of increased bone mineral density in habitual tea drinkers. *Arch Intern Med* 2002; 13;162(9):1001–6.

51. Morre, D.J., Morre, D.M., Sun, H., et al. Tea catechin synergies in inhibition of cancer cell prolifer-ation and of a cancer specific cell surface oxidase (ECTO-NOX). *Pharmacol Toxicol* 2003; 92(5):234–41. Weber, J.M., Ruzindana-Umunyana, A., Imbeault, L., Sircar, S. Inhibition of aden-ovirus infection and adenain by green tea catechins. *Antiviral Res* 2003; 58(2):167–173. Malik, A., Azam, S., Hadi, N., and Hadi, S.M. DNA degradation by water extract of green tea in the presence of copper ions: implications for anticancer properties. *Phytother Res* 2003; 17(4):358–63. Jatoi, A.,

Ellison, N., Burch, P.A., et al. A phase II trial of green tea in the treatment of patients with androgen independent metastatic prostate carcinoma. *Cancer* 2003; 15;97(6):1442–6. Demeule, M., Michaud-Levesque, J., Annabi, B., et al. Green tea catechins as novel antitumor and antiangiogenic compounds. *Curr Med Chem Anti-Canc Agents* 2002; 2(4):441–63. Li, N., Sun, Z., Han, C., and Chen, J. The chemopreventive effects of tea on human oral precancerous mucosa lesions. *Proc Soc Exp Biol Med* 1999; 220:218–24. Imai, K., Suga, K., Nakachi, K. Cancer-preventive effects of drinking green tea among a Japanese population. *Prev Med* 1997; 26(6):769–775.

52. Tokunaga, S., White, I.R., Frost, C., et al. Green tea consumption and serum lipids and lipoproteins in a population of healthy workers in Japan. *Ann Epidemiol* 2002; 12(3):157–65. Kono, S., Shinchi, K., Wakabayashi, K., et al. Relation of green tea consumption to serum lipids and lipoproteins in Japanese men. *J Epidemiol* 1996; 6(3):128–33. Imai, K., Nakachi, K. Cross sectional study of effects of drinking green tea on cardiovascular and liver diseases. *BMJ* Mar 1995; 310(6981):693–6. Stensvold, I., Tverdal, A., Solvoll, K., et al. Tea consumption. Relationship to cholesterol, blood pressure, and coronary and total mortality. *Prev Med* 1992; 21:546–53. Sagesaka-Mitane, Y., Milwa, M., and Okada, S. Platelet aggregation inhibitors in hot water extract of green tea. *Chem Pharm Bull* 1990; 38:790–3.

53. Vankemmelbeke, M.N., Jones, G.C., Fowles, C., et al. Selective inhibition of ADAMTS–1, –4 and –5 by catechin gallate esters. *Eur J Biochem* 2003; 270(11):2394–2403. Singh, R., Ahmed, S., Malemud, C.J., et al. Epigallocatechin–3-gallate selectively inhibits interleukin–1beta-induced activation of mitogen activated protein kinase subgroup c-Jun N-terminal kinase in human osteoarthritis chondrocytes. *J Orthop Res* 2003; 21(1):102–9. Mikuls, T.R., Cerhan, J.R., Criswell, L.A., et al. Coffee, tea, and caffeine consumption and risk of rheumatoid arthritis: results from the Iowa Women's Health Study. *Arthritis Rheum* 2002; 46(1):83–91. Ronday, H.K., Te Koppele, J.M., Greenwald, R.A., et al. Tranexamic acid, an inhibitor of plasminogen activation, reduces urinary collagen cross-link excretion in both experimental and rheumatoid arthritis. *Br J Rheumatol* 1998; 37(1):34–8.

54. Dulloo, A.G., Duret, C., Rohrer, D., et al. Efficacy of a green tea extract rich in catechin polyphenols and caffeine in increasing 24-h energy expenditure and fat oxidation in humans. *Am J Clin Nutr* 1999; 70(6):1040–5. For further experimental evidence in animals see also Murase, T., Nagasawa, A., Suzuki, J., et al. Beneficial effects of tea catechins on diet-induced obesity: stimulation of lipid catabolism in the liver. *Int J Obes Relat Metab Disord* 2002; 26(11):1459–64.

55. Haller, C.A., and Benowitz, N.L. Adverse cardiovascular and central nervous system events associated with dietary supplements containing ephedra alkaloids. *N Engl J Med* Dec 2000; 343(25):1833–8. See also Shekelle, P.G., Hardy, M.L., Morton, S.C., et al. Efficacy and safety of ephedra and ephedrine for weight loss and athletic performance: A meta-analysis. *JAMA* 2003; 289(12):1537–45. Bent, S., Tiedt, T.N., Odden, M.C., and Shlipak, M.G. The relative safety of ephedra compared with other herbal products. *Ann Intern Med* 2003; 138(6):468–71.

CHAPTER 6. FINDING BALANCE:
YOUR PERSONALIZED WEIGHT CONTROL PLAN

1. Howitz, K.T., Bitterman, K.J., Cohen, H.Y., et al. Small molecule activators of sirtuins extend Saccharomyces cerevisiae lifespan. *Nature* 2003; 425:191–6.

2. National Institutes of Health. National Heart, Lung, and Blood Institute. *Clinical Guidelines on the Identification, Education, and Treatment of Overweight and Obesity in Adults.* U.S. Department of Health and Human Services, 1998. Foster, G.D., Wadden, T.A., Vogt, R.A., and Brewer, G. What is a reasonable weight loss? Patients' expectations and evaluations of obesity treatment outcomes. *J Consul Clin Psychol* 1997; 65:79–85.

3. Willcox, B.J., Willcox, D.C., and Suzuki, M. *The Okinawa Program: How the World's Longest-Lived People Achieve Everlasting Health—and How You Can Too.* New York: Clarkson Potter, 2001.

4. The baseline calorie burn table works as an excellent rough tool to determine your daily calorie needs. Those who want a more precise way to calculate daily calorie needs should try the Harris-Benedict calorie formula. See Frankenfield, D.G., Rowe, W.A., Smith, J.S., and Cooney, R.N. Validation of several established equations for resting metabolic rate in obese and non-obese people. *J Am Diet Assoc* 2003; 103:1152–9.

5. All diets that induce fat loss will cause loss of lean tissue (muscle) as well. The key is to maximize the fat loss and minimize the muscle loss. A study by highly regarded sport science researcher William Fleck, Ph.D., at Penn State University showed that combining aerobic exercise, strength training, and low-cal eating works much better than dieting alone. Thirty-five overweight men were divided into one of three groups: diet only; diet and aerobics; or diet, aerobic exercise, *and* strength training. Twelve weeks later the subjects were evaluated for weight loss, muscle versus fat loss, and strength/power. The results were impressive and should be noted by anyone contemplating weight loss. All three groups had significant weight loss *but* the diet-only group had significant lean tissue (mostly muscle) loss as well. *Over 30 percent of the weight lost by the diet-only group was lean tissue.* The diet-only group also lost muscle power. The weight lost by the diet and aerobics group consisted of 25 percent lean tissue. However, the third group (diet, aerobics, and weight training) had excellent results and lost only 3 percent of their weight as lean tissue, the rest was fat. They were also the only group to show strength gains, and showed an increase in peak oxygen consumption, indicating better metabolic efficiency. Thus, by far the best weight-loss method for ensuring fat loss was a combination of low-cal eating, aerobic activity, and strength (weight) training. For further reading, see American College of Sports Medicine position stand. Progression models in resistance training for healthy adults. *Med Sci Sports Exerc* Feb 2002; 34:364–80. Also see Ballor, D. and Poehlman, T. Exercise-training enhances fat-free mass preservation during diet-induced weight loss: a meta-analytic finding. *Int J Obesity* 1994; 18:35–40.

6. Want to save time in the gym but still maintain your muscle as you lose fat? The technique, called slow speed or slow burn, involves lifting heavy weights at about one third of the usual speed for a single set. Lifting weights in slow motion has been proposed by some as the most efficient strength-training technique, because it's the fastest path to complete muscle fatigue. Pushing your muscles to their exercise limit in one set definitely saves time, but it doesn't appear to build muscle as effectively as two to four sets at normal speed. In slow-speed or slow burn, you must lift lighter weights to do a slow-speed set properly. Slow-speed advocates also sometimes claim that slow speed is the "best" way to optimal fitness. In other words, everything else, even flexibility and cardiovascular work, is not necessary. While it's true that the reduced speed can ease you into each exercise gradually so that you could theoretically do away with the warmups and stretching, it is not as good as a combination of aerobic activity balanced with strength training and stretching. So, how much strength training do we really need to do to gain the weight-loss/body-sculpting benefits? A recent meta-analysis (a study that combines the results of many other studies) of thirty years of strength training research found that the optimal training regimen for strength was four sets of several repetitions per body part, two to three times per week—twice a week for advanced and three times for beginners. But one set could still give you up a significant benefit. What were the key findings?

1. How many repetitions should be performed for maximum strength benefit? Those who are new to weight training should use a weight that is 60 percent of their one-repetition maximum (the most weight they are able to lift once for each exercise) for 15 to 17 repetitions per set (one group of exercises). People who have been weight-training regularly (three times per week for three to six months) should use a weight that is 80 percent of their one-rep maximum for six to eight repetitions per set.

2. How many sets should be performed to get the maximum strength benefit? Four sets per muscle group (not per exercise) elicited the biggest strength gains in both untrained and trained

individuals. One exercise per body part done very slowly results in significant muscle and strength gains but not as much as the conventional three to four sets. Muscle groups are defined as chest, back, arms, shoulders, thighs, calves, abdominals, and lower back. For further reading see Rhea, M.R., Alvar, B.A., Burkett, L.N., and Ball, S.D. A Meta-analysis to determine the dose response for strength development. *Med Sci Sports Exerc* 2003; 35:456–464.

7.   What is a healthy body weight? Most of the concern with a healthy weight has to do with body fat, which has been implicated as a risk factor for multiple diseases, particularly cardiovascular disease and cancer. Most large human studies that have used body mass index (BMI) or waist circumference as a surrogate measure for body-fat levels. These are crude measures for individuals but work well for large studies since they give you a rough measure of level of body fat. Few large studies have looked at body fat itself and its relationship to health and disease, which may be a much more important factor than body weight alone. What is the relationship between body fat and BMI and what level of body fat should we aim for? These questions need further research but expert bodies that have looked at the limited dataset make the following recommendations. The percentage of body weight that makes up essential fat is approximately 2 to 4 percent of body weight for men and 10 to 12 percent for women. Beyond that, there's a wide range of what is considered a healthy percentage of body fat for an individual, and this also varies somewhat with ethnicity. The American Dietetic Association recommends that men have 15 to 18 percent body fat and women have 20 to 25 percent body fat. Healthy male athletes might be as low as 5 to 12 percent body fat, and healthy female athletes could be as low as 10 to 20 percent. The American Council on Exercise suggests that men's body fat should be 6 to 25 percent and women's should be 14 to 31 percent. As you can see, these recommendations are close but are based on very little objective data.

8.   Body fat percentage is the amount of adipose (fat) tissue in your body as a percentage of total body weight. For example, if your total body weight is 200 pounds and you have 40 pounds of fat, your body fat percentage is 20 percent. There are two reasons why the percentage of body fat or adipose tissue is important with regard to weight. First, the higher your percentage of fat above average levels, the higher your health risk for weight-related illness, like coronary heart disease, other cardiovascular diseases, high blood pressure, gallstones, type 2 diabetes, osteoarthritis, and certain cancers. Second, the more fat you have in your body (and thus the less lean body tissue or muscle you have), the fewer calories you need to maintain your weight.

Because Body Mass Index (BMI) is only a rough measure of body fatness, some people, especially some highly trained athletes, have a high BMI but are not overfat. Similarly, there are people who have a normal weight according to BMI scales, especially the elderly, but who are overfat. BMI is a broad, general gauge of obesity and health risk. Since risk to health is believed to be due to excess body fat, then actually measuring body fat provides a more accurate picture.

Although muscular athletes or weight-lifting enthusiasts may decrease their body fat percentage when they gain weight (because their gain in weight is from adding extra muscle to their body), for most of us weight gain equals fat gain. Our body fat increases while our lean tissue or muscle remains fairly constant (actually about 75 percent of weight gain is fat). So for most people, their body fat percentage increases with every pound of weight gained.

Calculating BMI or waist measurement is an adequate gauge of weight-loss progress, but if you wish to measure your body fat, a professional body-fat monitor or a scale with a built-in body-fat calculator works well. For guidelines about normal body fat percentages, see below. Weight cycling, or yo-yo dieting, happens when you are constantly losing and regaining weight on different diets. Since you usually lose some muscle each time, particularly if you don't exercise, your body fat percentage tends to increase after each cycle. The bottom line? This means we need fewer calories (muscle uses more calories than fat) and weight gain becomes even easier. This is why it is so important to exercise when dieting.

A minimum amount of body fat is needed for energy reserves, bodily functions, and body protection, to cushion organs. Fat regulates body temperature, cushions and insulates organs and tissues, and is the main form of the body's energy storage. At present there is no clear consensus on what is a healthy body fat percentage. Here are two tables illustrating differing guidelines for healthy or normal body fat percentages.

Where your excess fat is located may be almost as important as the amount of body fat you carry. Many studies show that if you carry your extra fat around your waist (apple shape), you are at a higher risk for disease and death than if you carry the same amount of extra fat around your thighs and buttocks (pear shape).

BODY FAT GUIDELINES FROM THE AMERICAN COUNCIL ON EXERCISE

Classification	Women (% fat)	Men (% fat)
Essential Fat	10–12 percent	2–4 percent
Athletes	14–20 percent	6–13 percent
Fitness	21–24 percent	14–17 percent
Acceptable	25–31 percent	18–25 percent

BODY FAT GUIDELINES FROM THE AMERICAN DIETETICS ASSOCIATION

	Women	Men
Normal	15–25 percent	10–20 percent
Overweight	25.1–29.9 percent	20.1–24.4 percent
Obese	Over 30 percent	Over 25 percent

9. For those who are attempting to practice the art and science of caloric restriction, you will likely aim for even lower body fat levels. We suggest that you read the works of Dr. Roy Walford (see Recommended Readings) or visit some of the websites on caloric restriction on page 406.

Recommended Readings

Jennie Brand-Miller, et al. *The New Glucose Revolution: The Authoritative Guide to the Glycemic Index—the Dietary Solution for Lifelong Health.* New York: Marlow & Company, 2002.

Charles W. Fetrow and Juan R. Avila. *Professional's Handbook of Complementary and Alternative Medicines.* Springhouse, Penn.: Springhouse, 1999.

Donald D. Hensrud, ed., *Mayo Clinic on Healthy Weight: Answers to Help You Achieve and Maintain the Weight That's Right for You.* New York: Kensington Pub. Corp., 2000.

Hui O Laulima. *Okinawan Mixed Plate: Generous Servings of Culture, Customs and Cuisine.* Honolulu, Hawaii: Hui O Laulima, 2000.

George H. Kerr and Mitsugu Sakihara. *Okinawa: The History of an Island People.* New York: Charles E. Tuttle, 2000.

Barbara Rolls and Robert A. Barnett. *The Volumetrics Weight-Control Plan.* New York: HarperCollins, 2000.

Roy L. Walford. *Beyond the 120 Year Diet: How to Double Your Vital Years.* New York: Four Walls Eight Windows, 2000.

Andrew Weil. *Eating Well for Optimum Health: The Essential Guide to Bringing Health and Pleasure Back to Eating.* New York: Quill, 2001.

Bradley J. Willcox, D. Craig Willcox, and Makoto Suzuki. *The Okinawa Program: How the World's Longest-Lived People Achieve Everlasting Health—and How You Can Too.* New York: Crown, 2001.

Walter Willet. *Eat, Drink, and Be Healthy.* New York: Simon and Schuster, 2001.

Websites

OKINAWA CENTENARIAN STUDY
Okinawa Centenarian Study Website
www.okicent.org

HEALTH AND AGING ORGANIZATIONS
American Geriatrics Society
www.americangeriatrics.org/

American Institute for Cancer Research
www.aicr.org/index.lasso

Centers for Disease Control and Prevention's "Body and Mind"
www.bam.gov

Department of Health and Human Services' Healthfinder
www.healthfinder.gov

Gerontological Society of America
www.geron.org/

iVillage.com, Women's Health Forum
ivillage.com/

Mayo Clinic Health Oasis
www.mayoclinic.com

National Institute on Aging
www.nia.nih.gov/

See also the **Age Pages** at www.healthand
age.com/html/min/nih/content/
general.htm

DIET AND FOOD INFORMATION
American Dietetic Association
www.eatright.org

American Heart Association's Fish Oil Facts
www.americanheart.org

Cook's Thesaurus (Food Dictionary)
www.foodsubs.com/

Epicurious Food Dictionary
www.epicurious.com/run/fooddictionary/
home

International Food and Information Council
www.ificinfo.health.org

MSNBC's Diet and Nutrition Archive
www.msnbc.com/news/dieting_front.asp

Tufts University Nutrition Navigator
www.navigator.tufts.edu

University of Delaware's Trans Fatty Acid Database
napa.ntdt.udel.edu/trans/

University of Sydney's Glycemic Index Database
www.calvin.biochem.usyd.edu.au/GIDB/
searchD3.htm

USDA's Food and Nutrition Information Center
www.nal.usda.gov/fnic/index.html

USDA Nutrient Data Laboratory (to
search nutrients of your foods)
www.nal.usda.gov/fnic/cgi-
bin/nut_search.pl

WEIGHT CONTROL AND OBESITY
American Obesity Association
www.obesity.org/

Body Mass Index Calculator from National Center for Chronic Disease Prevention and Health Promotion
www.cdc.gov/nccdphp/dnpa/bmi/calc-
bmi.htm

Calorie Burn Calculator from Internetfit-ness.com
www.internetfitness.com/calculators/cal-
burncalc.htm

National Institutes of Health's Weight-Control Information Network
www.niddk.nih.gov/health/nutrit/win.htm

Tanita Body Fat Scales
www.tanita-body-fat-scales.com/

HEALTH STATISTICS
National Center for Health Statistics
www.cdc.gov/nchs/

The World Health Organization's Ranking of the World's Health Systems
www.photius.com/rankings/
healthranks.html

The World Health Organization's Statistical Information System (WHOSIS)
www3.who.int/whosis/menu.cfm

CALORIC RESTRICTION
Caloric Restriction Information Center at American Federation of Aging Research
www.infoaging.org/b-cal-home.html

CRON-WEB.org
www.cron-web.org/default.htm

CR Society
www.calorierestriction.org

Life Extension Foundation
www.lef.org

Sage KE—Science of Aging Knowledge Environment
http://sageke.sciencemag.org

Dr. Roy Walford's Site
www.walford.com/

University of Washington's Telemakus
www.telemakus.net/CR-aging/

SELECTION OF OKINAWA INFORMATION
Okinawa.com
www.okinawa.com/home.html

Okinawa Convention & Visitors Bureau
www.ocvb.or.jp/en/

JAPANESE FOOD STORES
Katagiri
www.katagiri.com/

Naniwa Foods
www.naniwafood.com/

Oriental Pantry
www.orientalpantry.com

Okinawan Restaurants

HAWAII
Hide-Chan Restaurant
2471 South King Street
Honolulu, HI 96826
(808) 942-7900

Kariyushi Restaurant
1436 Young Street
Honolulu, HI 96814
(808) 942-1137

Roy's (Hawaiian-Okinawan fusion cuisine)
6600 Kalanaianaole Highway
Honolulu, HI 96825
(808) 396-7697
www.roysrestaurant.com
Many other locations throughout the
nation

Sunrise Restaurant
525 Kapahulu Avenue
Honolulu, HI 96815
(808) 737-4118

Utage Restaurant & Lounge
1286 Kalani Street, B102
Honolulu, HI 96817
(808) 843-8109

EAST COAST
Oishii Japanese Foods
25 Preble Street
Portland, ME 04101
(207) 228-2050

Okinawa
496 LaGuardia Place
New York, NY 10012
(212) 253-8886/6794

Okinawa Japanese Restaurant
39-32 Bell Boulevard
Bayside, NY 11361
(718) 224-5622

Okinawa Japanese Restaurant
450 East College Avenue
State College, PA 16801
(814) 278-8689/8568

WEST COAST
Okinawa Restaurant
2306 East Main Street
Ventura, CA 93003
(805) 653-7336

Okinawa Teriyaki
1022 Alaskan Way
Seattle, WA 98104
(206) 447-2648

OUTSIDE THE UNITED STATES
Okinawa Japanese Restaurant
Regal Constellation Hotel
900 Dixon Road
Toronto, ON M9W1J7 Canada
(416) 798-1333

Yan-Baru
45 Crawford Street
London, UK W1H1Ha
017-17248780

General Index

Recipe Index

Visit us at our website at www.okicent.org. Let us know how you're doing on the program, or join us on one of our Okinawa Program retreats where you can learn the healing ways of the elders and perhaps even meet a few of them. Even if we don't see you in person, feel free to share any new and wonderful creations you come up with should you decide to experiment with our recipes. We would love to hear from you.